Ultrasound-Guided Regional Anesthesia and Pain Medicine

Ultrasound-Guided Regional Anesthesia and Pain Medicine

Edited by
Paul E. Bigeleisen, MD
Professor of Anesthesiology
University of Pittsburgh School of Medicine
Pittsburgh, Pennsylvania
Adjunct Professor of Anesthesiology and Biomedical Engineering
University of Rochester School of Medicine and Dentistry
Rochester, New York

Authors
Steven L. Orebaugh, MD
Nizar Moayeri, MD
Gerbrand J. Groen, MD, PHD
Stephen M. Breneman, MD
Jacques Chelly, MD, PHD, MBA

Illustrator/Videographer
Jooyeon Ha, MFA
Chris Bickel, BFA

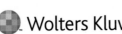 Wolters Kluwer | Lippincott Williams & Wilkins
Health

Philadelphia • Baltimore • New York • London
Buenos Aires • Hong Kong • Sydney • Tokyo

Acquisitions Editor: Frances DeStefano
Marketing Manager: Angela Panetta
Manufacturing Manager: Benjamin Rivera
Product Manager: Nicole Demoski
Design Coordinator: Stephen Druding
Production Service: Absolute Service/MDC

Library of Congress Cataloging-in-Publication Data

Ultrasound-guided regional anesthesia and pain medicine / editor, Paul Bigeleisen ; authors, Steven Breneman ... [et al.] ; illustrator/videographer, Jooyeon Ha, Chris Bickel.
   p. ; cm.
 Includes bibliographical references.
 ISBN 978-1-58255-849-3
 1. Nerve block—Atlases. 2. Conduction anesthesia—Atlases. 3. Ultrasonic imaging—Atlases. I. Bigeleisen, Paul. II. Breneman, Steven.
 [DNLM: 1. Anesthesia, Conduction—methods—Atlases. 2. Pain—therapy—Atlases. 3. Ultrasonography—methods—Atlases. WO 517 U47 2010]
 RD84.U48 2010
 617.9'64—dc22

2009030250

11 12 13
4 5 6 7 8 9 10

RRS1112

Acknowledgment

I began this atlas in Pittsburgh in 1988 with cadaver dissections, preserved in formalin tanks. In 1992, I created some simple ultrasound studies of the brachial plexus. By 1997, I was plastinating additional cadaver dissections at the University of Rochester and making simple line drawings of my dissections. Later, my colleagues and I created professional illustrations, animations, and three-dimensional virtual reality reconstructions. By 2002, I began ultrasound-guided nerve blocks. When I returned to Pittsburgh in 2006, I had the opportunity to work with an archive of micro-anatomical dissections of the brachial, thoracic, and lumbar plexuses.

During the next few years, Jacques Chelly and some outstanding fellows worked with me on new techniques in ultrasound-guided block. At the same time, Dr. Chelly introduced me to the editors at LWW and the formal foundation for this atlas was begun.

This atlas has been 20 years in the making; my colleagues from around the world and I have spent more than 8,000 hours working on these dissections, drawings, animations, and researches. I want to acknowledge the efforts of everyone involved:

- *Jooyeon Ha, Sara Bednarz, and Chris Bickel from the departments of animation and medical illustration at Rochester Institute of Technology;*

- *Nizar Moayeri, who, along with Gerbrand Groen (University of Utrecht), have created a large archive of micro-anatomical dissections;*

- *Pittsburgh fellows Alon Ben Ari, Melina Moreno, and David Burns;*

- *C.C. Li, James Chien, Steven Damelin, and Jung-Ha An who contributed new ideas in image processing;*

- *Phil Cory and Stuart Grant, who added new ideas in radio-frequency imaging and ultrasound;*

- *Assad Oberei, Robert Borcala, and Yun Jing who added new insights into needle design;*

- *Steve Orebaugh, who wrote many of the chapters; and*

- *Stephen Breneman and Meg Stanbury, who edited many of the chapters and images.*

I would also like to thank The Fulbright Foundation, National Institute of Health, National Science Foundation, Sleeping Gorilla, University of Pittsburgh, SonoSite, B Braun, Life Tech, and the Manipulative Therapy Foundation of Holland for their financial support.

I hope you enjoy the atlas.

Paul E. Bigeleisen
Summer 2009, Rochester, NY, and Pittsburgh, PA

Contents

ACKNOWLEDGMENT   V

CONTRIBUTOR LIST   XI

SECTION I   FUNDAMENTALS OF EQUIPMENT, ULTRASOUND, AND MICROANATOMY   1

1. Equipment   2
   Steven L. Orebaugh, Paul E. Bigeleisen

2. From Paresthesia to Neurostimulation and Ultrasound-Guided Regional Anesthesia   7
   Jacques Chelly

3. Principles of Sonography   10
   Paul E. Bigeleisen, Steven L. Orebaugh

4. Microanatomy of the Peripheral Nervous System and Its Implications
   for Paravertebral and Peripheral Nerve Blocks   26
   Andre P. Boezaart

5. Ultrasound-Guided Intraneural Injection: A Powerful Tool for Regional Anesthesia   34
   Meg A. Rosenblatt, Paul E. Bigeleisen

SECTION II   UPPER EXTREMITY   39

6. Ultrasound-Guided Interscalene Block Using the Posterior Approach   40
   David A. Burns, Patrik Filip

7. Ultrasound-Guided Interscalene Block   45
   Steven L. Orebaugh, Nizar Moayeri, Paul E. Bigeleisen

8. Ultrasound-Guided Supraclavicular Block   53
   Steven L. Orebaugh, Paul E. Bigeleisen

9. Ultrasound-Guided Infraclavicular Block   58
   Steven L. Orebaugh, Gerbrand J. Groen, Paul E. Bigeleisen

10. Ultrasound-Guided Axillary Block   65
     Steven L. Orebaugh, Paul E. Bigeleisen

11. Blocks at the Elbow and Forearm   71
     Steven L. Orebaugh, Paul E. Bigeleisen

SECTION III   LOWER EXTREMITY BLOCKS   80

12. Ultrasound-Guided Lumbar Plexus Block (Transverse Approach)   81
     Shinichi Sakura, Kaoru Hara, Jean-Louis Horn

13. Ultrasound-Guided Inguinal Nerve Block   89
     Urs Eichenberger

14. Ultrasound-Guided Transversus Abdominis Plane Block   93
     Kim Russon, Rafael Blanco

15. Ultrasound-Guided Femoral Nerve Block   97
     Stephen M. Breneman

16. Ultrasound-Guided Lateral Femoral Cutaneous Block   104
     Paul E. Bigeleisen, Milena Moreno, Steven L. Orebaugh

17. Ultrasound-Guided Saphenous Nerve Block   108
     Steven L. Orebaugh, Milena Moreno, Stephen M. Breneman, Paul E. Bigeleisen

18. Ultrasound-Guided Obturator Nerve Block   114
     Yoshihiro Fujiwara, Toru Komatsu

19. Ultrasound-Guided Parasacral Block   120
     Alon Ben-Ari, Bruce Ben-David

20. Ultrasound-Guided Anterior Sciatic Nerve Block   123
     Yasuyuki Shibata, Toru Komatsu, Laurent Delaunay

21. Subgluteal Sciatic Block   127
     Steven L. Orebaugh, Paul E. Bigeleisen

22. Ultrasound-Guided Popliteal Sciatic Block   132
     Steven L. Orebaugh, Paul E. Bigeleisen

23. Ultrasound-Guided Ankle Block   140
     Stephen M. Breneman

SECTION IV   CENTRAL BLOCKS   144

24. Ultrasound for Labor Epidural Placement   145
     Manuel C. Vallejo

25. Ultrasound-Guided Thoracic Paravertebral Block   150
     Paul E. Bigeleisen, Alon Ben-Ari

26. Ultrasound-Guided Thoracic Paravertebral Block: Classic Approach   156
     Andrea Fanelli, Mario I. Montoya, Daniela Elena Francesca Ghisi

SECTION V   PEDIATRIC ANESTHESIA   162

27. Fundamentals of Ultrasound-Guided Pediatric Regional Anesthesia   163
     Joseph D. Tobias

28. Ultrasound-Guided Brachial Plexus Blockade in Infants and Children   171
     Joseph D. Tobias, Stefan Lucas, Santhanam Suresh, Paul E. Bigeleisen

29. Ultrasound-Guided Regional Anesthesia of the Thorax, Trunk, and Abdomen
in Infants and Children   181
Joseph D. Tobias, Stefan Lucas, Santhanam Suresh, Jean-Louis Horn, Paul E. Bigeleisen

30. Ultrasound-Guided Lower Extremity Block in Children   195
Joseph D. Tobias, Stefan Lucas, Giovanni Cucchiaro, Paul E. Bigeleisen

SECTION VI PAIN BLOCKS   213

31. Ultrasound-Guided Maxillary Nerve Block   214
Paul E. Bigeleisen

32. Ultrasound-Guided Mandibular Nerve Block   217
Paul E. Bigeleisen, Milena Moreno

33. Stellate Ganglion Block   220
Yasuyuki Shibata, Toru Komatsu, Nizar Moayeri, Gerbrand J. Groen

34. Ultrasound-Guided Cervical Sympathetic Block   225
Michael Gofeld

35. Endoscopic Celiac Ganglion Block   232
Paul E. Bigeleisen

36. Ultrasound-Guided Superior Hypogastric Plexus Block   237
Paul E. Bigeleisen

37. Ultrasound-Guided Lumbar (L1–L4) Zygapophysial Medial Branch and L5 Dorsal Ramus Block   240
Yoshiro Fujiwara, Toru Komatsu, Michael Gofeld

38. Use of Ultrasonography in Rheumatology   252
Ralf Thiele

SECTION VII THE FUTURE OF ULTRASOUND   260

39. The Future of Sonography   261
Paul E. Bigeleisen

40. Identification of Nerves on Ultrasound Scans Using Artificial Intelligence and Machine Vision   263
Paul E. Bigeleisen, Jong-Chih Chien

41. Acoustic Radiation Force Imaging In Regional Anesthesia   272
Mark Palmeri, Stuart A. Grant

42. Impedance Neurography   276
Philip C. Cory, Paul E. Bigeleisen

43. Evaluation of Thoracic Paravertebral And Lumbar Plexus Anatomy Using a 3D Ultrasound Probe   280
Sanjib Das Adhikary, Sugantha Ganapathy

44. Optimum Design of Echogenic Needles for Ultrasound-Guided Nerve Block   283
Assad A. Oberai, Yun Jing, Robert E. Bocala, Paul E. Bigeleisen

45. Medical Image Segmentation Using Modified Mumford Segmentation Methods   289
Jung-Ha An, Steven Benjamin Damelin, Paul E. Bigeleisen

Index   295

Contributor List

Sanjib Das Adhikary, MD
Visiting Assistant Professor
Department of Anesthesiology
Milton S. Hershey Medical Center
College of Medicine
Hershey, Pennsylvania

Jung-Ha An, PhD
Assistant Professor
Department of Mathematics
California State University Stanislaus
Turlock, California

Alon Ben-Ari, MD
Visiting Instructor
Department of Anesthesiology
University of Pittsburgh
Attending Staff Anesthesiologist
Department of Anesthesiology
UPMC–Presbyterian
Pittsburgh, Pennsylvania

Bruce Ben-David, MD
Clinical Professor of Anesthesiology
Department of Anesthesiology
University of Pittsburgh Medical Center
Attending Faculty
Associate Director
Acute Interventional Pain Service
University of Pittsburgh Medical Center–Shadyside Hospital
Department of Anesthesiology
Pittsburgh, Pennsylvania

Paul E. Bigeleisen, MD
Professor of Anesthesiology
University of Pittsburgh School of Medicine
Pittsburgh, Pennsylvania
Adjunct Professor of Anesthesiology and Biomedical
Engineering
University of Rochester School of Medicine and Dentistry
Rochester, New York

Rafael Blanco, MD
Consultant Anaesthesiologist
Anaesthetic Department
University Hospital of Lewisham
London, United Kingdom

Robert E. Bocala, BS
Laboratory Assistant
Department of Mechanical
Aerospace & Nuclear Engineering
Rensselaer Polytechnic Institute
Troy, New York

Andre P. Boezaart, MD, PhD
Professor of Anesthesiology and Orthopaedic Surgery
Department of Anesthesiology
University of Florida College of Medicine
Gainesville, Florida

Stephen M. Breneman, MD
Assistant Professor,
Department of Anesthesiology
University of Rochester
Chief of Acute Pain Service
Department of Anesthesiology
Strong Memorial Hospital
Rochester, New York

David A. Burns, MD
Director Regional Anesthesia Fellowship
Assistant Professor
Department of Anesthesiology
Penn State University
Co-Director Acute Pain Services
Department of Anesthesiology
Penn State University Hershey Medical Center
Hershey, Pennsylvania

Jacques Chelly, MD, PhD, MBA
Professor of Anesthesiology (with Tenure) and Orthopedic
Surgery
Vice Chair of Clinical Research
Director of Regional and Orthopedic Fellowships
Director of Division of Acute Interventional and
Perioperative Pain and Regional Anesthesia
Department of Anesthesiology
UPMC Presbyterian-Shadyside Hospital
Pittsburgh, Pennsylvania

Jong-Chih Chien, PhD
Assistant Professor
Department of Computer Science and Information Engineering
Kainan University
Taoyuan, Taiwan

Philip C. Cory, MD
Chairman
Department of Anesthesia
St. James Healthcare
Butte, Montana

Giovanni Cucchiaro, MD
Associate Professor
Anesthesia and Critical Care Medicine
University of Southern California
Department of Anesthesia and Critical Care Medicine
Childrens Hospital Los Angeles
Los Angeles, California

Steven Benjamin Damelin, PhD
Full Processor
Department of Mathematical Sciences
Georgia State University
Statesboro, Georgia
Full Professor, School of Computational and Applied
Mathematics
Wits, South Africa

Laurent Delaunay, MD
Département d'anesthésiologie
Clinique Générale
Annecy, France

Urs Eichenberger, MD
Privatdozent
Department of Anesthesiology and Pain Therapy
University of Bern
Attending
Department of Anesthesiology and Pain Therapy
University Hospital of Bern
Inselspital
Bern, Switzerland

Andrea Fanelli, MD
Visiting Professor
Department of Anesthesiology
University of Pittsburgh
Fellow in Acute Pain Service
Department of Anesthesiology
UPMC Shadyside Hospital
Pittsburgh, Pennsylvania

Patrik Filip, MD
Attending/Staff Anesthesiologist
Department of Anesthesiology
West Penn Allegheny–Allegheny General Hospital
Pittsburgh, Pennsylvania

Yoshihiro Fujiwara, MD
Professor
Department of Anesthesiology
Aichi Medical University
Nagakute, Aichi, Japan

Sugantha Ganapathy, FRCPC, FRCA
Professor
Department of Anesthesiology & Perioperative Medicine
University of Western Ontario
Consultant, Director, Regional and Pain Research
Department of Anesthesiology & Perioperative Medicine
London Health Sciences Centre
London, Ontario
Canada

Daniela Elena Francesca Ghisi, MD
Visiting Professor
Department of Anesthesiology
University of Pittsburgh
Fellow in Acute Pain Services
Department of Anesthesiology
UPMC Shadyside Hospital
Pittsburgh, Pennsylvania

Michael Gofeld, MD
Assistant Professor
University of Washington School of Medicine
Director of Clinical Operations
Center for Pain Relief
Department of Anesthesiology and Pain Medicine
University of Washington Medical Center
Seattle, Washington

Stuart A. Grant, MBChB, FRCA
Professor
Department of Anesthesiology
Duke University
Durham, North Carolina

Gerbrand J. Groen, MD, PhD
Associate Professor
Department of Anesthesiology
University Medical Center Utrecht
Utrecht, The Netherlands

Kaoru Hara, MD
Lecturer
Department of Anesthesiology
Shimane University School of Medicine
Izumo City, Japan

Jean-Louis Horn, MD
Professor
Director of Regional Anesthesia
Department of Anesthesiology and Perioperative Medicine
Oregon Health Sciences University
Portland, Oregon

Yun Jing, PhD
Professional Staff
Department of Radiology
Brigham and Women's Hospital
Harvard Medical School
Boston, Massachusetts

Toru Komatsu, MD
Professor
Department of Anesthesiology
Aichi Medical University
Director
Department of Anesthesiology
Aichi Medical University Hospital
Aichi, Japan

Stefan Lucas, MD
Assistant Professor
Department of Anesthesiology
University of Rochester Medical Center
Chief of Anesthesia
URMC Ambulatory Surgery at Sawgrass
Rochester, New York

Nizar Moayeri, MD
Research Fellow
Department of Anesthesiology
Resident
Department of Neurosurgery
University of Medical Center Utrecht
Utrecht, The Netherlands

Mario I. Montoya, MD
Assistant Professor
Department of Anesthesiology
University of Pittsburgh
Presbyterian University Hospital
Pittsburgh, Pennsylvania

Milena Moreno, MD
Instructor in Anesthesiology
Department of Anesthesiology
Pontificia Javeriana University
Anesthesiologist
Department of Anesthesiology
San Ignacio Hospital
Bogota, Columbia, South America

Assad A. Oberai, PhD
Associate Professor
Mechanical Aerospace and Nuclear Engineering
Rensselaer Polytechnic Institute
Troy, New York

Steven L. Orebaugh, MD
Associate Professor of Anesthesiology
Department of Anethesiology
University of Pittsburgh School of Medicine
Staff Anesthesiologist
Department of Anesthesiology
University of Pittsburgh Medical Center–Southside
Pittsburgh, Pennsylvania

Mark Palmeri, MD, PhD
Assistant Research Professor
Biomedical Engineering
Duke University
Assistant Professor
Department of Anesthesiology
Duke University Medical Center
Durham, North Carolina

Meg A. Rosenblatt, MD
Professor, Director
Division of Orthopedic and Regional Anesthesia
Department of Anesthesiology and Orthopedics
Mount Sinai School of Medicine
New York, New York

Kim Russon, MRCP, FRCA
Consultant Anaesthetist
Anaesthetic Department
Rotherham Foundation Trust Hospital
Rotherham, England, United Kingdom

Shinichi Sakura, MD
Associate Professor
Department of Anesthesiology
Shimane University School of Medicine
Director
Surgical Center
Shimane University Hospital
Izumo City, Japan

Yasuyuki Shibata, MD
Assistant Professor
Department of Anesthesiology
Aichi Medical University
Aichi-gun, Aichi
Assistant Professor
Department of Anesthesiology
Nagoya University Hospital
Nagoya, Aichi, Japan

Santhanam Suresh, MD, FAAP
Professor of Anesthesiology and Pediatrics
Department of Anesthesiology
Feinberg School of Medicine
Northwestern University
Director
Pain Management Team
Director of Research
Department of Pediatric Anesthesiology
Children's Memorial Hospital
Chicago, Illinois

Ralf Thiele, MD
Department of Rheumatology
University of Rochester School of Medicine
Rochester, New York

Joseph D. Tobias
Vice-Chairman
Department of Anesthesiology
Chief
Division of Pediatric Anesthesiology
Professor of Anesthesiology and Pediatrics
Russell and Mary Sheldon Chair in Pediatric Critical Care
University of Missouri
Department of Anesthesiology
Columbia, Missouri

Manuel C. Vallejo, MD, DMD
Associate Professor
Department of Anesthesiology
University of Pittsburgh, Director
Obstetric Anesthesia
Department of Anesthesiology
Magee-Womens Hospital
Pittsburgh, Pennsylvania

Section *I*

Fundamentals of Equipment, Ultrasound, and Microanatomy

1   Equipment

2   From Paresthesia to Neurostimulation and Ultrasound-Guided Regional Anesthesia

3   Principles of Sonography

4   Microanatomy of the Peripheral Nervous System and Its Implications for Paravertebral and Peripheral Nerve Blocks

5   Ultrasound-Guided Intraneural Injection: A Powerful Tool for Regional Anesthesia

1

Equipment

STEVEN L. OREBAUGH, PAUL E. BIGELEISEN

Introduction: A variety of equipment is necessary for conducting ultrasound-guided peripheral nerve block. Some practitioners prefer to use nerve stimulation along with sonography to verify or confirm the nerve target before injection. Although both methods have proponents, it is not clear if either technique is superior; their efficacy appears similar.[1]

Equipment: Whether blocks are conducted in the operating room, the preoperative holding area, or a formal block area, patients should have an intravenous catheter initiated, monitors placed, and supplemental oxygen delivered prior to the block (Fig. 1-1). The induction of regional anesthesia has risks that are similar to those of general anesthesia. For this reason, a block cart stocked with equipment for regional block should also contain appropriate equipment and drugs for resuscitation in the event of an anesthetic catastrophe[2] (Fig. 1-2). Judicious sedation and analgesia, along with a kind bedside manner, will not only prepare most patients for regional anesthesia, but will also avoid a depth that precludes feedback to the anesthesiologist (Fig. 1-3).

Intravenous catheter and balanced salt solution
Blood pressure monitoring
Pulse oximetry monitoring
Electrocardiographic monitoring (necessary for patients with cardiac disease or dysrhythmias)
Supplemental oxygen by face mask or cannula
Medications for anxiolysis (e.g., midazolam, propofol, dexmetatomidine) and analgesia (fentanyl)
Equipment for airway management (larygoscopes, endotracheal tubes, bag and face mask, oral airways, laryngeal airways)
Pharmaceuticals for resuscitation (propofol, epinephrine, 20% intralipid, vasopressin, amiodarone)

The skin is prepared in sterile fashion, and subcutaneous local anesthetic solution is injected at the site at which the block needle is to be inserted. The ultrasound probe is covered with a sterile, transparent membrane for single-shot blocks, while the anesthesiologist dons sterile gloves. Most authors recommend the use of short-bevel needles, as it appears to be more difficult to penetrate the perineurium with this type of needle,[3] although clinical outcome data is lacking.

Antiseptic for skin preparation
Transparent, sterile membrane to cover ultrasound probe
Lidocaine in 3- or 5-mL syringe with 27- or 30-gauge needle for skin anesthesia
Short-bevel block needle, length appropriate to depth of nerve

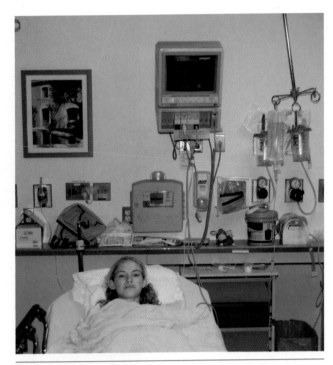

Figure 1-1. Equipment for monitoring, suction, and supplemental oxygen.

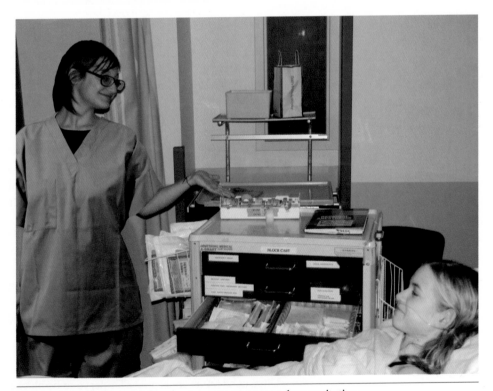

Figure 1-2. Equipment for airway management and resuscitation.

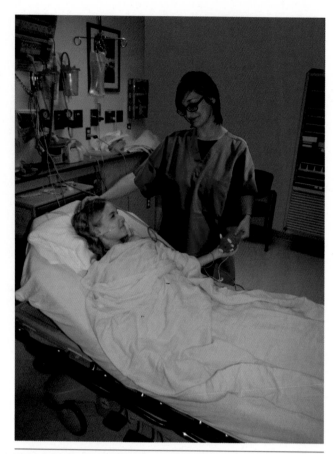

Figure 1-3. Nurse to assist with sedation and positioning.

The local anesthetic solution used will be dependent on the anesthesiologist's intent. Blocks intended for rapid onset and short duration may be conducted with mepivacaine, lidocaine, or chloroprocaine, whereas longer-acting blocks will require ropivacaine or bupivacaine. Mixtures probably add little to speed onset while significantly reducing the duration of long-acting agents. Although it is axiomatic that injection must not proceed when injection pressures are high, it is not yet clear whether pressure monitoring will influence the occurrence of nerve injury in the clinical setting.[4]

Appropriate volume of desired local anesthetic solution
Desired additives for local anesthetic (e.g., clonidine, dexamethasone, buprenorphine, epinephrine)
Peripheral nerve stimulator, attached to block needle and patient
Pressure-monitoring device in-line with injectate system, if desired

The choice of an ultrasound system depends on the resources and needs of the user. The system should be portable, with high definition and a choice of probes to allow imaging of both superficial (high-frequency probe) and deep (low-frequency probe) nerves[5] (Fig. 1-4).

Portable, high-fidelity ultrasound machine
Ultrasound gel, preferably sterile
Ultrasound probe appropriate for nerve to be blocked

For catheter insertion, a higher degree of sterility is necessary because it is an indwelling device with relatively high rates of colonization.[6] This should mandate the use of sterile gowns, masks, and drapes, as well as the catheter system itself (Fig. 1-5). The choice

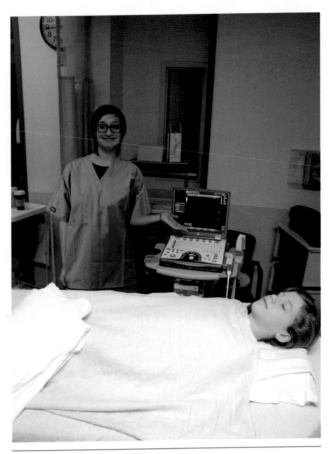

Figure 1-4. Ultrasound platform.

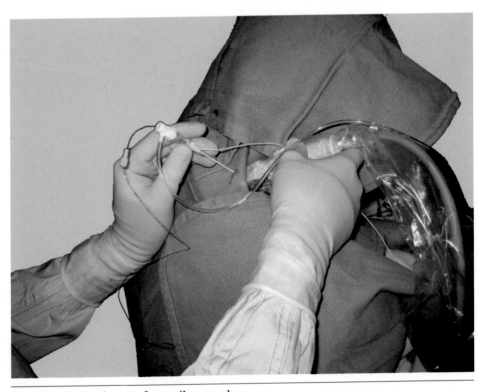

Figure 1-5. Equipment for sterile procedures.

remains for the individual anesthesiologist whether peripheral nerve stimulation is used for confirmation of the target nerve, and if so, whether a stimulating- or nonstimulating-type catheter is preferred.

Perineural needle/catheter set (stimulating or nonstimulating)
Sterile drapes
Sterile gown, mask, and gloves
Sterile adhesives to hold catheter in place
Sterile, transparent membrane to cover catheter site
Peripheral nerve stimulator, if desired

References

1. Chan VWS, Perlas A, McCartney CJL, et al. Ultrasound guidance improves success rate of axillary brachial plexus block. Can J Anaesth 2007;54:176–182.
2. Tucker MS, Nielsen KC, Steele SM. Nerve block induction rooms—physical plant setup, monitoring equipment, block cart, and resuscitation cart. Int Anesth Clin 2005;43(3):55–68.
3. Selander D, Dhuner KG, Lundborg G. Peripheral nerve injury due to injection needles used for regional anesthesia. An experimental study of the acute effects of needle point trauma. Acta Anaesth Scand 1977;21:182–188.
4. Hadzic A, Dilberovic F, Shah S, et al. Combination of intraneural injection and high injection pressure leads to fascicular injury and neurologic deficits in dogs. Reg Anesth Pain Med 2004;29:417–423.
5. Gray AT. Ultrasound-guided regional anesthesia: current state of the art. Anesthesiology 2007; 104:368–373.
6. Capdevila X, Pirat P, Bringuier S, et al. Continuous peripheral nerve blocks in hospital wards after orthopedic surgery: a multicenter prospective analysis of the quality of postoperative analgesia and complications in 1416 patients. Anesthesiology 2006;103:1035–1045.

From Paresthesia to Neurostimulation and Ultrasound-Guided Regional Anesthesia

JACQUES CHELLY

In 1911, Kulenkampf introduced the concept of locating a nerve with a paresthesia and blocking its conduction with local anesthetic. Paresthesia ruled as the technique of choice for another 50 years. Although the concept of neurostimulation was introduced around 1910, it took several decades for this technique to be recognized and used. In 1951, Sarnoff and Sarnoff also proposed the concept of a stimulating catheter. In the past 20 years, neurostimulation has gained popularity in the United States. Today it is considered the main technique for performing peripheral nerve blocks.

In the late 1980s, Ting and Sivagnanaratnam reported the use of ultrasound to confirm needle placement and observe local anesthetic spread during axillary nerve blocks. In the past 15 years, an increasing number of investigators have demonstrated the usefulness of ultrasound-guided techniques to perform regional anesthesia. In adults and children, the studies demonstrating the usefulness of ultrasound-guided techniques were initially conducted in patients undergoing upper extremity and superficial peripheral blocks. The use of ultrasound in the pediatric population has gained rapid recognition because of the quality of the images that can be generated in this patient population. The use of ultrasound was eventually extended to deeper peripheral blocks, especially sciatic and lumbar plexus blocks, when more powerful portable sonography platforms were developed. The basis defining the use of ultrasound for the performance of neuraxial blocks and for blocks traditionally used for the treatment of chronic pain was also developed in this time frame.

In the past few years, a number of authors have attempted to compare neurostimulation to ultrasound-guided techniques. A review of the literature revealed that several prospective randomized clinical trials comparing nerve stimulation and ultrasound have been conducted. In most cases, the number of patients included is very limited. Most of these studies have failed to show any significant difference in success rate when comparing the two techniques. The few studies in favor of the use of ultrasound-guided techniques were based on unusually low success rates achieved with the use of neurostimulation. For example, Dufour et al (2008) reported a difference of over 40% between the success rates of an interscalene performed using an ultrasound-guided technique versus neurostimulation. However, in this case the success rate reported with neurostimulation was only 16%. This is considerably lower than the usual 80% to 90% success published previously with the use of neurostimulation using the same approach. Other studies have reported smaller differences. In another study of interscalene block, ultrasound guidance achieved a success rate of 99% versus 91% for neurostimulation. However, in this case the authors not only compared an ultrasound-guided approach versus neurostimulation, but also a multi-injection technique (ultrasound) versus a single injection (neurostimulation) technique. In this regard, it is important to recognize that Casati et al established that the success rate associated with a multistimulation technique was much higher than with a single injection technique. The consensus among practitioners experienced in both techniques is that there is insufficient evidence to favor one technique over the other at the present time.

Recently, authors have compared the use of neurostimulation alone to the combination of ultrasound and neurostimulation. It seems that a combined approach is particularly useful in the case of deep blocks, such as block of the sciatic nerve or lumbar plexus. In these blocks, the limits of ultrasound imaging are exceeded in some patients. Another setting where combining ultrasound with stimulation appears effective is when the plexus is splayed out over a large area such as in the axilla. In these cases, the combination of neurostimulation and ultrasound has proven to be more reliable than the use of the neuro-stimulation alone.

There is no doubt that ultrasound guidance allows the practitioner to reduce the risk of intravascular puncture and intravascular injection. Marhofer et al reported 3 of 20 vascular punctures with neurostimulation versus 0 of 20 with the use of an ultrasound-guided approach while performing femoral nerve blocks. Sauter et al reported 33% of unintended blood aspiration with neurostimulation versus 5% with the use of ultrasound while performing infraclavicular blocks.

Another advantage of the ultrasound-guided technique included a reduction in the time to perform the block, possibly a faster onset of the block, and a lower cost to perform the block. Whether or not ultrasound can reduce the frequency of nerve injury associated with the performance of regional anesthesia is an important but complex question. Nerve injury following regional anesthesia and surgery is very uncommon and the etiology is multifactorial. Many of the injuries occurring after surgery have been shown to be related to the surgery; for example, compression of the tissues with a tourniquet, direct surgical injury of the nerve, and casting and positioning of the patient, rather than the performance of a regional technique. Even when the nerve block is suspected as the causative agent of injury, toxicity of the local anesthetic to the nerve may be the etiology rather than the needle or injection. At present, the forum is open to determine the relative indication of each technique or even the combination of both techniques in our goal to reduce the complications associated with regional anesthesia.

This is an exciting time for the use of ultrasound. The technology and equipment are constantly improving and declining in price, making access easier. Ultrasound training is widely available in most residencies and new techniques using ultrasound guidance are described in the literature on a regular basis. Prohibitions against the use of peripheral nerve block in anticoagulated patients have been liberalized when ultrasound is used to guide the block. The use of ultrasound in the pediatric populations has greatly facilitated nerve blocks because of the ability to visualize the area where the needle is placed and especially to decrease the amount of local anesthetic injected, which has been a critical limiting factor in the past. Nonetheless, the experience and skill of the practitioner are still paramount with this technique and will continue to be so in the near future. Advances in multiplanar sonography (three-dimension imaging), more echogenic needles, better needle guides, and machine identification of nerves will undoubtedly improve the efficiency of ultrasound in the future.

Suggested Reading

Brull R, Wijayatilake DS, Perlas A, et al. Practice patterns related to block selection, nerve localization and risk disclosure; a survey of the American Society of Regional Anesthesia and Pain Medicine. Reg Anesth Pain Med 2008;33:395–403.

Casati A, Baciarello M, Di Cianni S, et al. Effects of ultrasound guidance on the minimum effective anaesthetic volume required to block the femoral nerve. Br J Anaesth 2007;98:823–827.

Casati A, Danelli G, Baciarello M, et al. A prospective, randomized comparison between ultrasound and nerve stimulation guidance for multiple injection axillary brachial plexus block. Anesthesiology 2007;106:992–996

Casati A, Fanelli G, Beccaria P, et al. The effects of single or multiple injections on the volume of 0.5% ropivacaine required for femoral nerve blockade. Anesth Analg 2001;93:183–186.

Chan VW, Perlas A, McCartney CJ, et al. Ultrasound guidance improves success rate of axillary brachial plexus block. Can J Anaesth 2007;54:176–182.

Dufour E, Quennesson P, Van Robais AL, et al. Combined ultrasound and neurostimulation guidance for popliteal sciatic nerve block: a prospective, randomized comparison with neurostimulation alone. Anesth Analg 2008;106:1553–1558.

Kapral S, Greher M, Huber G, et al. Ultrasonographic guidance improves the success rate of interscalene brachial plexus blockade. Reg Anesth Pain Med 2008;33:253–258.

Kulenkampf D. Anesthesia of the brachial plexus. (German) Zentralbl Chir 1911;38:1337–1350.

Macaire P, Singelyn F, Narchi P, et al. Ultrasound-or nerve stimulation-guided wrist blocks for carpal tunnel release: a randomized prospective comparative study. Reg Anesth Pain Med 2008;33:363–368.

Marhofer P, Schrogendorfer K, Koinig H, et al. Ultrasonographic guidance improves sensory block and onset time of three-in-one blocks. Anesth Analg 1997;85:854–857.

Marhofer P, Schrogendorfer K, Wallner, T, et al. Ultrasonographic guidance reduces the amount of local anesthetic for 3-in-1 blocks. Reg Anesth Pain Med 1998;23:584–588.

Marhofer P, Sitzwohl C, Greher M, et al. Ultrasound guidance for infraclavicular brachial plexus anaesthesia in children. Anaesthesia 2004;59:642–646.

Orebaugh SL, Williams BA, Kentor ML. Ultrasound guidance with nerve stimulation reduces the time necessary for resident peripheral nerve blockade. Reg Anesth Pain Med 2007;32:448–454.

Perlas A, Brull R, Chan VW, et al. Ultrasound guidance improves the success of sciatic nerve block at the popliteal fossa. Reg Anesth Pain Med 2008;33:259–265.

Sauter AR, Dodgson MS, Stubhaug A, et al. Electrical nerve stimulation or ultrasound guidance for lateral sagittal infraclavicular blocks: a randomized, controlled, observer-blinded, comparative study. Anesth Analg 2008;106:1910–1915.

Sia S, Bartoli M. Selective ulnar nerve localization is not essential for axillary brachial plexus block using a multiple nerve stimulation technique. Reg Anesth Pain Med 2001;26:12–16.

3

Principles of Sonography

PAUL E. BIGELEISEN, STEVEN L. OREBAUGH

The frequency of medical ultrasound ranges between 2 and 13 MHz. The speed of sound in tissues is about 1500 m/sec. The average wavelength of the ultrasound beam in this band is less than 1 mm. This limits the use of ultrasound to structures that are 1 mm in diameter or larger (Fig. 3-1). Most nerves of interest range in size from 2 to 10 mm. Veins and arteries of interest are typically 3 to 15 mm.

Many factors contribute to the quality and resolution of the ultrasound image. In general, higher frequency probes generate higher resolution images. Unfortunately, the signal strength or intensity (I) of high-frequency ultrasound waves (10–13 MHz) is rapidly attenuated in tissue. Thus, high-frequency probes are best suited for structures less than 4 cm deep from the skin. For deeper structures, probes in the 2- to 5-MHz range are more useful (Fig. 3-2).

The ultrasound beam may be refracted as it passes through tissue. When this occurs, a nerve or other organ may appear at a different anatomical location than its actual site. This is the same phenomenon responsible for the apparent bending of your forearm when you place it in a bucket of water (Fig. 3-3). Fat globules below the skin, in the muscle, and around nerves are about 1 mm in diameter. These globules (Fig. 3-4A) serve as scattering and diffraction sites for the incident and reflected ultrasound beam and cause a speckled appearance in the image (Fig. 3-4B,C). This is called *speclation*. For these reasons, obese patients can be very difficult to image (Fig. 3-5A,B).

The image formed on ultrasound is very sensitive to the angle of incidence of the beam relative to the nerve. This is referred to as the *angle of insonation*. Sometimes, changing the angle of insonation by only a few degrees can bring the nerve into focus.

Diffraction and scattering, as well as the heterogeneous three-dimensional structure of the nerves and their surrounding tissues, are thought to cause this phenomenon. An analogy is shown in Figure 3-6A. Here, light is shown on a three-dimensional ikon. Varying the direction of the incident light beam by only a few degrees will result in a radically different shadow in any direction. To obtain the optimal ultrasound image, the image should be centered on the screen by sliding or rotating the probe on the patient's skin. For deep structures, compressing the tissue with pressure may improve the image. Once these maneuvers have been completed, toggling will produce the best image (Fig. 3-6B through F).

Modern platforms allow the user to adjust the brightness (gain) of the entire image or more superficial (near field) and deep (far field) structures. Increasing the gain makes the entire image whiter. Increasing the gain too much creates a snowy background in which all of the structures become indistinguishable. In general, the gain should be set so that most of the background is black and only the structures of interest, such as nerves and vessels, are easily seen. Many machines have an autogain button that adjusts the gain for the user.

What We See on Ultrasound Will Depend Upon

1) The frequency of the sound wave:

$$\lambda = c/\nu = (1.5 \times 10^3 \text{ m/sec}) / 5 \times 10^6 \text{ Hz} = 0.3 \text{ mm}$$

Resolution = 1 mm

Figure 3-1. Relationship between wavelength and resolution.

$$I(\mu,r) = I_0 e^{-\mu r}$$
$$\mu = \mu_1 \nu$$

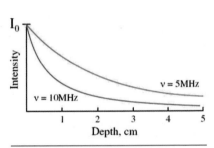

Figure 3-2a. Equation for beam attenuation as a function of frequency. R, tissue depth; ν, frequency; μ, amplitude attenuation constant.

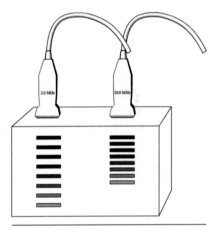

Figure 3-2b. Beam attenuation as a function of frequency.

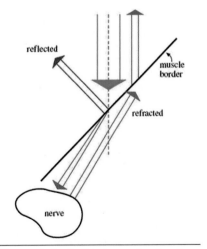

Figure 3-3. Reflection and refraction of ultrasound beam.

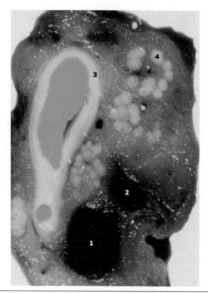

Figure 3-4a. Cross section through the axilla. *1*, axillary vein; *2*, basilic vein; *3*, wall of axillary artery; *4*, nerve fascicles.

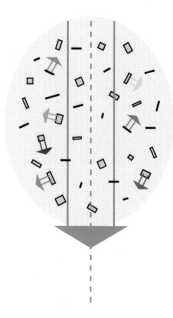

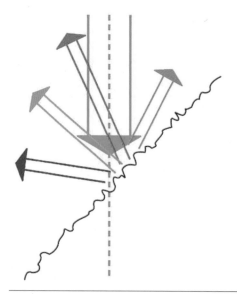

Figure 3-4b. Scattering from an irregular surface.

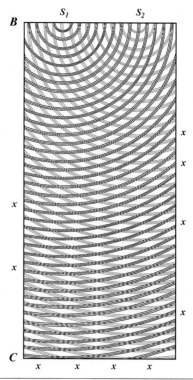

Figure 3-4c. Diffraction of ultrasound beam causing speclation.

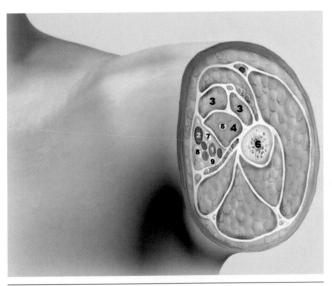

Figure 3-5a. Schematic through the axilla. *1*, axillary artery; *2*, axillary vein; *3*, biceps muscle; *4*, coracobrachialis muscle; *5*, branch of musculocutaneous nerve; *6*, humerus; *7*, median nerve; *8*, ulnar nerve; *9*, radial nerve.

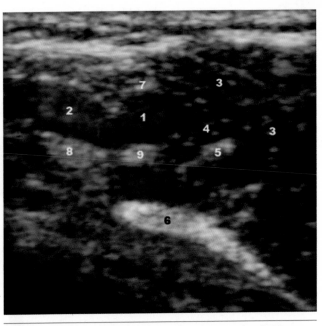

Figure 3-5b. *1*, axillary artery; *2*, axillary vein; *3*, biceps muscle; *4*, coracobrachialis muscle; *5*, branch of musculocutaneous nerve; *6*, humerus; *7*, median nerve; *8*, ulnar nerve; *9*, radial nerve.

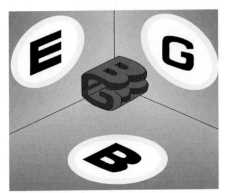

Figure 3-6a. Relationship between beam direction and image.

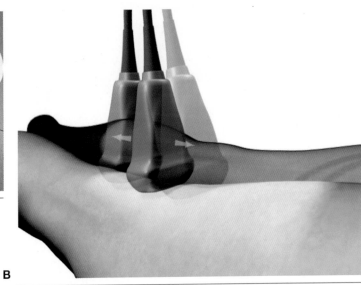

B

Figure 3-6b–f. Different probe movements (*not mentioned in text*).

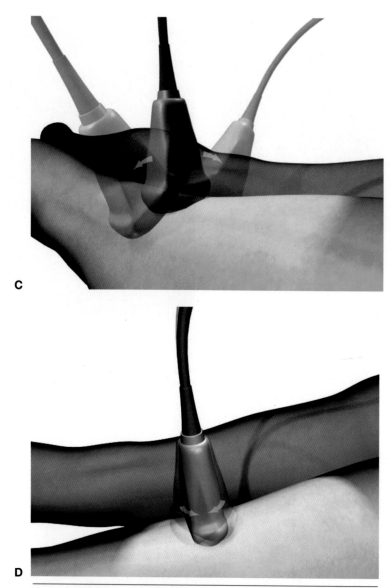

Figure 3-6c,d. *(continued).*

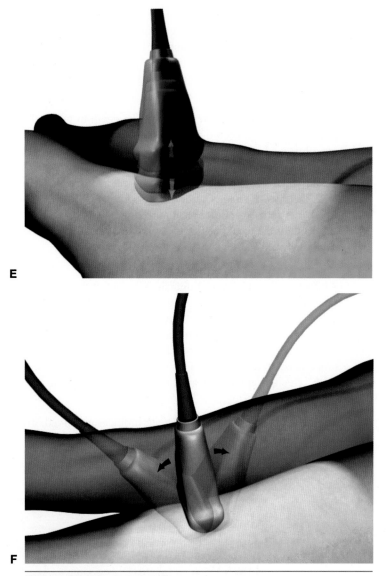

Figure 3-6e,f. *(continued).*

Modern machines also allow the user to adjust the contrast. The formal term for contrast is *dynamic range compression*. Increasing the dynamic range compression makes the white images whiter and the black images blacker (Fig. 3-7A). This may bring the edges of an anatomic structure into better view. Decreasing the dynamic range compression makes everything in the image a more homogeneous gray.

All machines allow the user to adjust the depth to which the probe penetrates. Whenever possible, the depth should be set to the shallowest setting in which the structures of interest are all imaged. Some machines come with a preset focal zone, and some machines allow the user to set multiple focal zones. In general, the focal zone should encompass the area of greatest interest in the image. The near focal zone has the greatest resolution and is referred to as the *Fresnel zone*. The deeper focal zone (far field) is referred to as the *Fraunhofer zone*. This zone has poorer resolution (Fig. 3-8A). Most machines allow the user to adjust the depth of the focal zone or to set multiple focal zones (Fig. 3-8B) by adjusting the time delays between transducer elements in the probe.

Arteries can usually be distinguished by their pulsatile nature. Veins can be distinguished by their compressibility. Pressing on the skin with the probe will usually cause the vein to collapse. Color flow Doppler imaging can also be used to identify and distinguish arteries and veins. Blood flowing perpendicular to the probe is black (Fig. 3-9A). By convention, blood flowing toward the probe is colored red (Fig. 3-9B). Blood flowing away from the probe is colored blue (Fig. 3-9C). Velocity gates can be set to measure the flow velocity. High velocities are usually arteries; low velocities are usually veins.

Transducer elements can be arranged in linear or curved arrays (Fig. 3-10). Linear arrays create rectangular images and are most useful for superficial structures. Curved arrays create wedge-shaped images and are most useful for deeper structures. When a curved array is used,

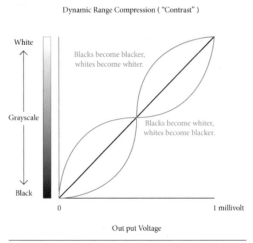

Figure 3-7a. Schematic for contrast adjustment (dynamic range compression) of the supraclavicular fossa.

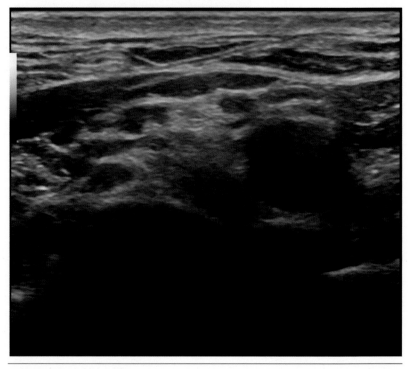

Figure 3-7b. Normal contrast.

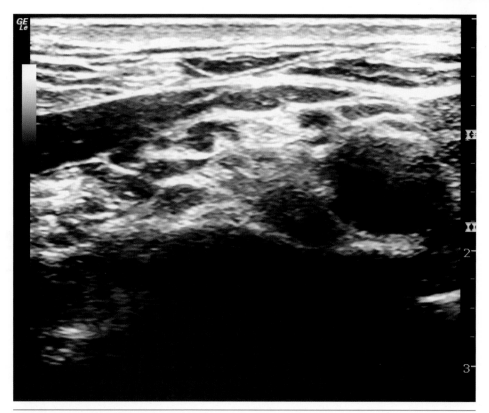

Figure 3-7c. High contrast.

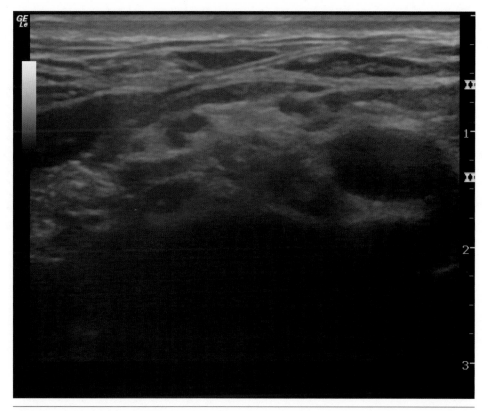

Figure 3-7d. Low contrast.

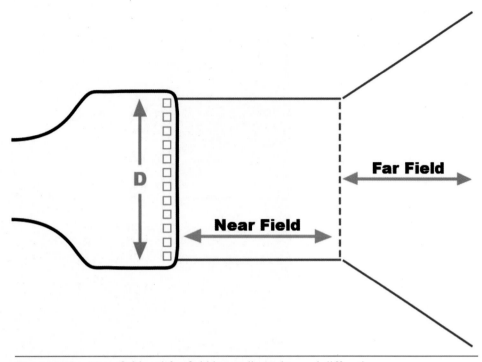

Figure 3-8a. Near-field and far-field beam dispersion and diffraction.

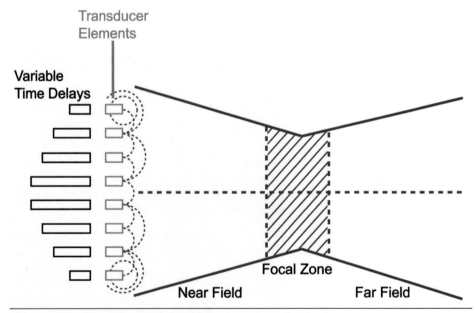

Figure 3-8b. Use of variable time delays to change the focal zone.

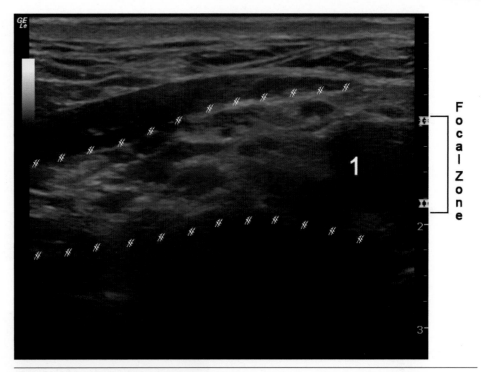

Figure 3-8c. Supraclavicular fossa in focus.

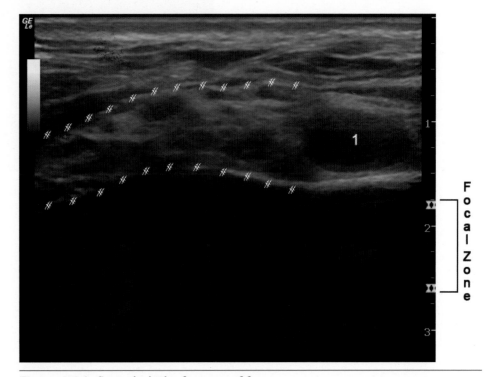

Figure 3-8d. Supraclavicular fossa out of focus.

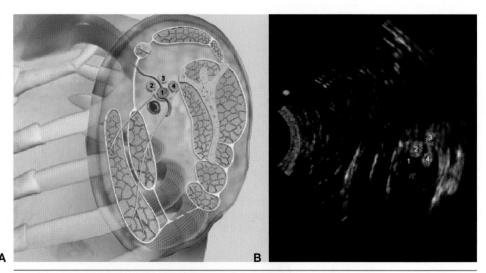

Figure 3-9a,b. Schematic of the infraclavicular fossa. *1*, axillary artery; *2*, *3*, and *4*, lateral, posterior, and medial cords.

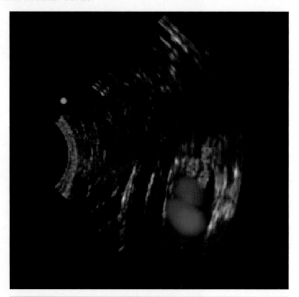

Figure 3-9c. Color flow Doppler. *Red*, flow toward the probe; *blue*, flow away from the probe.

The type of array used in the transducer;

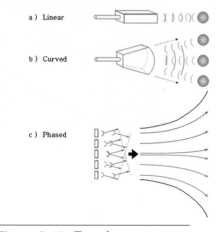

a) Linear

b) Curved

c) Phased

Figure 3-10. Transducer types.

the beam disperses laterally, resulting in a lower resolution than a linear array. A phased array retains the transducer elements in a linear arrangement, but the elements fire in sequence creating a phase delay between each element. The net result is a wedge-shaped image from a set of linear transducers. Because this signal is averaged, its resolution is also lower than a standard linear array. The array in a transducer can also be programmed to fire with multiple phase delays. This creates a simple two-dimensional tomogram called a *compound beam image*. This signal can be processed to highlight nerves (Fig. 3-11A). The image formed is less sensitive to the angle of incidence, because the beam comes from many directions. Thus, even though transducer alignment may not be optimal, a recognizable image may still be produced (Fig. 3-11B). The resolution in the compound beam mode is blurred compared with a standard linear or curved array without this type of signal averaging.

Most probes have transducers that emit the highest amplitude of their ultrasound wave at a specific fundamental frequency. Higher harmonics of this frequency are also emitted at lower amplitudes (Fig. 3-12). By listening for the echo at these higher harmonic frequencies, image resolution can be enhanced. Because the harmonics are very low amplitude, only transducers that have sufficient power output can be used for harmonic imaging. This type of image enhancement is referred to as *tissue harmonic imaging*. It is very useful in cardiac imaging, but it has not been shown to be useful in nerve imaging at this time. Compound beam imaging negates most of the advantages of tissue harmonic imaging.

Modern probes operate in pulsed mode. The transducer elements in the probe are used as both transmitters and receivers. The transducer elements emit a short ultrasound burst and then wait for the echo before emitting another ultrasound burst. This allows the probe to be smaller compared with continuous wave probes in which there are separate emitters and transducers (Fig. 3-13).

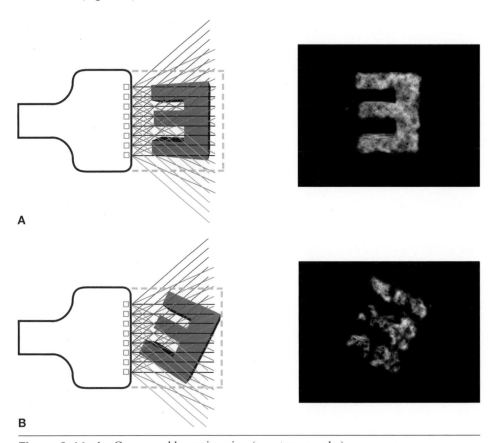

A

B

Figure 3-11a,b. Compound beam imaging (sonotomography).

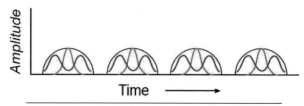

Figure 3-12. Frequency band in transducer.

When a needle is inserted into tissue perpendicular to the ultrasound beam, it is a good reflector and easy to image. Ghosts on the deep side of the needle are caused by continued needle vibration after the ultrasound wave strikes the needle (Fig. 3-14A,B). These reverberations return to the receiver later than the first volley of echoes. Consequently, they are seen as deeper in the tissue. In some cases, it may be necessary to insert the needle nearly parallel to the beam to reach the targeted organ. In this case, most of the echo is lost, and the needle image is much fainter (Fig. 3-15A,B).

Above the collar bone, nerves are usually dark (hypoechoic) (Fig. 3-16A,B). Nerves located below the collar bone are usually white (hyperechoic) (Fig. 3-5B). The reasons for this dichotomy are not known but are thought to be related to the depth of the nerves, the amount of fat around the nerves, and the relative amounts of fat and stroma within the nerves themselves. On ultrasound cross section, nerves are round, hypo- or hyperechoic, reticulated structures. When imaged along their long axis, nerves appear as linear, hypo- or hyperechoic streaks. Bones are hyperechoic (Fig. 3-5B) and usually very bright white. Arteries and veins are black unless color flow Doppler imaging is used (Fig. 3-9). If the transducer is perpendicular to the blood flow, arteries and veins will be black even with color flow Doppler imaging.

Most nerves have some fascia around them. There is usually a potential space between the fascia and the epineurium. When a needle punctures the fascia, local anesthetic can usually be deposited between the fascia and nerve (Fig. 3-17A). This creates a black (hypoechoic) ring around the nerve. In some cases, the fascia adheres to the epineurium or is missing. In that case, the needle may puncture the nerve, and the nerve will swell as the local anesthetic is injected (Fig. 3-17B).

 Tips

1. Stimulation with a peripheral nerve stimulator is not necessary if the operator is certain of the nerve's identity on ultrasound. When a stimulator is used, it should only be used to confirm the target nerve; then it can be turned off. Because the local anesthetic is injected around the target nerve under ultrasound visualization, there is no need to "titrate" the current to the twitch.
2. It is challenging to keep the needle perfectly parallel to the long axis of the transducer. Frequent fine adjustment of the transducer may be necessary along with switching the

The signal processing

a) Continuous   (separate transmitter and receiver)
))))))))))

b) Pulsed   (may have a single transmitter and receiver)
)))   )))   )))

c) Harmonic   (increased power requirement but better resolution)
) ((( ) ((( ) ((( ) ((( ) ((( ) ((( ) (((●

Figure 3-13. Signal-processing modes.

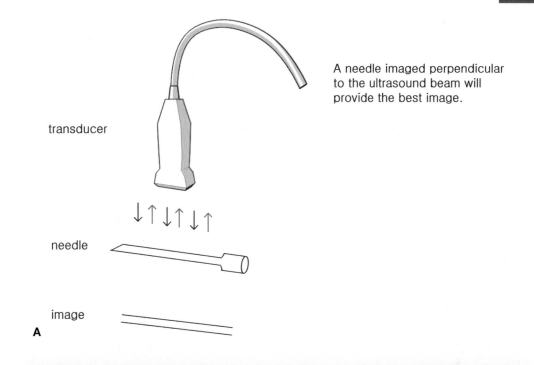

A needle imaged perpendicular to the ultrasound beam will provide the best image.

transducer

needle

image

A

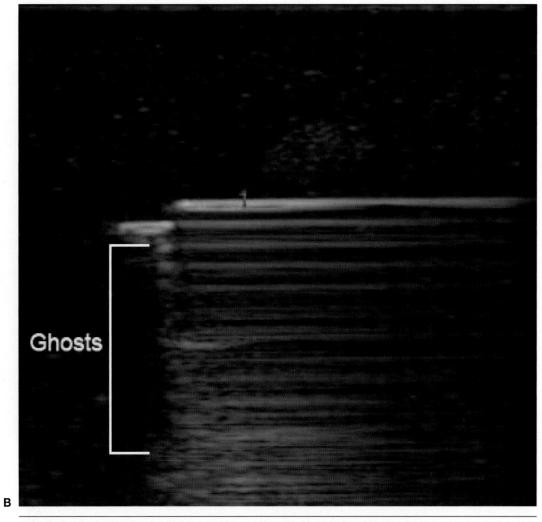

Ghosts

B

Figure 3-14a,b. Reflection from needle at perpendicular angle of insonation.

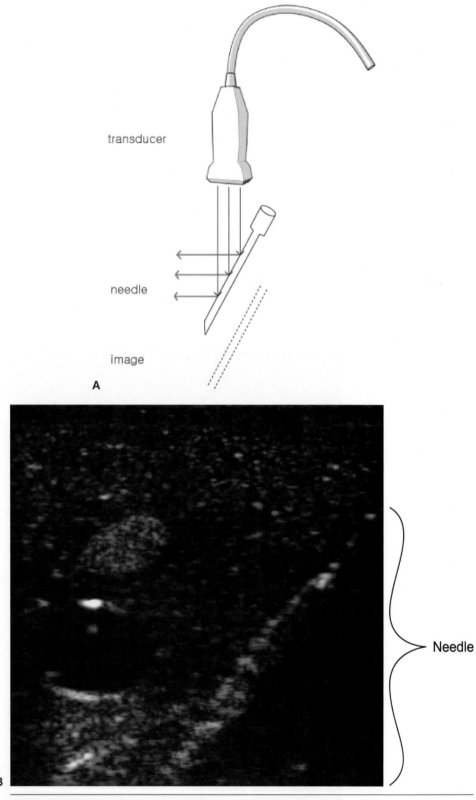

Figure 3-15a,b. Reflection from needle at oblique angle of insonation.

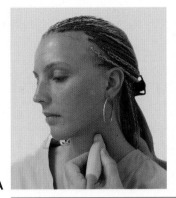
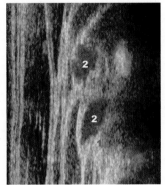

Figure 3-16a,b. Ultrasound scan of nerve roots. *1*, transverse process; *2*, nerve root.

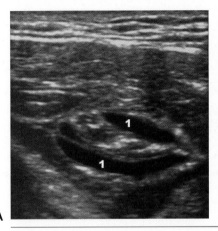
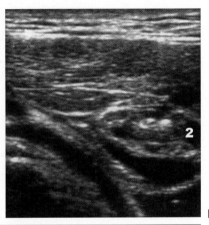

Figure 3-17a,b. Ultrasound scan of musculocutaneous nerve. *1*, local anesthetic around nerve; *2*, local anesthetic injected into nerve.

line of site of the operator from the ultrasound screen to the site of needle insertion. Some people prefer to use a needle guide to help keep the needle aligned with the ultrasound beam. Other practitioners have had some success with a laser guide.

3. As local anesthetic is injected, each increment should cause visible expansion of the tissues at the tip of the needle. This provides evidence that the tip of the needle is neither intravascular nor intraneural.

4. If all of the local anesthetic solution seems to accumulate on only one side of the target nerve, the needle should be gently advanced or moved to another site around the nerve to allow accumulation of the solution around the entire nerve (the "halo" effect). This minimizes block set-up time. It should be clear that each aliquot of local anesthetic injected should cause distension of the tissues at the tip of the needle. It is not necessary to restimulate when the needle is moved around the nerve, but the patient should be assessed for paresthesia or pain in the territory of the stimulated nerve.

5. As with any block guided by the nerve stimulator, mild injection paresthesias may occur during injection of local anesthetic in blocks carried out by ultrasound guidance. This should be differentiated from the severe pain that is more likely indicative of intrafascicular injection.

Suggested Reading

Jan J. Medical Image Processing, Reconstruction, and Restoration. New York: Taylor and Francis; 2006.

4

Microanatomy of the Peripheral Nervous System and Its Implications for Paravertebral and Peripheral Nerve Blocks

ANDRE P. BOEZAART

Introduction: The use of ultrasound has provided anesthesiologists a deeper understanding of the location of peripheral nerves, as well as a powerful tool to anesthetize these nerves. The wavelength of medical ultrasound used for nerve blocks ranges from 0.1 to 1 mm. In most cases, the nerves that we wish to image range from 3 to 15 mm in diameter. Under optimal conditions, we may therefore be able to "look" inside large nerves or a nerve plexus and "see" individual fascicles. Unfortunately, the resolution provided by ultrasound does not allow us to view the perineurium, a protective sheath that surrounds the fascicles as the nerve root emerges from the lateral recess of the spinal canal and travels toward the periphery as a peripheral nerve. However, in small patients and children, we may be able to image the dura mater where it surrounds the cauda equina, although this is of little use when performing peripheral nerve blocks. Some anesthesiologists may not be familiar with the ultrastructure of nerve roots and nerves and, for this reason, may not appreciate the risks involved with paravertebral nerve blocks—even with ultrasound guidance.

Catastrophic outcomes following paravertebral blocks at the cervical,[1-4] thoracic,[5] and lumbar levels[6-8] have been reported, some of which were reversible cases of extensive epidural/subdural block or total spinal anesthesia. Unfortunately, other cases resulted in paraplegia, quadriplegia, and death. The explanation for these catastrophes focused on intracord injection, which complicated the blocks performed on patients under general anesthesia. Interscalene block has also been blamed for disastrous outcomes.[9-14] The report of four cases of spinal injury after interscalene block by Benumof[9] attracted much attention and generated a fierce debate on the safety of performing blocks on patients under general anesthesia. The conclusions reached by Benumof, that blocks should not be performed under general anesthesia, were regrettably largely incorrect, particularly in the case of pediatric patients. These tragic outcomes, like many others, were most likely caused by intraroot injection and had nothing to do with the fact that the patients were under general anesthesia when the blocks were placed. Benumof's conclusions were largely based on a misunderstanding of the microanatomy of the connective tissue framework of the nervous system. All of these cases have two things in common: root level nerve blocks and thin, relatively sharp needles.[15-17]

Microanatomy of the Peripheral Nervous System: Our understanding of the microanatomy of the peripheral nervous system is already more than 130 years old. Key and Retzius[18] in 1876 (Richardson stain) and Horster and Whitman[19] in 1931 (trypan blue)

26

studied the spread of intraneurally injected solutions. In 1948, French[20] repeated this work with radiopaque contrast medium in dogs. In 1952, Moore[21] used methylene blue-stained exocaine, and in 1978, Selander[22] used radioactive local anesthetic with fluorescent dye to study the microanatomy of the sciatic nerve in rabbits. In the interval, electron microscopy[23] was used to confirm what was already known.[24]

According to conventional teaching, (including many modern anatomy and anesthesia textbooks), the cerebrospinal fluid (CSF) originates in the choroid plexus, is discharged into the cerebral ventricles, and exits through the foramina of Luschka and Magendie. The CSF then gathers in the cisterns at the base of the brain, where it flows to the villi or pacchionian bodies, and then into the peripheral venous circulation.

In 1948, Hassin[25] proposed a new depiction of how the CSF courses through the circulation.

In summary:

The CSF is the extracellular fluid of the brain and spinal cord.

1. The circulation of the CSF involves the Virchow-Robin spaces that surround the arterioles in the brain; these spaces form the blood–brain barrier.
2. Absorption of the CSF is not through the villi or pacchionian bodies, but mostly through the perineurial spaces of the cranial nerves and spinal roots.
3. The CSF acts as the "lymph fluid" of the central nervous system and carries away waste.
4. There is no central force per se that drives the CSF into the circulation. The cardiac cycle causes expansion and contraction of the brain and spinal cord, which are encased in a rigid compartment. During systole, the entire brain and spinal cord expand, and pressure in the CSF increases. Following a pressure gradient, the CSF flows from the central space out into the perineural spaces of the cranial and spinal nerve roots.

Peripheral Nerves and Plexuses: The tissue fluid deep to the epineurium, but outside of the perineurium, in a peripheral nerve is lymph and drains to the regional lymph nodes.[25] The axons of peripheral nerves are extensions of nerve cells in the central nervous system. These axons, which are surrounded by perineurium, form fascicles, and are bathed by CSF. Under normal conditions, the longitudinal flow of the CSF within the fascicle is minimal.[22] Lateral extension (centrifugal) of the perineurium is minimal even under high pressure. As the nerve approaches dural penetration, resistance to lateral extension increases, and a peripherally injected medium comes to lie in the clefts of the perineurium. Final emergence into the subarachnoid space appears to occur, first, by way of the subdural space and, subsequently, by breaking through the arachnoid barrier into the subarachnoid space. Injection into peripheral nerve fascicles, which is difficult to achieve under clinical conditions, provides direct access to the CSF and interstitium of the spinal cord. Conversely, penetration and injection into a spinal root is relatively easy under clinical conditions, and this injectate similarly has direct access to the CSF and spinal cord interstitium (Fig. 4-1). The clinical consequence of an injection into a spinal root will depend on the volume, rate, and pressure of the injectate.

Peripheral nerves are composed of numerous fascicles that contain axons. Each fascicle is bounded by a dense perineurium, and a fine epineurial membrane holds the fascicles together (Fig. 4-2). The epineurium consists of a condensation of areolar connective tissue that surrounds the perineural ensheathment of the fascicles on unifascicular and multifascicular nerves. The attachment of the epineurium to surrounding connective tissue is loose, so that the nerve is relatively mobile except where tethered by entering blood vessels or

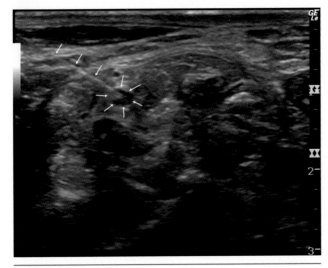

Figure 4-1a. Ultrasound scan at C5 showing intraneural injection.

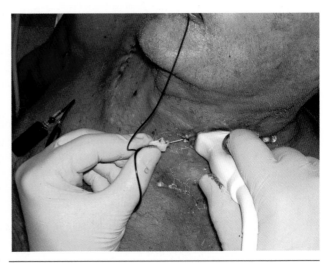

Figure 4-1b. Needle and probe position during injection in **A**.

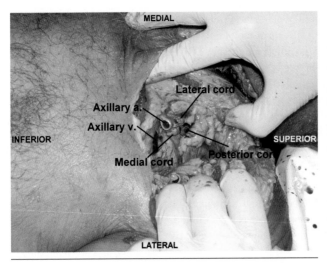

Figure 4-1c. Cadaver dissection in the infraclavicular region after injection of C5.

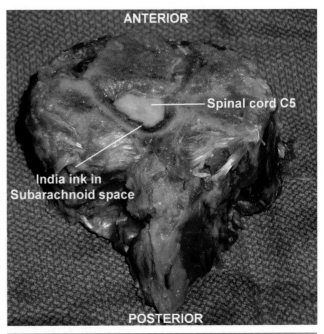

Figure 4-1d. Cross section through spine at C5 after injection of C5.

nerve branches. Greater amounts of connective tissue are normally present where nerves cross over joints, and nerves usually carry sensory signals from branches from those joints. In general, the more fascicles within a nerve, the thicker the epineurium would be. Variable quantities of fat are also present in the epineurium, particularly in larger nerves. This fat cushions the fascicles against injury by compression; and, thus, large multifascicular nerves are less susceptible to injury by compression than smaller or unifascicular nerves. The vaso nervorum enter the epineurium where they communicate with a longitudinal anastomotic network of arterioles and venules. The epineurium also contains lymphatic vessels, which are not present within the fascicles. These lymphatic channels accompany the arteries of the peripheral nerves and pass into the regional lymph nodes.[25]

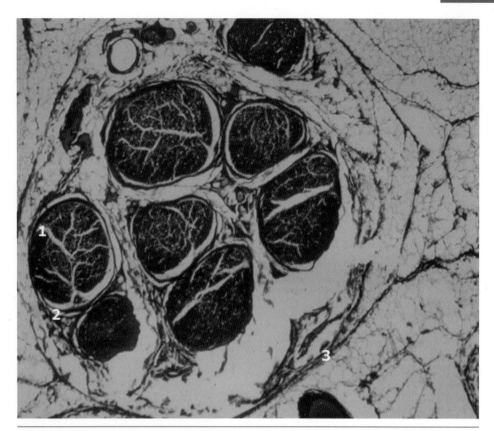

Figure 4-2. Cross section of peripheral nerve. *1*, endoneurium; *2*, perineurium; *3*, epineurium.

The essential structure of the perineurium is a lamellated arrangement of flattened cells separated by layers of collagenous connective tissue.[18] It provides ensheathment for both the somatic and peripheral autonomic nerves and their ganglia. The cellular lamellae are composed of concentric sleeves of flattened polygonal cells. These cells are equipped to function as a metabolically active diffusion barrier, although they do not have the morphologic features of a true epithelium. The *endoneurium* refers to intrafascicular connective tissue, excluding the perineurial portions that may subdivide fascicles. About 40% to 50% of the intrafascicular space is occupied by nonneural elements, and about 20% to 30% of this is the endoneural fluid (CSF) and connective matrix, which we call the endoneurium.[24]

The injection of local anesthetic deep to the epineurium, but outside the perineurium in humans and pigs causes a centrifugal expansion of the epineurium—referred to as a *subepineurial injection*. The injection of several millimeters of local anesthetic deep to the epineurium will cause the diameter of the nerve to double. When 10 to 20 mL of local anesthetic is injected into the subepineurial space, the epineurium ruptures (neurolysis), causing the local anesthetic to surround the nerve. The injection of several milliliters of local anesthetic into the subepineurial space over a few seconds may cause the pressure within the subepineurial space to rise to 15 lb/in². Once the injection is stopped, the pressure inside the epineurium returns to baseline pressure within seconds.

When Selander[22] injected blue tracer into a fascicle (subperineurial injection) of rabbit sciatic nerves, the tracer spread rapidly, both proximally and distally, within the fascicle. The injection within the fascicle (0.05–0.1 mL) created pressures between 435 mm Hg and 675 mm Hg. These pressures remained above capillary perfusion pressure (50 mm Hg) for at least 10 minutes. In all cases, the injection reached the sacral plexus. Distally, the tracer colored the tibial

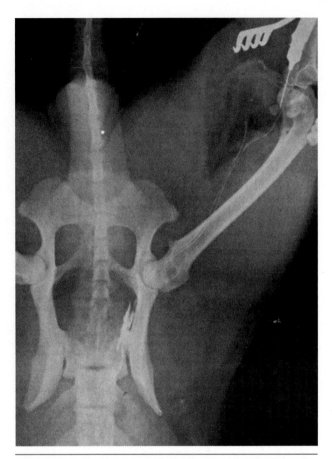

Figure 4-3. Radiocontrast injection into the fascicle of a dog sciatic nerve.

nerve, sometimes reaching the foreleg. If the injection was made into a small fascicle, the injectate did not extend beyond the sacral plexus. If the tracer was injected into a large fascicle, the injectate passed the sacral plexus and reached the spinal medulla; during slow injection, it spreads in the medulla superficially, under the pia mater. In some animals, the spread was into the CSF, and the dura and arachnoid were also colored with the tracer. In one animal, the blue stain extended to the cerebellum, and the animal died shortly after injection.[22] In cross-sections of the spinal medulla, the tracer was noted in the dorsal root–medulla junction area, extending into the substantia gelatinosa and into the anterior median fissure. In the canine studies of French,[20] the radiopaque tracer reached the lumbar plexus via the injected fascicle, and then tracked distally via an entirely different nerve (Fig 4-3). The contrast injected intrathecally under high pressure also spread peripherally into the fascicles of peripheral nerves.

Plexus Trunks and Spinal Roots: The distal roots and trunks of the plexuses should be seen as transitional areas where the fascicles are no longer ensheathed by the perineurium. At the trunk level, the perineurium has split into septae (Fig. 4-4). Functionally, the trunks should be regarded as a zone between peripheral nerves with clearly defined fasciculi and rigid perineuria, and the root area is where perineurial septae have joined to form the dura mater. The perineuria of peripheral nerves, therefore, are continuations of the dura mater. The axons inside roots are no longer protected by the perineurium, and the tissue fluid inside the root is the CSF (Fig. 4-4). When Bigeleisen[26] injected 2 mL of India ink over 2 seconds into the C5 nerve root of a fresh cadaver, the pressure exceeded 30 lb/in^2. The tracer stained the subarachnoid space at the C5 level and traveled distally into a fascicle of the posterior cord (Fig. 4-1).

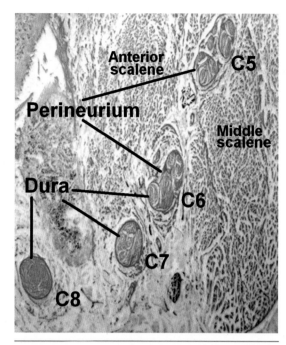

Figure 4-4. Cross setion through the roots of the brachial plexus. C5 and C6 with epineurium and septae. C7 and C8 with dura/perineurium.

The mesothelial cells of the arachnoid membrane become hyperplastic at the point where the nerve leaves the spinal cord and form a cuff around the roots, just after they penetrate the dura mater. Beyond this cuff, no tissue that is recognized as arachnoid can be seen. The connective tissue framework of the peripheral nervous system, therefore, appears to arise entirely from a continuation of the perineurium, starting at the dura mater. As the nerve progresses peripherally, it is further subdivided by perineural septations until each fascicle eventually has its own perineural sheath. This most likely gives rise to the well-known dictum that the more distal a nerve block is placed, the safer it is to block it.

Practical Matters and Clinical Consequences: With the recent increase in ultrasound utilization, it has become apparent to practitioners that nerves can range from hypoechoic to hyperechoic in appearance.[27] In most cases, the closer the nerve lies to the spine, the more likely it is to be hypoechoic. With the insight of microanatomy, this is easy to understand. At the root level, there are mostly axons interspersed with CSF, which, similar to the fluid within the axons, is hypoechoic. In the periphery, the nerve has stroma and fat outside the perineurium, which is hyperechoic. The perineurium itself, which divides the nerve into fascicles, is also hyperechoic. This architecture, gives rise to the honeycomb appearance of peripheral nerves.[27]

Recent ultrasound work on axillary nerve blocks has also confirmed our clinical impressions. Intraneural injections have no bad consequences as long as the injection is deep to the epineurium but outside the perineurium.[28] Intrafascicular injections are difficult when blunt needles are used. Nonetheless, the work of French[20] showed that contrast medium injected into fascicles lingered for up to 5 weeks. This finding makes the occasional numb finger that we encounter in our patients from time to time, several weeks after an interscalene or supraclavicular block, more comprehensible.

Injections at the root level and trunk level in some individuals should be regarded as epidural injections because the injection is made directly outside the dura or peridural space. All of the time-tested rules for epidural injections should, thus, apply for root level or paravertebral injections. This should include the avoidance of sharp thin needles as well as incorporation of large bore Tuohy needles for continuous and single injections.[29] Fractionation of the dose, with frequent aspiration for vascular and intrathecal injection, should also be performed; perhaps it also would be wise to follow the anticoagulation guidelines for epidural placement.

All of the tragic cases referred to previously can reasonably be attributed to intraroot injections with relatively thin, sharp needles that can easily penetrate the dura. These blocks were performed with needles that should never be used for an epidural block, and yet, they were used for a form of epidural block—the paravertebral or paraspinal block. The differences in the ultimate clinical presentations were merely a function of the volume, rate, and pressure of the injection. All or most of these tragic outcomes may have been avoided by using large bore Tuohy needles, test dosing, and perhaps the use of ultrasound. An understanding of the functional microanatomy would have gone a long way toward understanding what was happening to these unfortunate patients.

Sadly, many cases of total spinal anesthesia and permanent nerve damage continue to occur in the anesthesia community because of a lack of understanding of the ultrastructure of nerves. Because these injuries, as well as the risk of monetary and legal punishment to practitioners and hospitals, have previously been reported in the literature, these additional cases no longer reach the standard anesthesia community as case reports. It is the author's hope that the information in this chapter will diminish this problem.

References

1. Voermans NC, Crul BJ, de Bondt B, et al. Permanent loss of cervical spinal cord function associated with the posterior approach. Anesth Analg 2006;102:330–331.
2. Aramideh M, van den Oever HL, Walstra GJ, et al. Spinal anesthesia as a complication of brachial plexus block using the posterior approach. Anesth Analg 2002;94:1338–1339.
3. Grefkens JM, Bürger K. Total spinal anaesthesia after an attempted brachial plexus block using the posterior approach. Anaesthesia 2006;61(11)1105–1108.
4. Gentili M, Aveline C, Bonnet F. Total spinal anesthesia after posterior plexus block [in French]. Ann Fr Anesth Reanim 1998;17(7)740–742.
5. Lekhak B, Bartley C, Conacher ID, et al. Total spinal anaesthesia in association with insertion of a paravertebral catheter. Br J Anaesth 2001;86(2)280–282.
6. Houten JK. Paraplegia after lumbosacral nerve root block: report of three cases. Spine J 2002; 2(1)70–75.
7. Pousman RM, Mansoor Z, Sciard D. Total spinal anesthetic after continuous posterior lumbar plexus block. Anesthesiology 2003;98(5)1281–1282.
8. Litz R, Vicent O, Wiessner D. Misplacement of a psoas compartment catheter in the subarachnoid space. Reg Anesth Pain Med 2004;29(1)60–64.
9. Benumof JL. Permanent loss of cervical spinal cord function associated with interscalene block performed under general anesthesia. Anesthesiology 2000;93(6)1541–1544.
10. Ross S, Scarborough CD. Total spinal anesthesia following brachial-plexus block. Anesthesiology 1973;39(4)458.
11. Dutton RP, Eckhardt WF III, Sunder N. Total spinal anesthesia after interscalene blockade of the brachial plexus. Anesthesiology 1994;80:939–941.
12. Tetzlaff JE, Yoon HJ, Dilger J, et al. Subdural anesthesia as a complication of an interscalene brachial plexus block. Case report. Reg Anesth 1994;19(5)357–359.
13. Dutton RP, Eckhardt WF III, Sunder N. Total spinal anesthesia after interscalene blockade of the brachial plexus. Anesthesiology 1994;80(4)939–941.
14. White JL. Catastrophic complications of the interscalene nerve block. Anesthesiology 2001;95(5)1301.
15. Capdevila X, Macaire P, Dadure C, et al. Continuous psoas compartment block for postoperative analgesia after total hip arthroplasty: new landmarks, technical guidelines, and clinical evaluation. Anesth Analg 2002;94:1606–1613.

16. Boezaart AP, Koorn R, Rosenquist RW. Paravertebral approach to the brachial plexus: an anatomic improvement in technique. Reg Anesth Pain Med 2003;28:241–244.

17. Boezaart AP, de Beer JF, Nell ML. Early experience with continuous cervical paravertebral block using a stimulating catheter. Reg Anesth Pain Med 2003;28:406–413.

18. Key A, Retzius G. Studien in der Anatomie des Nervensystems und des Bindegewebes (2.Hafte). Stockholm: Samson & Wallin, 1876:187.

19. Horster H, Whitman L. Die Methode der intraneuralen injektion. Z Hygiene 1931;13:113.

20. French JD, Strain WH, Jones GE. Mode of extension of contrast substances injected into peripheral nerves. J Neuropathol Exp Neurol 1948;7:47–58.

21. Moore DC, Hain RF, Ward A, et al. Importance of the perineural spaces in nerve blocking. J Am Med Assoc 1954;156:1050–1053.

22. Selander D, Sjöstrand J. Longitudinal spread of intraneurally injected local anesthetics. An experimental study of the initial neural distribution following intraneural injections. Acta Anaesthesiol Scand 1978:22:622–634.

23. Rohlich P, Knoop A. Elektronenmikroskopische Untersuchenen an den Hullen des N. Ischiadicus der Ratte. Z Zellforsch Mikrosk Anat 1961:53:288–305.

24. Thomas PK, Berthold CH, Ochoa J. Microscopic anatomy of the peripheral nervous system. In: Dyck PJ, Thomas PK, eds. Peripheral Neuropathy. 3rd ed. Philadelphia, PA: WB Saunders, 1993:28–91

25. Hassin GB. Cerebrospinal fluid, its origin, nature and function. J Exp Neuropathol Exp Neurol 1948;7(1):172–181.

26. Bigeleisen PE. Intra-root injection of India ink and contrast dye in fresh cadaver. Where does the dye go and what does it mean? Submitted to Anesthesiology.

27. Chan VWS. The use of ultrasound for peripheral nerve blocks. In: Boezaart AP, ed. Anesthesia and Orthopaedic Surgery. New York: McGraw-Hill, 2006:283–290.

28. Bigeleisen PE. Nerve puncture and apparent intraneural injection during ultrasound-guided axillary block does not invariably result in neurologic injury. Anesthesiology 2006;105:779–783.

29. Boezaart AP, Franco CD. Thin sharp needles around the dura. Reg Anesth Pain Med 2006;31:388–389.

5

Ultrasound-Guided Intraneural Injection: A Powerful Tool for Regional Anesthesia

MEG A. ROSENBLATT, PAUL E. BIGELEISEN

Intraneural injections were once considered harbingers for neural injury, and the practice of regional anesthesia focused on their avoidance. Stimulation techniques centered on maximizing proximity of needles and catheters to nerves without piercing them[1,2] while studies examined the risks to nerves involved with elicitation of paresthesias.[3] The use of ultrasound for regional anesthesia has offered new insights into the relationship between intraneural (into the epineurium) and intrafascicular (within the perineurium) injections of local anesthesia and their relationship with postoperative neurological complications.

Bigeleisen promoted the idea that intraneural injections of local anesthesia did not necessarily yield postoperative neural dysfunction. He performed ultrasound-guided axillary nerve blocks on 26 patients undergoing surgery on the base of the thumb. Using a 22-gauge short-beveled needle under direct visualization, he attempted to inject each of the four nerves (radial, median, ulnar, musculocutaneous) with 2 to 3 mL of local anesthetic. Nerve swelling was considered evidence of an intraneural injection and was observed in 72 of the 104 injections, whereas the remaining injections occurred immediately outside the epineurium (Fig. 5-1). Complete surgical anesthesia was achieved in 100% of patients. Postoperatively and at 6-month follow-up examinations, none of the patients reported paresthesias or dysesthesias in the distribution of the four injected nerves. Bigeleisen offers the explanation that fascicles in the axillary nerves are separated by large amounts of stroma between the fascicles. Intraneural injections performed with blunt needles then do not result in neurologic damage because the nerves are able to swell and because the needles do not readily penetrate the perineurium, which is much stronger than the epineurium (Fig. 5-2).[4,5] There are other reports of intraneural injections without neurologic sequelae. Upon review of video ultrasound images of an axillary block, Russon[6] noted that an intraneural injection of 7 mL of levobupivacaine into the musculocutaneous nerve had occurred. That patient reported no subjective or objective neurologic deficit 6 months after the event. An inadvertent intraneural injection of 35 mL of local anesthesia into the femoral nerve, with no adverse sequelae, has also been published.[7] In a separate study, 34 patients received ultrasound-guided intraneural supraclavicular blocks. Included in this cohort were seven patients with long-standing diabetes, three of whom had polyneuropathy. All of these patients also had successful blocks without any measurable neurological injuries at 6 months.[8]

A pig study by Chan[9] supports the potential safety of intraneural injections. Needles inserted into 28 brachial plexus nerves (equivalent to the cords) of anesthetized pigs, and injected with 5 mL of dextrose 5% and Sennelier Black India Ink (50:50) under direct ultrasound

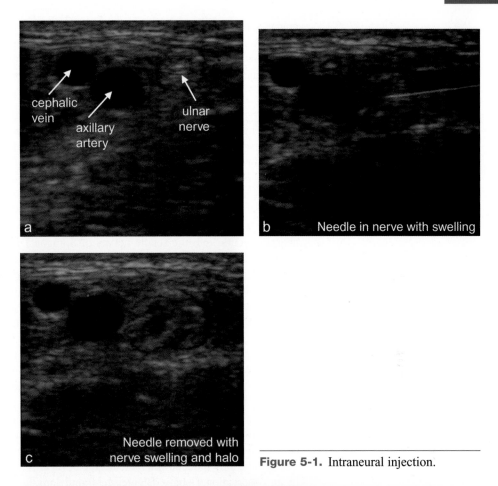

Figure 5-1. Intraneural injection.

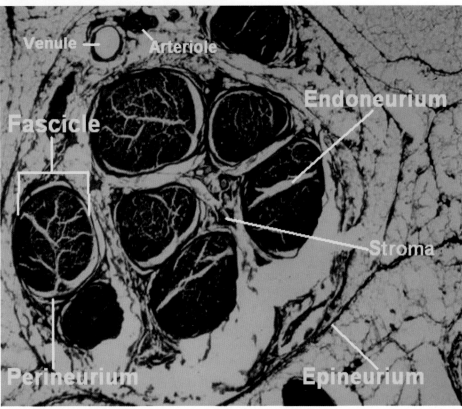

Figure 5-2. Peripheral nerve.

guidance revealed nerve expansion in 24 of the 28 nerves. Although histologic examination of the 24 ink-stained segments revealed that ink had penetrated the epineurium in 22 nerves and minimally penetrated the perineurium in the remaining two (intrafascicular injections), no evidence of dysplasia of any nerve fascicles was appreciated on histologic studies.

Needle type, or more specifically bevel type, may affect the incidence of nerve injury when in intraneural injection occurs. In 1977, Selander injected Evans blue dye into rabbit sciatic nerves using needles with 14- (long) and 45-degree (short) bevel angles, placed parallel or perpendicular to fibers. He evaluated fascicular injury and found that (1) nerve fascicles slide or roll away from needle points especially with the short-beveled needles, (2) short-beveled needles significantly diminish the risk of fascicular injury, and (3) the degree of injury with long-beveled needles varies with orientation of the bevel.[10] These findings were confirmed by Macias who looked at injury 7, 14, and 21 days after intraneural injection into the sciatic nerves of Sprague Dawley rats, with 14- and 45-degree bevel needles. He confirmed that the longer beveled needles were associated with greater injury.[11] Rice showed that when intrafascicular penetration occurred, short-beveled needles were associated with more frequent and more severe injury of longer duration than long-beveled ones. However, he used needles with 12 and 27 degree bevels for comparison.[12] In 1997, Maruyama looked at the amount of axonal damage caused by different 21-gauge needles. He placed beveled needles with the face of the bevel transverse to the nerve fibers; beveled needles with the face of the bevel longitudinal to the nerve fibers; short-tapered needles (Whitacre type); and long-tapered needles (Sprotte type) into rabbit sciatic nerves and then performed histomorphologic studies of the stained longitudinally sectioned nerves at the needle puncture point. The number of transected axons was counted. He found that axonotmesis with interruptions in the myelin sheath occurred with all needles. Importantly, the mean number of transected axons was significantly less with the tapered needles than the beveled ones, and the amount of damage produced by the beveled needles was significantly reduced when the needle bevel was inserted parallel to the nerve fibers.[13] In an observational study, Bigeleisen found long-lasting nerve injuries in 4 out of 20 patients when a long-bevel, 22-gauge needle was used to perform ultrasound-guided intraneural injections during axillary brachial plexus block. Three of these injuries resolved within 3 months and the fourth injury resolved within 12 months.[14]

It has been hypothesized that nerve damage is a result of mechanical injury and ischemia caused by high pressures generated during intraneural injections. Hadzic et al[15] placed 25-gauge needles both within the fascicles and epineurium in the sciatic nerves of seven anesthetized dogs. He used manometry to look at the pressures achieved during the injection of 4 mL of lidocaine 2% delivered by an automated infusion pump. All of the intraneural injections resulted in low pressures (≤4 psi), whereas the intrafascicular injections were associated with much higher pressures (25–45 psi). On postinjection day 7, the nerves were excised and studied. Those nerves subjected to high pressure injections displayed mechanical disruption, demyelination, and cellular infiltration, which were not observed in the nerves subjected to low injection pressures. In a second study of 15 dogs, needles were inserted into the sciatic nerve and local anesthetic was delivered through an injection pump. All of the injections at low injection pressures (>12 psi) were intraneural and were not associated with loss of neural function. All of the injections requiring high pressures (20–38 psi) resulted in intrafascicular injections and these animals had clinical deficits (paresis and moderate disability) as well as fascicular anxiolysis and cellular infiltration on histological examination.[16]

Little is known about the effect of the specific agents that are injected intraneurally. The blood supply to peripheral nerves is dual. The extrinsic system, which is responsive to adrenergic stimuli, is in the epineurium and perineurium, while the intrinsic system is nutritive and lies within the endoneurium. This intrinsic system is not under adrenergic control but may potentially be influenced by agents used during peripheral nerve block.[17] Both local anesthetics and vasoconstrictors have been shown to reduce blood flow to nerves in rat models.[18] Iohom et al[19] dissected the sciatic nerves of 52 Sprague Dawley rats and the animals were randomized to receive intraneural 0.2 cc injections of normal saline, ropivacaine 0.2%, ropivacaine 0.75%, or formalin 15%. The nonoperative leg served as the control for each animal. Walking track analysis was performed preprocedural and intermittently until the 67th postprocedure day. Although it took until day 67 for the formalin group to return to baseline, there was no detectable impairment of motor function in the saline group or in the groups that received ropivacaine in concentrations that are in clinical use. This supports the concept that intraneural injection of agents we use clinically may not themselves contribute to postoperative neural dysfunction; however, data do not exist to confirm this when vasoconstrictors are used.

The use of ultrasound offers the ability to visualize what has historically been performed blindly, but with a low incidence of complications. Although it is premature to conclude that intraneural injections are without neurologic sequelae, ultrasound is helping to elucidate the multifactorial etiology of postoperative neurologic dysfunction. This appears not only to depend on the location of the needle with respect to the nerve, but potentially also on the type of needle, the pressure achieved during the injection, the agents injected, and the microarchitecture of the nerve at the site where the nerve block is performed. Our own registry at Rochester and Pittsburgh now includes an observational database of over 2300 ultrasound-guided intraneural injections at the supraclavicular, infraclavicular, axillary, sciatic, and femoral sites without any apparent motor injuries when blunt needles were used. Within the same cohort, sensory injuries (2.7%) were limited in duration to 3 months. We have not performed any paravertebral nerve root or interscalene nerve root injections because of the risk of damaging the nerve root or spinal cord. A much larger prospective study will be needed to determine an outcome-based approach to ultrasound-guided intraneural injection.

References

1. Gurnaney H, Ganesh A, Cucchiaro G. The relationship between current intensity for nerve stimulation and success of peripheral nerve blocks performed in pediatric patients under general anesthesia. Anesth Analg 2007;105:1605–1609.
2. Pham-Dang C, Kick O, Collet T, et al. Continuous peripheral nerve blocks with stimulating catheters. Reg Anesth Pain Med 2003;28:83–88.
3. Liguori GA, Zayas VM, YaDeau JT, et al. Nerve localization techniques for interscalene brachial plexus blockade: a prospective, randomized comparison of mechanical paresthesia versus electrical stimulation. Anesth Analg 2006;103:761–767.
4. Bigeleisen PE. Nerve puncture and apparent intraneural injection during ultrasound-guided axillary block does not invariably result in neurologic injury. Anesthesiology 2006;105:779–783.
5. Moayeri N, Bigeleisen PE, Groen G. Quantitative architecture of the brachial plexus and surrounding compartments: their possible implications for plexus blocks. Anesthesiology 2008;108(2):299–305.
6. Russon K Blanco R. Accidental intraneural injection into the musculocutaneous nerve visualized with ultrasound. Anesth Analg 2007;105:1504–1505.
7. Schafhalter-Zoppoth I, Zeitz ID, Gray AT. Inadvertent femoral nerve impalement and intraneural injections visualized by ultrasound. Anesth Analg 2004;99:627–628.
8. Bigeleisen PE, Moayeri N, Groen GJ. Extraneural versus intraneural stimulation thresholds during ultrasound-guided supraclavicular block. Anesthesiology 2009;110(6):1229–1234.
9. ChanVW, Brull R, McCartney CJ, et al. An ultrasonic and histological study of intraneural injection and electrical stimulation in pigs. Anesth Analg 2007;104:1281–1284.
10. Selander D, Dhunér KG, Lundborg G. Peripheral nerve injury due to injection needles used for regional anesthesia. An experimental study of acute effects of needle point trauma. Acta Anaesth Scand 1997;21:182–188.
11. Macias G, Razza F, Peretti GM, et al. Nervous lesions as neurological complications in regional anesthesiologic block: an experimental model [in Italian]. Chir Organi Mov 2000;85:265–271.
12. Rice AS, McMahon SB. Peripheral nerve injury caused by injection needles in regional anesthesia: influence of bevel configuration, studied in a rat model. Br J Anaesth 1992;69:433–438.

13. Maruyama M. Long-tapered double needle used to reduce needle stick nerve injury. Reg Anesth 1997;22:157–160.

14. Bigeleisen PE. L'influence du biseau d'aiguille sur le risqué de belssure d'un nerf. J d'Echo en rad 2009;110(6):1229–1234.

15. Hadzic A, Dilberovic F, Shah S, et al. Combination of intraneural injection and high injection pressure leads to fascicular injury and neurologic deficits in dogs. Reg Anesth Pain Med 2004;29:417–423.

16. Kapur E, Vuckovic I, Dilberovic F, et al. Neurologic and histologic outcome after intraneural injections of lidocaine in canine sciatic nerves. Acta Anaesthesiol Scand 2007;51:101–107.

17. Neal JM. Effects of epinephrine in local anesthetics on the central and peripheral nervous systems; neurotoxicity and neural blood flow. Reg Anesth Pain Med 2003;28:124–134.

18. Myers RR, Heckman HM. Effects of local anesthesia on nerve blood flow: studies using lidocaine with and without epinephrine. Anesthesiology 1989;71:757–762.

19. Iohom G, Lan GB, Diarra DP, et al. Long-term evaluation of motor function following intraneural injection of ropivacaine using walking track analysis in rats. Br J Anaesth 2005;94:524–529.

Section II

Upper Extremity

6 Ultrasound-Guided Interscalene Block Using the Posterior Approach

7 Ultrasound-Guided Interscalene Block

8 Ultrasound-Guided Supraclavicular Block

9 Ultrasound-Guided Infraclavicular Block

10 Ultrasound-Guided Axillary Block

11 Blocks at the Elbow and Forearm

6

Ultrasound-Guided Interscalene Block Using the Posterior Approach

DAVID A. BURNS, PATRIK FILIP

 Introduction and Indications: The posterior approach to the roots of the brachial plexus was originally described by Kappis[1] in 1923 who argued that a posterior approach was safest because the carotid, internal jugular, vertebral vessels, sympathetic ganglia, phrenic nerve, and recurrent laryngeal nerves are located anterior to the brachial plexus. Studies by Sandefo et al[2] and Pere[3] showed an overall success rate of 97% including 100% block of the axillary and radial nerves, 97% block of the median and musculocutaneous nerves, and 68% block of the ulnar nerve. They also showed a 0.5% phrenic nerve block compared to the near 100% rate of phrenic nerve block with the lateral approach and only a 7% superior sympathetic ganglion block. The technique was little used before it was revised by Pippa[4] in 1990 and again by Boezaart[5] in 2003, with modifications to make it less painful by directing the needle between muscle groups. The block is used for surgery of the shoulder and proximal arm when an indwelling catheter that is distant from the surgical site is desired.

 Anatomy: The brachial plexus is composed of the ventral roots of spinal nerves C5-T1. The roots exit the lateral foraminal spaces and pass between the anterior and middle scalene muscles to innervate the upper limb (Fig. 6-1). At the root level, the fascicles are surrounded by dura/perineurium. Within the perineurium, there is little or no stroma so care must be taken not to position the needle within the nerve root itself. For this reason, the authors recommend using an 18-gauge Tuohy needle even for single-injection techniques. The carotid artery and jugular vein should be identified as well to prevent their puncture (Fig. 6-2).

 Patient Position: Sitting or lateral decubitus.

 Transducer: Linear (25 mm or 38 mm) oscillating at 13 MHz. Curved (11 mm) oscillating at 10 MHz.

 Transducer Orientation: Transverse, over the sternocleidomastoid at the level of the thyroid cartilage.

 Needle: 5- or 10-cm, 18-gauge Tuohy needle with a 20-gauge catheter.

 Local Anesthetic: 10 mL of 0.2% ropivacaine or 0.25% bupivacaine.

 Technique: The patient is positioned in either lateral or sitting position, with the neck flexed and the face turned away from the block side. Some practitioners choose to use

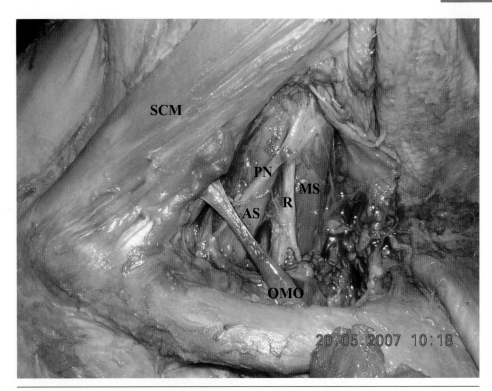

Figure 6-1. Gross anatomy of the brachial plexus. *AS*, anterior scalene muscle; *MS*, middle scalene muscle; *OMO*, omohyoid muscle; *PN*, phrenic nerve; *R*, roots of the brachial plexus; *SCM*, sternocleidomastoid muscle.

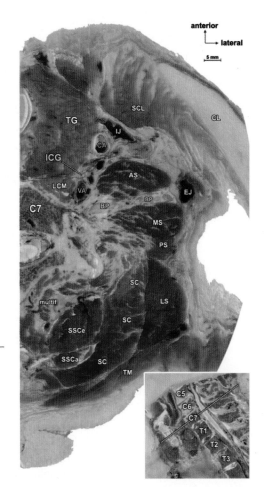

Figure 6-2. Transverse section through C7. *AS*, anterior scalene muscle; *BP*, brachial plexus; *CA*, carotid artery; *IJ*, jugular vein; *LS*, levator scapulae; *MS*, middle scalene muscle; *Multi*, multifidus muscle; *PS*, posterior scalene; *SC*, splenius capitis; *SSCA*, semispinalis capitis; *SSCE*, semispinalis cervicis; *TM*, trapezius muscle.

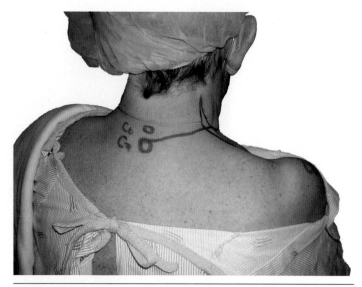

Figure 6-3a. Traditional landmarks for posterior cervical block.

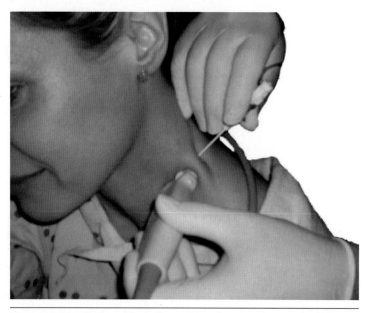

Figure 6-3b. Probe and needle position for posterior cervical block.

electrostimulation along with ultrasound. The anesthesiologist stands behind the patient with the ultrasound machine placed in front of the patient. The interscalene brachial plexus is located with the ultrasound probe and the needle entry site identified. Historically, the posterior spinous process of C7 was identified by palpation and the space between the trapezius and levator scapulae muscles was used as the point of entry (Fig. 6-3A). With the advent of ultrasound, it is usually easier to place the probe in the supraclavicular fossa and then trace the plexus cephalad to the level where the roots are readily visible (Fig. 6-3B).

The skin over the supraclavicular fossa and neck are washed with sterile solution. A 25- or 38-mm, 13-MHz probe covered with a sterile sheath is placed in the supraclavicular fossa and the subclavian artery and brachial plexus are identified. The probe is then moved in a cephalad direction until the roots of C5, C6, and C7 are identified as three round hypoechoic spheres (Fig. 6-4). In most cases, the carotid artery and jugular vein can also be seen. In some cases, the roots C8 and T1 may also be identified in the same image. With proper toggling of the probe, the sulcus of the transverse process can also be identified (Fig. 6-4).

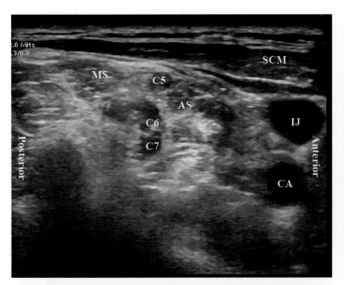

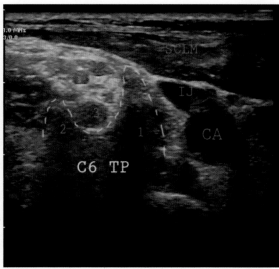

Figure 6-4a. *1*, C5 nerve roots; *2*, C6 nerve roots; *3*, C7 nerve roots; *4*, carotid artery; *5*, internal jugular vein; *6*, sternocleidomastoid muscle; *7*, middle scalene muscle; *8*, anterior scalene muscle.

Figure 6-4b. *1*, anterior tubercle of C6 transverse process; *2*, posterior tubercle of C6 posterior process; *3*, C6 nerve root; *4*, C5 nerve root; *C6 TP*, C6 transverse process; *CA*, carotid artery; *IJ*, internal jugular artery; *SCLM*, sternocleidomastoid muscle.

A 25-gauge, 4-cm needle is used to anesthetize the skin as well as the path to the brachial plexus under ultrasound guidance using an entrance point immediately posterior to the probe. This makes the subsequent placement of the 18-gauge Tuohy needle painless. The infiltration needle is removed and a 5-cm, 18-gauge Tuohy needle is advanced along the same path until the tip of the needle lies immediately posterior to the 5th and 6th nerve roots (Fig. 6-5). To make sure that the needle tip is neither intraneural nor intravascular, a small dose of anesthetic is injected. Ten to 25 mL of local anesthetic is then injected in aliquots of 5 mL with care taken. At the end of the injection, the roots should be surrounded with local anesthetic. Once the injection is complete, the catheter is inserted through the needle and then the needle is withdrawn over the catheter (Fig. 6-6). The catheter is then fixed in place with Steri-Strips and bio-occlusive dressings. Some catheters may be visible on ultrasound (Fig. 6-6). Some practitioners prefer to insert the catheter next to the plexus before injecting any local anesthetic around the nerve roots. In some cases, the catheter may be visualized on ultrasound. If the catheter cannot be visualized, local anesthetic is injected through the catheter to ensure proper

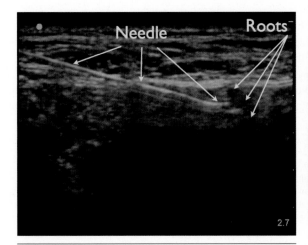

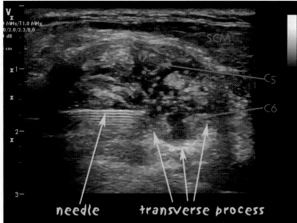

Figure 6-5a. Ultrasound scan showing needle and nerve roots.

Figure 6-5b. C5, C6 nerve roots; *green dots*, local anesthetic spread; *SCM*, sternocleidomastoid muscle. *Note* C6 bifasicular nerve root.

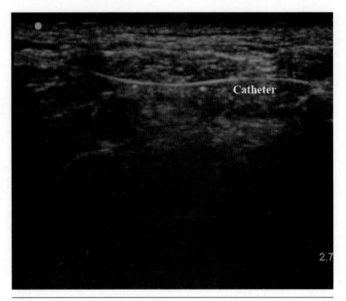

Figure 6-6. Catheter in place.

location. As local anesthesia is injected, the pooling of local anesthesia around the nerve roots can be visualized on color flow Doppler imaging. The catheter is secured in place and covered with a sterile occlusive dressing.

The catheter is then connected to a pump for continuous postoperative infusion. For most brachial plexus catheters, an infusion of 8 mL/h results in adequate spread of local anesthetic. An infusion of lidocaine 0.5% or ropivacaine 0.2% provides adequate analgesia with a minimum of motor blockade. Patient-controlled regional anesthesia (PCRA) is a very safe and effective means of providing adequate analgesia and excellent patient satisfaction through a peripheral nerve catheter. In this case, the infusion is run at 6 mL/h with a 2-mL bolus available every 30 to 60 minutes. Anesthesia to the phrenic nerve, recurrent laryngeal nerve, and the sympathetic ganglia resulting in dyspnea, hoarseness, and Horner syndrome may occur as side effects. If the catheter is used to deliver the dose of local anesthetic as described above, instead of a large bolus through the needle, the incidence of phrenic nerve, recurrent laryngeal nerve, and the sympathetic ganglia being anesthetized is greatly diminished. Occasionally, the catheter may migrate into a vessel and the staff must remain vigilant for this complication.

Tips
1. Some practitioners prefer to insert the catheter into the Tuohy needle before inserting the needle into the skin. Once the needle is in the proper position, the catheter can then be inserted beyond the end of the needle after which the needle is removed.
2. Spiral-bound or Flex Tip catheters can usually be visualized on ultrasound.
3. For surgery of the shoulder, it is best to position the catheter next to C5. When surgery or analgesia of the forearm is desired, it is best to position the catheter at the level of C7.

References

1. Kappis M. Weitere Erfahrungen mit der Sympathektomie. Klin Wehr 1923;2:1441.
2. Sandefo I, Iohom G, Van Elstraete A, et al. Clinical efficacy of the brachial plexus block via the posterior approach. Reg Anesth Pain Med 2005;30(3):238–242.
3. Pere P, Pitkänen M, Rosenberg PH, et al. Effect of continuous interscalene brachial plexus block on diaphragm motion and on ventilatory function. Acta Anaesthesiol Scand 1992;36(1):53–57.
4. Pippa P, Cominelli E, Marinelli C, et al. Brachial plexus block using the posterior approach. Eur J Anaesthesiol 1990;7:411–420.
5. Boezaart, A. Paravertebral approach to the brachial plexus: an anatomic improvement in technique. Reg Anesth Pain Med 2003;28(3):241–244.

7

Ultrasound-Guided Interscalene Block

STEVEN L. OREBAUGH, NIZAR MOAYERI, PAUL E. BIGELEISEN

Background and Indication: Winnie[1] first described the interscalene block in 1970. This block is ideal for surgery of the shoulder, distal clavicle, or proximal humerus because it provides anesthesia to the superior elements of the brachial plexus, including the suprascapular nerve as well as the supraclavicular nerve (C4). It frequently spares the ulnar nerve completely and preserves some motor and sensory function of the radial and median nerves of the forearm and hand.

Anatomy: Block of the brachial plexus at this level requires placement of local anesthetic in the interscalene groove, a potential space between the anterior and middle scalene muscles, which is occupied by the nerve elements of the plexus, as well as the subclavian artery. This space typically lies just posterior to the lateralmost extent of the sternocleidomastoid muscle and is exposed when the patient turns the head to the contralateral side (Fig. 7-1). The groove between the anterior and middle scalene muscles can be palpated in most thin patients. It may be difficult to palpate in obese patients and in those patients with limited neck mobility.

In the interscalene space, the roots of C5-T1 coalesce to form the superior (C5-C6), middle (C7), and inferior (C8-T1) trunks, which proceed laterally and inferiorly toward the space between the clavicle and first rib and then into the axilla (Fig. 7-2). Several important branches are released from the brachial plexus at this level, including the suprascapular nerve, the dorsal scapular nerve, and the long thoracic nerve.

On ultrasound, an appreciation of the anatomy at the level of the roots begins with imaging of a reliable landmark at the base of the neck, that is, the subclavian artery and the brachial plexus, which lies dorsolateral to the artery and superior to the rib (Fig. 7-3). This requires placement of the transducer first in the supraclavicular fossa, in a sagittal oblique orientation (Fig. 7-3). At this level, the nerves appear as a cluster of grapes dorsal and lateral (posterior) to the artery. Upon establishing these landmarks, the transducer should be moved slowly cephalad, tilting the probe more horizontally and following the nerve plexus proximally. This position will reveal the nerve elements (roots) aligning vertically between the scalene muscles (Figs. 7-4 through 7-6). The sternocleidomastoid muscle at this position is usually very attenuated and is visible as a triangular slip of muscle lying superficial to the plexus and scalene muscles. At this level, the practitioner may be imaging trunks (Fig. 7-4) or roots (Figs. 7-5 and 7-6). In a few patients, the C5 nerve root may pass anterior to or directly through the anterior scalene muscle (Fig. 7-7).

The interscalene space is lined by evaginated prevertebral fascia, which proceeds distally with the plexus as a sheath[1] (Fig. 7-1). This fascia is not typically evident on ultrasound imaging;

45

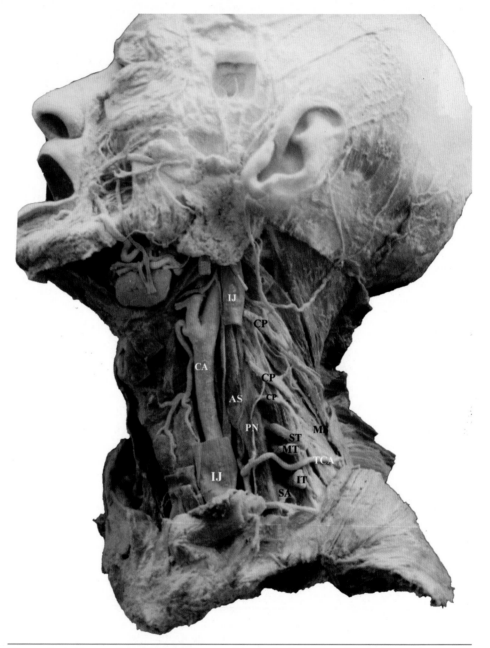

Figure 7-1. Roots of the brachial plexus. *CP*, cervical plexus; *IT*, inferior trunk; *MT*, middle trunk; *Phren*, phrenic nerve; *SA*, anterior scalene; *SM*, middle scalene; *ST*, superior trunk; *TCA*, transverse cervical artery.

rather, the nerve roots and trunks are sandwiched between the scalene muscles and appear as hypoechoic nodules[2] (Fig. 7-6). In most patients, roots C5, C6, and C7 are readily visible in the same image. In some patients, all five roots are visible (Fig. 7-6). The nerves, which are separated from the carotid sheath by the anterior scalene muscle, are relatively superficial in most subjects and lie at a mean depth of 5.5 mm from the skin surface[3] (Fig. 7-1).

Superficial to the muscles, just beneath the skin, the external jugular vein is often apparent, but is easily compressed. Gentle "bobbing" up and down with the transducer may be required to demonstrate this small vein. Fortunately, it is seldom in the path of the blocking needle with this technique. Another vessel of importance in this region,

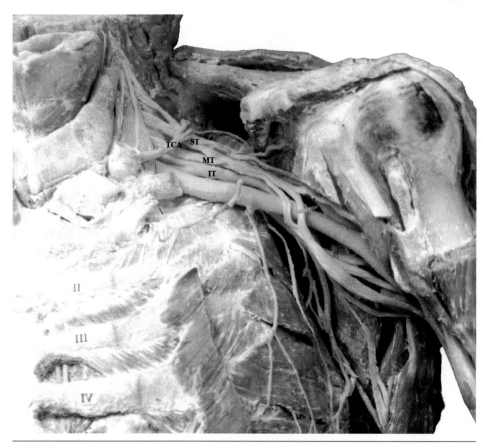

Figure 7-2. Trunks of the brachial plexus. *AS*, anterior scalene; C5, C6, C7, C8, cervical roots 5, 6, 7, 8; *IT*, inferior trunk; *MT*, middle trunk; *PN*, phrenic nerve; *ST*, superior trunk; *SA*, subclavian artery; *TCA*, transverse cervical artery.

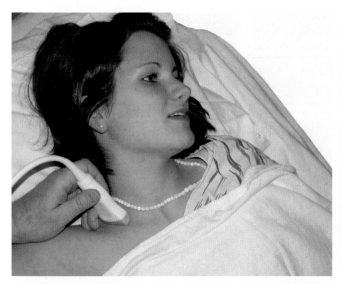

Figure 7-3a. Probe position in the supraclavicular fossa

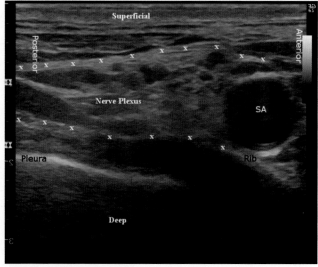

Figure 7-3b. Ultrasound scan of supraclavicular brachial plexus. *SA*, subclavian artery.

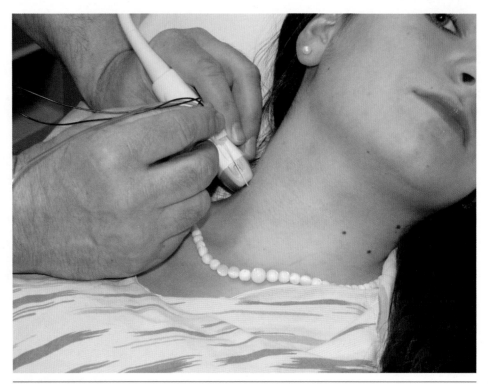

Figure 7-4. Probe and needle position for anterior interscalene block.

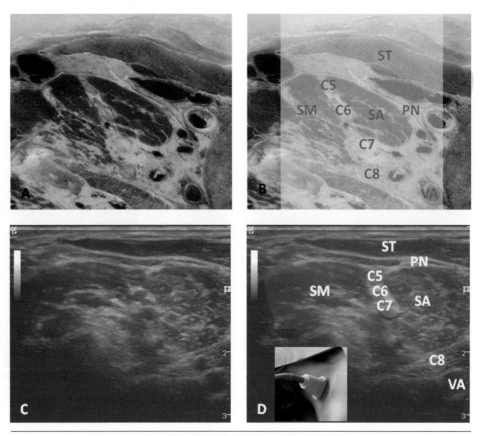

Figure 7-5. Micro-anatomy of the brachial plexus. C5,C6,C7,C8, cervicle nerve roots of the brachial plexus; *PN*, peripheral nerve; *SA*, anterior scalene muscle; *SM*, middle scalene muscle; *ST*, sternocleidomastoid muscle; *VA*, vertebral artery.

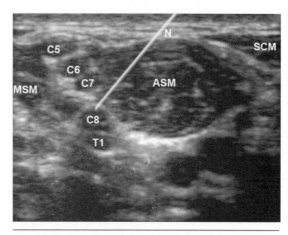

Figure 7-6. Ultrasound scan with 5 nerve roots. *ASM*, anterior scalene muscle; C5,C6,C7,C8,T1, nerve roots of the brachial plexus; *MSM*, middle scalene muscle; *N*, needle.

coursing transversely across the space, is the transverse cervical artery and associated vein[4] (Fig. 7-1). A muscular structure in this space, which may be confused with a vessel, is the inferior belly of the omohyoid muscle.

 Patient Position: Supine with the head turned away from the practitioner, lateral decubitus position.

 Transducer Type: 25- or 38-mm linear probe oscillating at 13 MHz.

 Transducer Orientation: Transverse over the sternocleidomastoid muscle at the level of the thyroid.

 Needle: 50-mm, 22-gauge blunt needle. 18-gauge Tuohy needle for continuous blocks and when the posterior approach is used.

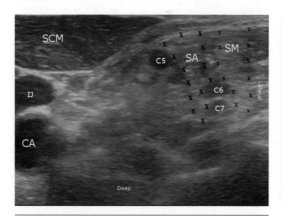

Figure 7-7a. Ultrasound of inter scalene region. *CA*, carotid artery; *SA*, anterior scalene muscle; C5, C5 nerve root medial to anterior scalene muscle; C6, C7, C6, C7, nerve roots between anterior and middle scalene muscles; *IJ*, internal jugular vein; *SM*, middle scalene muscle.

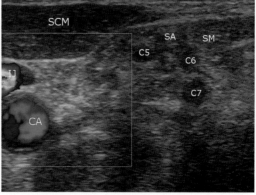

Figure 7-7b. Color flow Doppler of interscalene region. *CA*, carotid artery; C5, C5 nerve root medial to anterior scalene muscle; C6, C7, C6, C7 nerve roots between anterior and middle scalene muscles; *IJ*, internal jugular vein; *SA*, anterior scalene muscle; *SM*, middle scalene muscle.

Local Anesthetic: 10 to 20 mL of 0.5 % ropivacaine or bupivacaine.

Technique: Oxygen by face mask is initiated. The patient monitors are placed and sedation is administered. A brief preprocedural "time out" is conducted at the bedside, and the anesthesiologist marks the patient's operative extremity. Antiseptic is used to prepare the skin of the block area.

Given the relatively superficial nature of the nerves to be imaged, a high-frequency transducer (10–13 MHz) is desired. The transducer is placed in the supraclavicular fossa in the coronal oblique position. The subclavian artery, brachial plexus, and first rib are identified, and the transducer is used to follow the nerve plexus proximally up the neck until it lies in an axial oblique position. An optimal image of the brachial plexus roots is obtained by toggling the transducer, usually with slight caudad tilt (Fig. 7-4).

Ultrasound-guided interscalene block may be conducted with or without nerve stimulator confirmation. The needle may be inserted either posterior (Fig. 7-8) or anterior to the transducer (Fig. 7-4) using an in-plane approach. One may also use an out-of-plane approach, in which the transducer position is identical, but the needle is introduced from a position superior or inferior to the midpoint of the transducer.

After establishing an appropriate image of the nerve roots, the skin is anesthetized, along with the subcutaneous tissues. The author prefers a 5-cm needle using the in-plane approach. The block needle is then introduced along the predicted pathway, with subtle transducer adjustments to maintain an image of both the nerve and needle. The nerve stimulator, if used, is turned on before needle introduction, or later, as the needle approaches

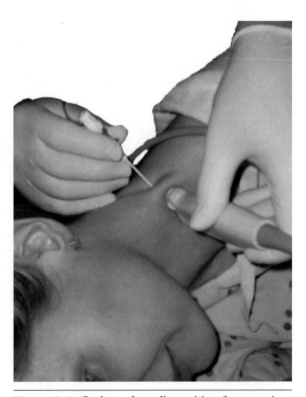

Figure 7-8. Probe and needle position for posterior interscalene block.

the nerves. The threshold for stimulation has not been found to be of importance in this technique.[5] After appropriate positioning of the needle and obtaining the desired motor response, local anesthetic solution, typically 20 mL, ensuring that the injectate surrounds the visible nerve elements. If necessary, the needle position may be shifted to ensure that all of the nerve roots are surrounded by local anesthetic.

For indwelling catheter placement, an out-of-plane technique is desirable. In addition, a sterile sheath should be used for placement of an indwelling device, along with sterile gloves, cap, mask, and drapes. After establishing an optimal view of the nerve roots, the skin is anesthetized with a subcutaneous wheal of local anesthetic. If the nerves lie at a depth of 2 cm, then a needle introduced 2 cm proximal to the midpoint of the transducer will require an angle of insertion of 45 degrees to encounter the target. The needle is then guided to the nerve roots, and nerve stimulation is used for confirmation if desired. For nonstimulating catheters, a bolus of local anesthetic, saline, or dextrose solution is used to confirm accurate needle tip placement, and the catheter is then inserted. If the catheter to be placed is of the stimulating variety, then the stimulator is attached to the catheter after needle localization, and placement is confirmed by continued stimulation as the catheter is inserted. By either technique, after catheter placement, ultrasound imaging can be used to confirm that the solution injected through the catheter is deposited in juxtaposition to the nerves of interest. Color flow Doppler may improve the ability to image in this situation.

Summary of Clinical Evidence: Data on the conduct of interscalene block with ultrasound guidance is largely descriptive. Chan[6] describes the use of ultrasound-guided interscalene block to rescue a block that failed after nerve stimulation was used for guidance. In a study of 15 volunteers, Perlas et al[2] described the anatomy of the brachial plexus at several levels, including the interscalene groove. The authors used the axial oblique plane to visualize the plexus. They described it as consisting of hypoechoic nodules, which may be visualized between the scalene muscles, deep to the posterior border of the sternocleidomastoid muscle. Nearby vascular structures, including the internal jugular vein and vertebral artery, are well visualized.

Kessler and Gray[7] conducted a study of volunteers in which the plexus and its surrounding anatomy were visualized in the interscalene region with ultrasonography. In 13% of plexuses, variations from the typical relationship of the scalene muscles and brachial plexus roots were present, the most common being the C5 nerve root running through or outside the anterior scalene muscle. The authors postulate that this arrangement may be responsible for occasional incomplete interscalene blocks.

To evaluate the existence of a brachial plexus "sheath" at proximal levels, Yang et al[4] inserted catheters into the interscalene space under real-time ultrasound guidance. Injection of contrast under fluoroscopy was used to confirm catheter position, and the movement of contrast was studied as evidence of the conformation and integrity of the sheath enveloping the brachial plexus at this region. Injected contrast not only collected in the interscalene space, but also made its way out of the apparent fascial confines of this space, enveloping the scalene muscles in 90% of the volunteers and abutting the carotid sheath in half. The authors concluded that the connective tissue sheath surrounding the brachial plexus is discontinuous.

References

1. Winnie AP. Interscalene brachial plexus block. Anesth Analg 1970;49:455–466.
2. Perlas A, Chan VW, Simons M. Brachial plexus examination and localization using ultrasound and electrical stimulation. Anesthesiology 2003;99:429–435.

3. Yang WT, Chui PT, Metreweli C. Anatomy of the normal brachial plexus revealed by sonography and the role of sonographic guidance in anesthesia of the brachial plexus. AJR Am J Roentgenol 1998;171:1631–1636.
4. Demondion X, Herbinet P, Boutry N, et al. Sonographic mapping of the normal brachial plexus. AJNR Am J Neuroradiol 2003;24:1303–1309.
5. Sinha SK, Abrams JH, Weller RS. Ultrasound-guided interscalene needle placement produces successful anesthesia regardless of motor stimulation above or below 0.5 mA. Anesth Analg 2007;105: 848–852.
6. Chan VW. Applying ultrasound imaging to interscalene brachial plexus block. Reg Anesth Pain Med 2003;28:340–343.
7. Kessler J, Gray AT. Sonography of scalene muscle anomalies for brachial plexus block. Reg Anesth Pain Med 2007;32:172–173.

8

Ultrasound-Guided Supraclavicular Block

STEVEN L. OREBAUGH, PAUL E. BIGELEISEN

Background and Indications: Supraclavicular brachial plexus block was originally described by Kulenkampff[1] in 1911. After initial popularity, the block fell into disfavor because of the relatively high risk of pneumothorax. The compact structure of the plexus is an advantage to nerve block at this level. With the advent of ultrasound, supraclavicular block has become the most popular and common technique to provide anesthesia and analgesia to the entire upper extremity distal to the shoulder.

Anatomy: After traversing the interscalene groove, the trunks of the brachial plexus cross the supraclavicular fossa and divide into anterior and posterior divisions at, or distal to, the level of the clavicle (Fig. 8-1). With ultrasound, the most important landmark for the supraclavicular block is the subclavian artery, which is readily imaged in cross-section as it lies atop the bright, hyperechoic first rib (Figs. 8-2 and 8-3). Below the rib, a lack of echoes represents the air-filled lung. In some patients, the hyperechoic line of the pleura may be seen as well (Fig. 8-3). Adjacent to the subclavian artery are the elements of the brachial plexus, arrayed as a group of hypoechoic nodules posterior to the vessel, frequently described as a "cluster of grapes." While the fascicles may be distinct, the epineurium (Fig. 8-3), which lines and separates the trunks or divisions, is not readily discernable. In some patients, it may be difficult to image the inferior trunk, which lies immediately superior to first rib.

The brachial plexus has a fascial investment as it courses laterally to the arm, usually referred to as a "sheath," though its existence as such has been challenged.[2,3] Nevertheless, a connective tissue investment around the plexus is common, and has been described as an evagination of the prevertebral fascia at cervical levels.[4] This connective tissue covering is not a simple, continuous tube, nor is it impermeable to leakage of contrast or local anesthetic.[5]

Just anterior to the artery, a hypoechoic structure is seen, which may be mistaken for a vessel but does contain some internal echoes. This represents the anterior scalene muscle, which descends from the neck to insert on the first rib (Fig. 8-3). Further anteriorly, the subclavian vein is seen at its confluence with the internal jugular vein. This vein can be difficult to visualize with a linear probe, as it lies anterior to the artery and deep to the clavicle. If the practitioner wishes to visualize the vein, a small, curved transducer is the best choice. In some patients, valves can be imaged within the vein, whereas in other patients the omohyoid muscle can be visualized as well (Fig. 8-2).

Patient Position: Supine with the head turned away from the patient.

Transducer: 25- or 38-mm linear transducer oscillating at 13 MHz; 11-mm curved transducer oscillating at 10 MHz.

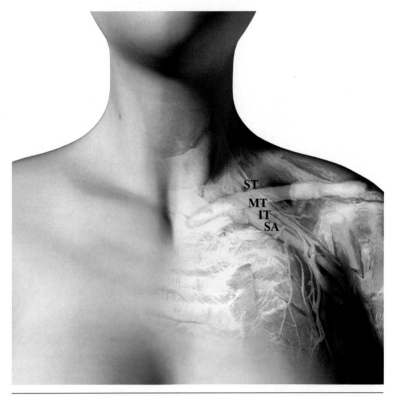

Figure 8-1. Position of the trunks relative to the subclavian artery and the clavicle. *IT*, inferior trunk; *MT*, middle trunk; *ST*, superior trunk.

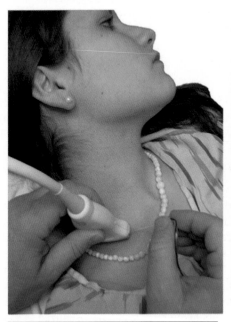

Figure 8-2a. Needle and probe position.

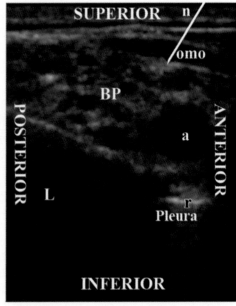

Figure 8-2b. *a*, subclavian artery; *BP*, brachial plexus; *L*, lung; *n*, needle; *omo*, omohyoid artery.

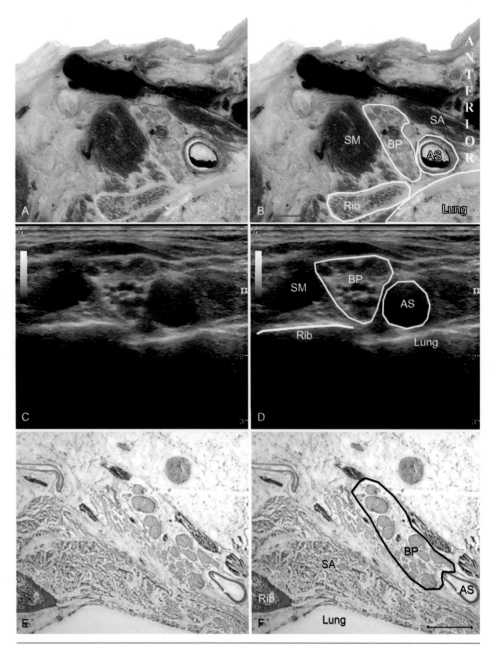

Figure 8-3. Microanatomy at the level of the supraclavicular block. *AS*, subclavian artery; *BP*, brachial plexus; *SA*, anterior scalene muscle; *SM*, middle scalene muscle.

Transducer Orientation: Coronal oblique position just anterior to the clavicle.

Needle: 50-mm, 22-gauge blunt needle.

Local Anesthetic: 15 to 25 mL of 0.5% ropivacaine or 0.5% bupivacaine with epinephrine.

Technique: The patient monitors are placed, and oxygen and sedation are administered to the patient. The operative arm is marked by the anesthesia team after an appropriate time-out to identify the correct surgical site. An antiseptic is utilized to prepare the skin of the block area.

For supraclavicular block, the transducer is placed in a coronal oblique position, just anterior to the clavicle (Fig. 8-2). Usually, the transducer must be held relatively vertically to obtain transverse images of the subclavian artery and optimal images of the nearby nerve plexus.

Because of the proximity of the needle to the lung and pleura in supraclavicular block, an in-plane approach to this ultrasound-guided block is desirable. After establishing the ideal imaging plane for the subclavian artery and the nerves lying next to it, the skin either anterior or posterior to the transducer is anesthetized with a subcutaneous needle. The author prefers to utilize a 5-cm needle, while imaging, to establish the insertion trajectory of the block needle. If desired, peripheral nerve stimulation may be used to confirm needle contact with appropriate motor stimulation. Local anesthetic solution is injected upon confirmation of the appropriate needle-tip position. It is essential that the needle tip be imaged at all times to avoid pneumothorax. Although surrounding the nerve structure in question is always desirable, it is important to inject some of the local anesthetic solution between the nerve cluster and the first rib.[6] This causes the nerves to rise up and "float" in the liquid, ensuring anesthesia of the inferior trunk.

For placement of an indwelling catheter, an out-of-plane technique makes threading the catheter easier. As the needle contacts the nerves of the plexus, the catheter is inserted, with or without stimulation guidance. As in other levels, the physician may choose to combine ultrasound with a stimulating needle and stimulating catheter. Injection of dextrose or local anesthetic solution may then be used to confirm appropriate catheter placement under ultrasound visualization.

Summary of Evidence: To quantify the relationships of the brachial plexus to the surrounding anatomy at the level of the supraclavicular block, Apan et al[7] performed sonographic examinations in 30 patients, along with coronal magnetic resonance imaging (MRI) images in a subset of these. The authors found that the depth of the brachial plexus from the skin at this level, with the transducer in the coronal oblique position, averaged 1.65 cm in men and 1.45 cm in women.

Several authors have used sonography in attempts to simplify the supraclavicular block and improve its safety profile. Kapral et al[8] evaluated 40 patients for forearm or hand surgery, comparing the supraclavicular approach with the axillary approach to ultrasound-guided brachial plexus block. Blocks were conducted as single injections of 30 mL of 0.5% bupivacaine. In both the axillary and the supraclavicular block groups, 95% successful surgical anesthesia was achieved. However, 5 of the 20 patients in the axillary block group did not achieve block of the musculocutaneous nerve.

Chan et al[9] evaluated ultrasound-guided supraclavicular block in 40 outpatients for arm or hand surgery. The authors localized the plexus at supraclavicular levels with ultrasound and confirmed the needle position with nerve stimulation, then injected 40 mL of a mixture of 2% lidocaine and 0.5% bupivacaine. The needle was repositioned as necessary to facilitate complete surrounding of the elements of the brachial plexus with local anesthetic solution. Overall, 95% of blocks were successful, with one failure because of subcutaneous injection and another because of a partial intravascular injection. The average time required to complete the block in these patients was 9 minutes, with a mean time to complete sensory and motor blockade of 16.7 minutes.

In a comparative study, Williams et al[10] performed either ultrasound-guided supraclavicular block with nerve stimulation (for confirmation) or landmark-guided supraclavicular block with peripheral nerve stimulation in 80 patients for hand or forearm surgery. Successful surgical block, with no requirement for supplementation or conversion to general anesthesia, was reported in 85% of the ultrasound-guided blocks and 78% of peripheral nerve stimulation-guided blocks, an insignificant difference. However, the time required to perform the block was significantly shorter with use of ultrasound (5 versus 9.8 minutes). An average of 21 seconds was required to obtain an adequate ultrasound image of the supraclavicular brachial plexus. No significant complications occurred; two patients (one in each group) developed respiratory discomfort from diaphragmatic paresis. Five patients reported altered sensation in the affected extremity after the block and surgery, and all resolved by 1 week.

References

1. Kulenkampff D. Brachial plexus anesthesia: Its indications, technique, and dangers. Ann Surg 1928;87:883–891.
2. Partridge BL, Katz J, Benirschke K. Functional anatomy of the brachial plexus sheath: implications for anesthesia. Anesthesiology 1987;66:743–747.
3. Cornish PB, Leaper C. The sheath of the brachial plexus: fact or fiction? Anesthesiology 2006;105: 563–565.
4. Winnie AP. Interscalene brachial plexus block. Anesth Analg 1970;49:455–466.
5. Yang WT, Chui PT, Metreweli C. Anatomy of the normal brachial plexus revealed by sonography and the role of sonographic guidance in anesthesia of the brachial plexus. AJR Am J Roentgenol 1998;171:1631–1636.
6. Soares LG, Brull R, Lai J, et al. Eight ball, corner pocket: the optimal needle position of ultrasound-guided supraclavicular block. Reg Anesth Pain Med 2007;32:94–95.
7. Apan A, Baydar S, Yylmaz S, et al. Surface landmarks of brachial plexus: ultrasound and magnetic resonance imaging for supraclavicular approach with anatomical correlation. Eur J Ultrasound 2001;13:191–196.
8. Kapral S, Krafft P, Eibenberger K, et al. Ultrasound-guided supraclavicular approach for regional anesthesia of the brachial plexus. Anesth Analg 1994;78:507–513.
9. Chan VW, Perlas A, Rawson R, et al. Ultrasound-guided supraclavicular brachial plexus block. Anesth Analg 2003;97:1514–1517.
10. Williams SR, Chouinard P, Arcand G, et al. Ultrasound guidance speeds execution and improves the quality of supraclavicular block. Anesth Analg 2003;97:1518–1523.

9

Ultrasound-Guided Infraclavicular Block

STEVEN L. OREBAUGH, GERBRAND J. GROEN, PAUL E. BIGELEISEN

Background and Indications: Infraclavicular brachial plexus block permits anesthesia of the plexus where most of the major motor and sensory nerves to the arm are anesthetized. In addition, anesthesia of the phrenic nerve with resultant diaphragmatic paralysis is unlikely.[1] Infraclavicular block is used to provide anesthesia and analgesia for procedures involving the distal arm and elbow, wrist, forearm, and hand.

Anatomy: Beneath the clavicle, the cervicoaxillary canal is formed, bounded by the first rib below and the clavicle above. Through this passageway, the vessels and brachial plexus enter the apex of the axilla. Overlying this region, the infraclavicular fossa is formed between the pectoralis major muscle and the deltoid muscle. Needle insertion for infraclavicular block at this point will traverse the pectoralis major and pectoralis minor muscles en route to the plexus (Fig. 9-1). Posterior to the neurovascular bundle is the rib cage and, posteromedially, the pleura and lung.

The cords of the brachial plexus are closely aligned with the axillary artery at the infraclavicular region, and derive their names from their position with respect to the vessel: posterior, lateral, and medial. Because the plexus spirals around the vessel, this relationship may not be apparent until cords reach the second or third part of the artery (Fig. 9-2). Utilizing magnetic resonance imaging (MRI), Sauter et al[2] evaluated the relative positions of the cords in volunteers. The authors found that the cords consistently lay within 2.5 cm of the center of the artery, in a range from directly inferior to the vessel, to cephalo-anterior, arranged circumferentially around the artery. The connective tissue investment, or "sheath," that defines the space through which the neurovascular bundle passes has multiple interdigitations and septations which may sequester solutions injected near the nerves[3] (Fig. 9-3).

The infraclavicular plexus lies deeper than at other sites of the brachial plexus. Wilson et al[4] evaluated the plexus at the pericoracoid region with MRI and found a mean depth of the plexus elements of 4.2 cm for men and 4.0 cm for women, although the relationship to body mass index was not explored. On ultrasound, this greater depth is readily appreciated and may require use of a lower frequency transducer setting to provide adequate imaging.[5] The cords of the plexus typically appear hyperechoic, or bright, in the infraclavicular region (Fig. 9-1).

During ultrasound imaging in the infraclavicular fossa, the structures that appear superficial to the nerves include the skin and subcutaneous tissues, the pectoralis major and minor muscles, and the clavipectoral fascia (Fig. 9-1). Deep to this fascia, the second part of the axillary artery and the axillary vein are apparent. The artery lies cephalad

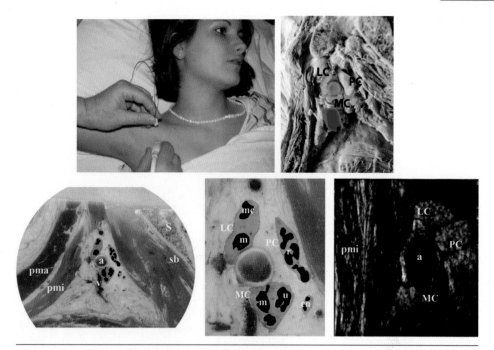

Figure 9-1. Lateral infraclavicular block. *PMA*, pectoralis major muscle; *PMI*, pectoralis minor muscle; *A*, axillary artery; *V*, axilllary vein; *S*, scapula; *SB*, subscapularis; *LC*, lateral cord; *PC*, posterior cord; *MC*, medial cord; *MC*, musculocutaneous nerve; *M*, median nerve; *R*, radial nerve; *U*, ulnar nerve; *CN*, cutaneous nerve.

to the vein. The vein is usually compressible, even at this depth. The hyperechoic cords of the plexus lie close to the artery, typically reflecting their named positions (Fig. 9-1). Posteromedial and caudad to the nerves and vessels, the hypoechoic region represents the lung. The pleura may at times be evident because of its hyperechoic nature and its motion during respiration.

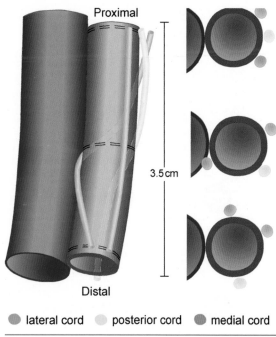

Figure 9-2. Anatomic path of the cords from proximal to distal.

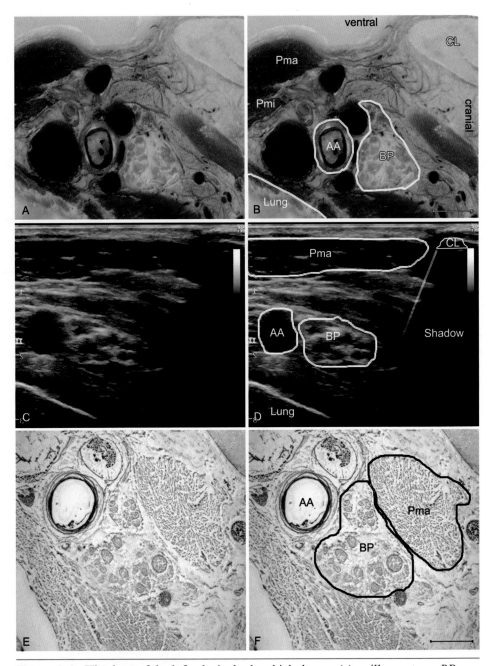

Figure 9-3. Histology of the infraclavicular brachial plexus. *AA*, axillary artery; *BP*, brachial plexus; *PMA*, pectoralis major muscle; *PMI*, pectroralis minor muscle.

Patient Position: Supine with arm at the side or with the arm abducted and elbow flexed.

Transducer: 11-mm curved array oscillating at 8 to 10 MHz or 25-mm linear transducer oscillating at 10 MHz.

Transducer Orientation: In or lateral to the deltopectoral groove with a parasagittal orientation.

Needle: 22-gauge, 5-cm blunt-tip needle.

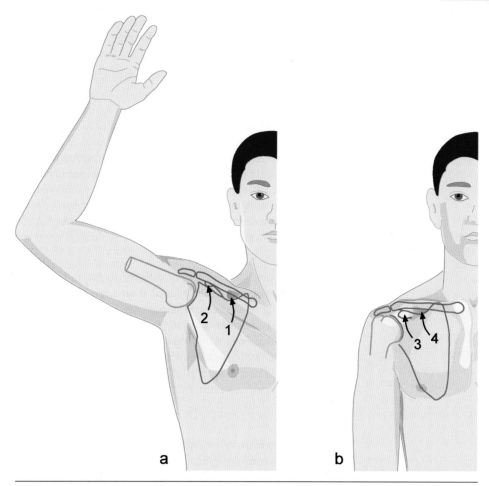

Figure 9-4. Different positions for infraclavicular block. *1, 4,* deltopectoral groove; *2, 3,* coracoid process.

Local Anesthetic: 15 to 30 mL of 0.5% ropivacaine or 0.5% bupivaciane with epinephrine.

Technique: Patient monitors are placed, and sedation is introduced. Oxygen by face mask is administered. A brief preprocedural "time out" is conducted at the bedside, and the operative extremity is marked by the anesthesiologist. An antiseptic is utilized to prepare the skin of the block area.

The transducer is placed in the deltopectoral groove between the pectoralis major and deltoid muscles with a parasagittal orientation (Fig. 9-4). The transducer may be moved laterally, medially, or toggled to provide the optimal images of the nerves and vessels. The arm may be placed at the side or with arm abducted and the elbow flexed (Fig. 9-4).

Because of the proximity of the tip of the needle to the lung and pleura during ultrasound-guided infraclavicular block, an in-plane approach is preferred. A subcutaneous needle is utilized to anesthetize the skin at the cephalad end of the transducer and to establish the tract that the block needle will follow under ultrasound guidance. If desired, a peripheral nerve stimulator is utilized and attached to an insulated block needle. In most cases, a 22-gauge, 5-cm blunt-tip needle may be used. In larger patients, a 10-cm, 18-gauge Tuohy needle will be required to reach the target.[6] As the needle is introduced, the transducer is adjusted to obtain a view of the tip during its progress. It is essential to maintain imaging of the tip of the needle at all times to avoid vascular or pleural puncture.

The needle is then advanced under continuous observation toward each of the cords in turn. It is frequently easiest to guide the needle to the lateral cord first, using nerve stimulation if desired for confirmation (a musculocutaneous or median nerve-type motor stimulation would be expected). Local anesthetic of 5 to 10 mL is then deposited next to the nerve. Posterior to the artery, the posterior cord is frequently apparent but must not be confused with artifact that is uniformly present behind the vessel. Once again, when the needle tip is adjacent to the cord, 5 to 10 mL of local anesthetic is deposited. It is important to ascertain that local anesthetic is placed posterior to the vessel, and not just on each side of it, to ensure adequate anesthesia of the posterior cord. Finally, the needle is brought into position next to the medial cord and a similar volume of the local anesthetic injected. In each case, the physician may elect to utilize peripheral nerve stimulation to confirm the target.

To place an indwelling catheter in the infraclavicular region, a 5- to 10-cm, 18-gauge Tuohy needle is introduced at the same site as used for the single-injection technique, utilizing an in-plane technique. Again, nerve stimulation may be utilized for confirmation of needle position and catheter position. After anesthetizing the skin and subcutaneous tract, the needle is introduced and its tip brought into position next to one of the nerve targets. Some authors recommend that the catheter be placed next to the posterior cord for optimal analgesia.[6] Appropriate catheter position may be confirmed by injecting saline, dextrose, or local anesthetic solution while observing with ultrasonography. Ideally, the solution will spread to encompass all three of the cords.

The Medial or Midinfraclavicular Approach: Some practitioners prefer to perform an ultrasound-guided infraclavicular block at a more proximal position where the cords are grouped together cephalad to the artery (Figs. 9-4 and 9-5). This allows for access to all three cords along one needle path. Using this technique, the onset time is faster, the axillary nerve is more reliably anesthetized, and the intercostal brachial nerve is often blocked as well when compared with a more lateral approach.[7] The drawback is that the cords lie close to the first and second ribs so that pleural puncture is more likely if the user does not have a thorough understanding of the anatomy and good technical skills (Fig. 9-4).

The upper extremity is positioned in the same position used for axillary block. This pulls the plexus cephalad and away from the rib cage and pleura. At the same time, it rotates the plexus anteriorly so that it is closer to the skin. The deltopectoral goove is palpated and the transducer is sited with a sagittal orientation in the groove, or 1 to 2 cm medial to the groove (Fig. 9-5). Occasionally, toggling the transducer medially may be necessary. The axillary artery is identified, and the plexus can be seen cephalo-anterior to the artery. A small curved transducer (11 mm, 8–10 MHz) is very useful for this block, because there is very little space between the clavicle and transducer. The needle (5 cm, 22 gauge) is introduced in-line cephalad to the transducer at an angle that is nearly perpendicular to the skin (Fig. 9-5). The needle is passed through the skin, and pectoral muscles while injecting local anesthetic to anesthetize the skin and muscles. Once the clavipectoral fascia is pierced, 5 to 10 mL of local anesthetic is injected into or around each of the three cords. The plexus may appear as a single cord before injection, but once injection is begun, the cords begin to separate.

If the practitioner plans to use a catheter, the same technique is used except that a 5- or 10-cm, 18-gauge Touhy needle is used to guide the catheter to the plexus. In this case, the practitioner must anesthetize the skin and muscles with local anesthetic using a small-gauge needle before inserting the Tuohy needle.

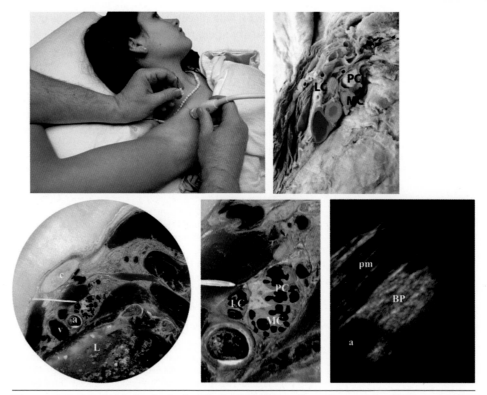

Figure 9-5. Medial infraclavicular block. *PM*, pectoralis major muscle; *PMI*, pectoralis minor muscle; *A*, axillary artery; *V*, axillary vein; *C*, clavicle; *L*, lung; *BP*, brachial plexus; *LC*, lateral cord; *PC*, posterior cord; *MC*, medial cord.

Summary of Evidence: Ootaki et al[8] utilized a 7-MHz transducer for ICB with ultrasound guidance. The authors reported a 95% success rate for surgical block of the arm, with sensory block of all nerves in more than 95% of patients and motor block in over 90%. The technique involved injection of 15 mL of 1.5% lidocaine medial to the artery, and 15 mL lateral to it, with real-time US guidance.

Sandhu and Capan[6] reported on their experience of infraclavicular block with ultrasound guidance in 126 patients undergoing hand surgery. The authors utilized a 2 to 5 MHz transducer, and injected 7 to 11 mL of a solution of 2% lidocaine with epinephrine and sodium bicarbonate around each of the three cords at the second part of the axillary artery, deep to the pectoralis minor muscle. Ninety percent of patients developed a surgical block, with three requiring conversion to general anesthesia and seven necessitating local supplementation to complete the block. One vascular puncture occurred. The mean onset time of the blocks, which required an average time of 10 minutes to complete, was 6.3 minutes.

Klaasted et al[9] have described a "lateral and sagittal" technique for ICB, in which the needle is inserted along the medial border of the coracoid process, aiming inferior and posterior to contact the cords, in the parasagittal plane. This approach, which is similar to that described in this section, has been corroborated by Brull et al.[9] These authors utilized real-time sonographic needle guidance with this approach, consistently contacting the cords at a depth of 4 to 6 cm. By report, this has resulted in improved block success and reduced morbidity in their practice.

Dingemans et al[11] have characterized the necessary distribution of local anesthetic solution during ICB with US guidance by randomizing 72 patients for hand or forearm surgery to one group with placement of the solution in a U shape, posterior to, and on both sides of the axillary artery, or a second group in which local anesthetic was injected at one site, guided by ultrasound imaging and detection of a distal motor stimulation in the wrist or hand. Patients in the group with ultrasound spread around the artery as the endpoint for the block required less time for block (3.1 minutes versus 5.2 minutes) and had a higher likelihood of complete sensory block (86% versus 57%). In addition, successful attainment of surgical block, with no requirement for supplementation, was significantly higher in the group in which local was deposited around the artery, without guidance by nerve stimulation (92% versus 72%).

References

1. Rettig HC, Gielen MJM, Boersma E, Klein J, Groen GJ. Vertical infraclavicular block of the brachial plexus: effects on hemidiaphragmatic movement and ventilatory function. Reg Anesth Pain Med 2005;30:529–535.
2. Sauter AR, Smith HJ, Stubhaug A, Dodgson MS, Klaasted Ø. Use of magnetic resonance imaging to define the anatomic location closest to all three cords of the infraclavicular brachial plexus. Anesth Analg 2006;103:1574–1576.
3. Partridge BL, Katz J, Benirschke K. Functional anatomy of the brachial plexus sheath: implications for anesthesia. Anesthesiology 1987;66:743–747.
4. Wilson JL, Brown DL, Wong GY, et al. Infraclavicular brachial plexus block: parasagittal anatomy important to the coracoid technique. Anesth Analg 1998;87:870–873.
5. Perlas A, Chan VW, Simons M. Brachial plexus examination and localization using ultrasound and electrical stimulation. Anesthesiology 2003;99:429–435.
6. Sandhu NS, Capan LM. Ultrasound-guided infraclavicular brachial plexus block. Br J Anaesth 2002;89:254–259.
7. Bigeleisen PE, Wilson M. A comparison of two techniques of ultrasound guided infraclavicular block. Br J Anaesth 2006;96:502–507.
8. Ootaki C, Hayashi H, Amano M. Ultrasound-guided infraclavicular brachial plexus block: an alternative technique to anatomic landmark-guided approaches. Reg Anesth Pain Med 2000;25:600–604.
9. Klaasted O, Smith HJ, Smedby O, et al. A novel infraclavicular brachial plexus block: the lateral and sagittal technique, developed by magnetic resonance imaging studies. Anesth Analg 2004;98:252–256.
10. Brull R, McCartney CJL, Chan VW. A novel approach to the infraclavicular brachial plexus block: the ultrasound experience. Anesth Analg 2004;99:950–952.
11. Dingemans E, Williams SR, Arcand G, et al. Neurostimulation in ultrasound-guided infraclavicular block: a prospective, randomized trial. Anesth Analg 2007;104:1275–1280.

10

Ultrasound-Guided Axillary Block

STEVEN L. OREBAUGH, PAUL E. BIGELEISEN

 Background and Indications: Traditionally, axillary block was the most commonly performed of the brachial plexus blocks because of the ease of locating the plexus relative to the axillary artery by palpation. It does have some draw backs. The arm must be abducted and the elbow flexed to access the axilla. This can be painful for patients with fractures and impossible for people with contractures or arthritis. In addition, it was often difficult to anesthetize the musculocutaneous nerve with a blind or stimulation technique. The addition of ultrasound allows the user to identify all four nerves (median, radial, ulnar, musculocutaneous) necessary for a successful block. Those, coupled with the safety of the block, make it an attractive procedure when ultrasound is used. The block is used for surgery of the elbow, forearm, and hand. A separate block of the intercostal brachial nerve is required when the incision is along the medial aspect of the extremity.

 Anatomy: The biceps muscle lies anterosuperior to the neurovascular bundle, whereas the coracobrachialis muscle is superior to the neurovascular bundle, and the triceps muscle is inferior to the neurovascular bundle. The humerus lies deep to the neurovascular bundle. The brachial artery and one to two brachial veins are evident in the neurovascular bundle. The radial, median, and ulnar nerves are found within the neurovascular bundle (Fig. 10-1). Most commonly, the median nerve is anterior or cephaloanterior to the artery. The radial nerve is most commonly posterior or posteroinferior to the artery, whereas the ulnar nerve is most commonly found inferior or anteroinferior to the artery. Proximal in the axilla, the musculocutaneous nerve may be found cephaloposterior to the artery. In more distal sites in the axilla, the musculocutaneous nerve is usually found in the fascia between the biceps and coracobrachialis muscles 1 to 2 cm cephaloposterior to the artery. Cutaneous nerves of the arm or forearm may also be visualized.

 Patient Position: Supine, with ipsilateral arm abducted, externally rotated, and flexed at the elbow.

 Transducer: 25- or 38-mm linear transducer oscillating at 13 MHz.

 Transducer Position: Transverse across the axilla (sagittal oblique), placed at the intersection of the pectoralis and biceps muscles.

 Needle: 22-gauge, 50-mm insulated needle.

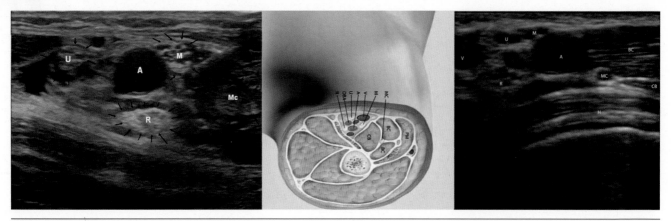

Figure 10-1a. Cross-section of the axilla. *A*, axillary artery; *V*, axillary vein; *BC*, biceps muscle; *MC*, musculocutaneous nerve; *CB*, coracobrachialis muscle; *M*, median nerve; *U*, ulnar nerve; *R*, radial nerve; *H*, humerus.

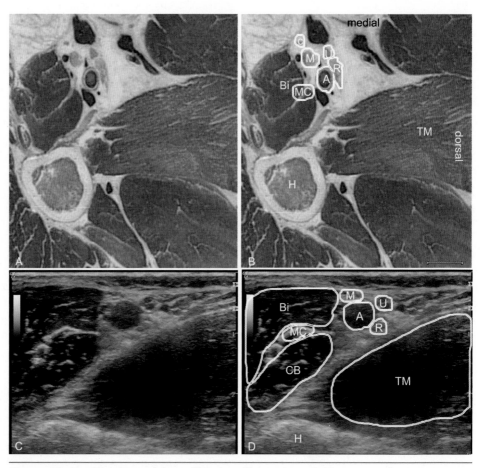

Figure 10-1b. Histology of the axilla. *A*, axillary artery; *B*, biceps muscle; *MC*, musculocutaneous nerve; *C*, cutaneous nerve; *M*, median nerve; *U*, ulnar nerve; *R*, radial nerve; *TM*, triceps muscle; *H*, humerus.

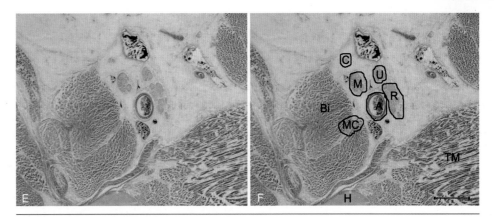

Figure 10-1b. *(continued).*

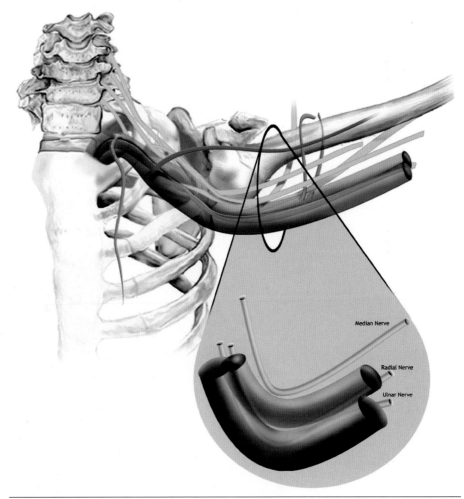

Figure 10-1c. Median, radial, and ulnar nerves.

Local Anesthetic: 15 to 25 mL of 0.5% ropivacaine or 0.5% bupivacaine with epinephrine.

Technique: The skin is cleansed with sterile solution and the transducer is covered with a sterile cover. A wheel of local anesthetic should be injected beneath the skin along a 5-cm arc from medial to lateral to the brachial artery pulsation (Fig. 10-2). This allows needle placement from either side of the artery, without repeatedly injecting subcutaneous local anesthetic, as well as providing anesthesia for the intercostobrachial nerve and the medial brachial cutaneous nerve. The artery should be localized with the transducer, and the hyperechoic nerves sought at its periphery. Initially, the block needle is inserted in-plane, along the long axis of the transducer, from the superior side of the artery (Fig. 10-2). In the posterocephalad region, the musculocutaneous nerve is sought. The peripheral nerve stimulator may be left on throughout the procedure, with a current level of 0.5 to 1 mA, or it may be switched on as each nerve is approached, then turned off after confirmation. When elbow flexion occurs, the nerve is localized. The stimulator can be switched off, and incremental injections of 2 to 3 mL of local anesthetic are begun. A "halo" of local anesthetic should be created around the nerve. A total of 5 mL is injected here (Fig. 10-3).

The needle is then withdrawn and redirected toward the median nerve, if evident, or to the region anterior and/or superior to the artery. The nerve stimulator may be left on throughout the procedure, or turned on at this time. When appropriate motor or cutaneous stimulation confirms contact with the nerve, local anesthetic is incrementally injected (5 mL) until a halo appears around the nerve. The needle is then directed to the ulnar nerve, if evident, or to the inferior edge of the artery. When motor or sensory stimulation of the ulnar nerve occurs, 5 mL of local anesthetic is injected as described above. Finally, the needle is redirected more posterior, and guided to the radial nerve. After confirmation of the nerve with motor or sensory stimulation, 5 mL of local anesthetic is injected incrementally, following the procedure outlined above. In some patients, it may necessary to push the artery out of the way with needle to anesthetize all four nerves from the same entry point.

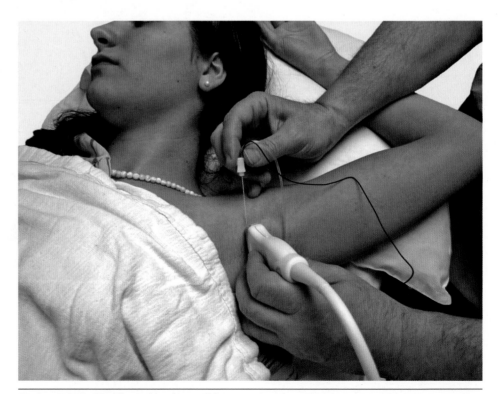

Figure 10-2. Needle and probe position.

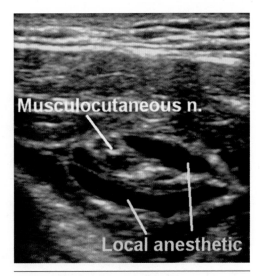

Figure 10-3. Musculocutaneous nerve surrounded with local anesthetic.

 Tips

1. Veins may vary in number, with one, two, or even more being present. They are easily compressed, and care must be taken to note their position because even mild pressure with the transducer can obliterate the lumen on the ultrasound image. Five to ten percent of patients will have an accessory axillary artery located deep or posterior to the primary axillary artery (Fig. 10-4).

2. It is difficult to contact and anesthetize all four nerve blocks from one needle insertion site because of the location of the nerves around the circumference of the artery and the variable location of the musculocutaneous nerve. Some practitioners prefer to block the musculocutaneous and median nerves from a cephalad approach and to block the ulnar and radial nerves by introducing the needle inferior to the probe.

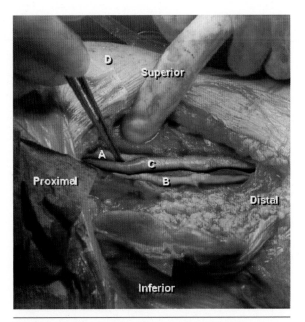

Figure 10-4a. Bifid axillary artery and vein.
a, superficial/ superior branch of the axillary artery;
b, deep branch/ inferior branch of the axillary artery;
c, axillary vein.

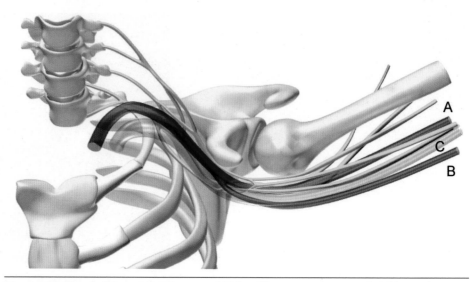

Figure 10-4b. Axillary plexus between bifid axillary artery. *a*, superficial/ superior branch of the axillary artery; *b*, deep branch/ inferior branch of the axillary artery; *c*, axillary vein.

Suggested Reading

Bigeleisen PE. The bifid axillary artery. J Clin Anesth 2004;16:224–225.

Kovacs P, Gruber H, Bodner G. "Interventional Techniques" in Peer S, Bodner G, eds. High Resolution Sonography of the Peripheral Nervous System. Berlin: Springer-Verlag, 2003:94–104.

Retzl G, Kapral S, Greher M, et al. Ultrasonographic findings of the axillary part of the brachial plexus. Anesth Analg 2001;92:1271–1275.

Schafhalter-Zoppoth I, Gray AT. The musculocutaneous nerve: ultrasound appearance for peripheral nerve block. Reg Anesth Pain Med 2005;30:385–390.

11

Blocks at the Elbow and Forearm

STEVEN L. OREBAUGH, PAUL E. BIGELEISEN

Background and Indications: Axillary or infraclavicular blocks sometimes fail to provide anesthesia in all of the nerve territories required for surgery on the forearm or hand. When this occurs, anesthesiologists may choose to provide a more distal block to supplement the brachial plexus block, selectively placing local anesthetic around the nerve that was not adequately anesthetized. Selective block of more distal nerves under ultrasound guidance may also be useful for limited surgical procedures of the forearm or hand, such as open reduction and fixation of a finger, carpal tunnel release, tendon repair, or ganglion cyst removal.[1]

Anatomy: The ulnar nerve may be followed with ultrasound from the axilla to the sulcus ulnaris, where it travels through the bony groove between the medial epicondyle of the radius and the olecranon process of the ulna. Most authors recommend providing the block 5 cm proximal to the sulcus ulnaris (Fig. 11-1). Here, the nerve is subcutaneous and amenable to block. As one moves closer to the elbow, the nerve lies within the sulcus ulnaris (Fig. 11-2). Performing the block within the boney canal (sulcus ulnaris) may lead to high pressures deep to the retinaculum that confines the nerve to the boney canal in most patients. Injection at the level of the sulcus ulnaris may also lead to a higher probability of intraneural injections because the nerve is less mobile.[2] Immediately below the elbow, the nerve is also superficial and easily blocked where it lies between the flexor digitorum superficialis and the flexor carpi ulnaris (Fig. 11-3). More distally, in the forearm, the ulnar nerve courses between the flexor tendon layers. Nearby lies the ulnar artery and median nerve.[3,4] At the level of the wrist, the artery and nerve can be seen passing distally into the hand, medial to the carpal tunnel (Fig. 11-4).

The median nerve remains with the brachial artery in its course through the medial aspect of the arm to the elbow. At the elbow, it can be located quite readily with ultrasonography adjacent to the brachial artery (Fig. 11-5). As the median nerve travels distally, into the forearm, it initially remains close to the ulnar artery. It can be followed with ultrasound scanning into the wrist, where it is seen in the carpal tunnel, among the flexor tendons (Fig. 11-6). Voluntary motion by the patient of his or her fingers causes the tendons to "dance," moving about quite actively while the nerve is less mobile, which may help distinguish these structures from one another.

The radial nerve can be difficult to follow with ultrasound imaging from the axilla to the elbow, because its course requires one to "spiral" the transducer around the humerus. However, the nerve is quite apparent in most patients because it emerges from the posterior aspect of the humerus, piercing the lateral intermuscular septum and arriving at the elbow on the lateral aspect of the arm (Fig. 11-7). In the antecubital region, the nerve lies between the biceps tendon and the brachioradialis muscle lateral to the brachial artery. The nerve bifurcates at this point, giving rise to the superficial radial nerve and the posterior interosseous nerve (deep radial nerve). The former is quite small and difficult to trace into the forearm (Fig. 11-8), whereas the latter is deep and provides innervation to all of the dorsal (extensor) forearm musculature.

A

B

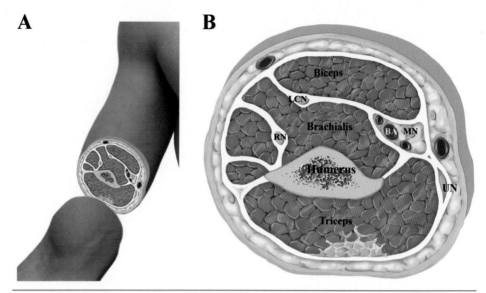

Figure 11-1a. Gross anatomy above the elbow. *RN*, radial nerve; *LCN*, lateral antebrachial cutaneous nerve; *MN*, median nerve; *UN*, ulnar nerve; *BA*, brachial artery.

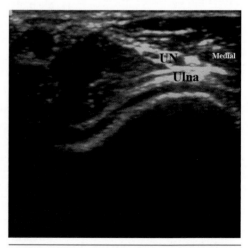

Figure 11-1b. Needle and probe position for ulnar nerve block above the elbow.

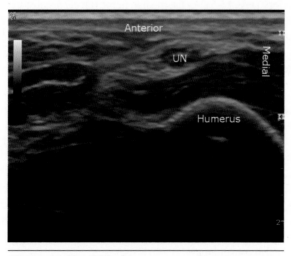

Figure 11-2a. *UN*, ulnar nerve.

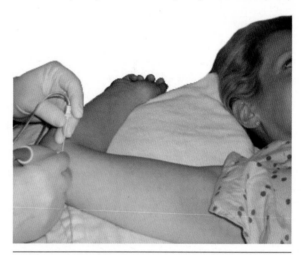

Figure 11-2b. *U*, ulna, *UN*, ulnar nerve.

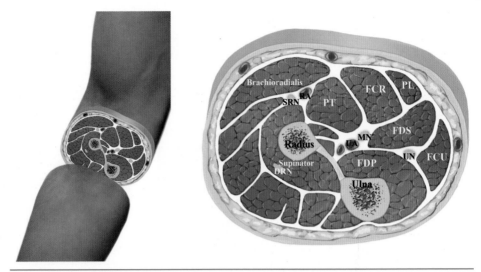

Figure 11-3a. Gross anatomy below the elbow. *UA*, ulnar artery; *MN*, median nerve; *UN*, ulnar nerve; *SRN*, superficial radial nerve; *DRN*, deep radial nerve; *PT*, pronator teres; *FCR*, flexor carpi radialis, *PL*, palmaris longus; *FDS*, flexor digitorum superficialis; *FCU*, flexor carpi ulnaris; *FDP*, flexor digitorum profundus.

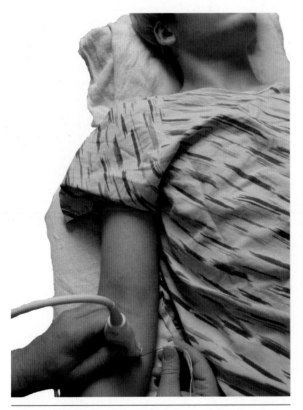

Figure 11-3b. Needle and probe position for ulnar block below the elbow.

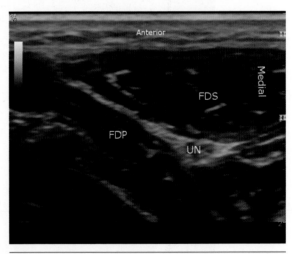

Figure 11-3c. *UN*, ulnar nerve; *FDS*, flexor digitorum superficialis; *FDP*, flexor digitorum profundus.

A   **B**

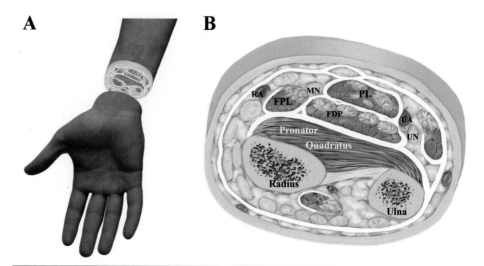

Figure 11-4a. Gross anatomy at the wrist. *UA*, ulnar artery; *UN*, ulnar nerve; *MN*, median nerve; *PL*, palmaris longus tendon; *FPL*, flexor policis longus; *FDP*, flexor digitorum profundus.

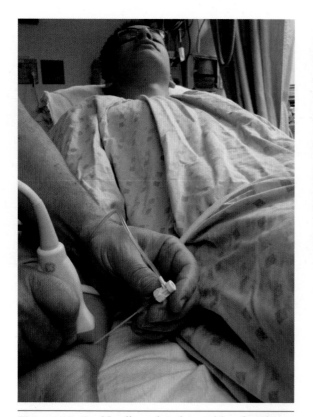

Figure 11-4b. Needle and probe position for ulnar nerve block at wrist (missing).

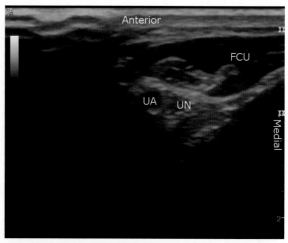

Figure 11-4c. Ultrasound scan of ulnar nerve at wrist. *UN*, ulnar nerve; *UA*, ulnar artery; *FCU*, flexor carpi ulnaris.

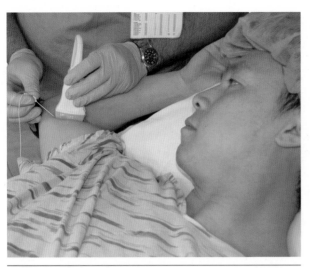

Figure 11-5a. Needle and probe position for median nerve block above the elbow.

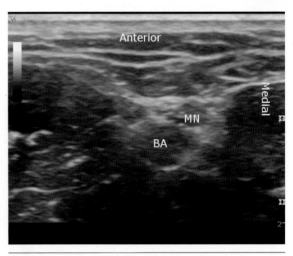

Figure 11-5b. Median nerve above the elbow. *MN*, median nerve; *BA*, brachial artery.

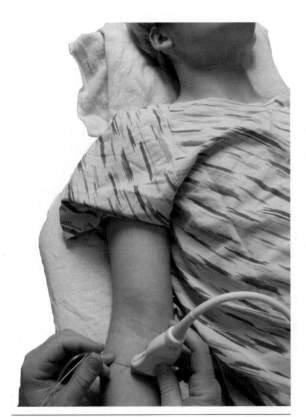

Figure 11-5c. Needle and probe position for median nerve block below the elbow.

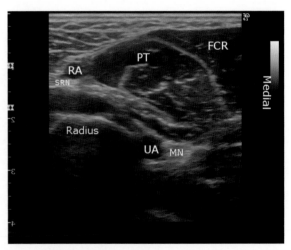

Figure 11-5d. Ultrasound scan showing ulnar artery and median nerve. *UA*, ulnar artery; *MN*, median nerve; *FCR*, flexor carpi radialis; *PT*, pronator teres; *RA*, radial artery; *SRN*, superficial radial nerve.

A

B

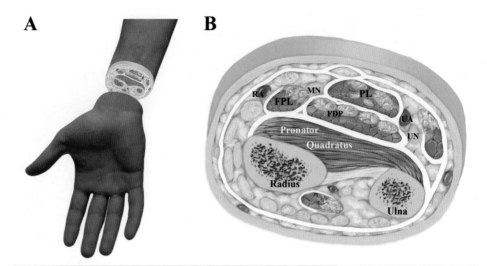

Figure 11-6a. Gross anatomy at the wrist. *UA*, ulnar artery; *UN*, ulnar nerve; *MN*, median nerve; *PL*, palmaris longus tendon; *FPL*, flexor policis longus; *FDP*, flexor digitorum profundus.

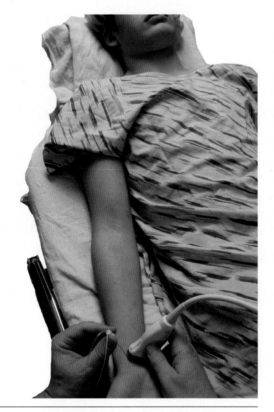

Figure 11-6b. Needle and probe position for median nerve block at wrist.

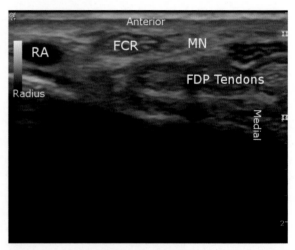

Figure 11-6c. Ultrasound scan at the wrist. *FCR*, flexor carpi radialis; *FDP* tendons, flexor digitorum profundus tendons; *MN*, median nerve; *PL*, palmaris longus; *MN*, median nerve; *RA*, radial artery.

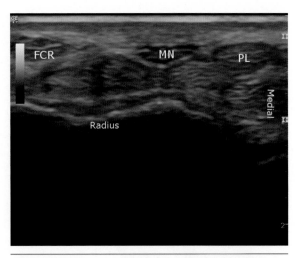

Figure 11-6d. Ultrasound scan at the wrist. *MN*, median nerve; *FCR*, flexor carpi radialis; *PL*, palmaris longus.

A   **B**

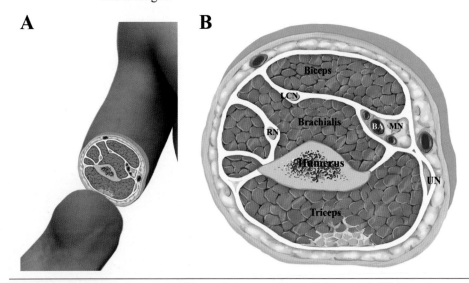

Figure 11-7a. Gross anatomy of the radial nerve. *RN*, radial nerve; *LCN*, lateral antebrachial cutaneous nerve; *MN*, median nerve; *UN*, ulnar nerve; *BA*, brachial artery, *RN*, radial nerve.

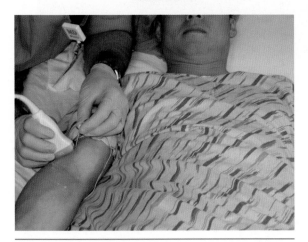

Figure 11-7b. Needle and probe position for radial nerve block above elbow.

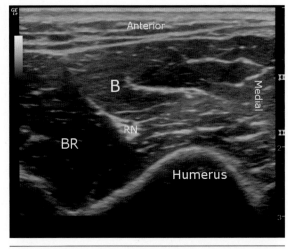

Figure 11-7c. *RN*, radial nerve; *BR*, brachioradialis; *B*, brachialis.

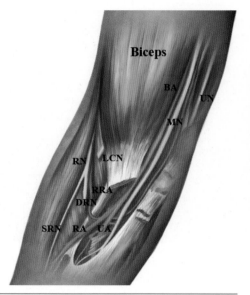

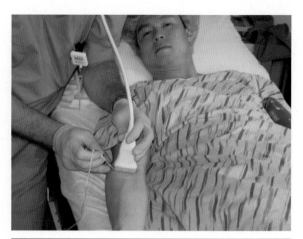

Figure 11-8a. Gross anatomy of the radial nerve. *BC*, biceps; *BA*, brachial artery; *RN*, radial nerve; *RRA*, radial recurrent artery; *DRN*, deep radial nerve; *SRN*, superficial radial nerve; *RA*, radial artery; *UA*, ulnar artery; *MN*, medial nerve; *UN*, ulnar nerve; *LCN*, lateral cutaneous nerve.

Figure 11-8b. Needle and probe position for radial nerve block below the elbow.

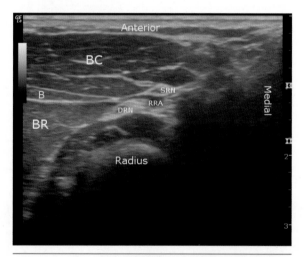

Figure 11-8c. *SRN*, superficial radial nerve; *DRN*, deep radial nerve; *RRA*, radial recurrent artery; *BR*, brachioradialis; *B*, brachialis; *BC*, biceps.

Patient Position: Supine with the arm supinated. For ulnar block above the elbow, the arm is abducted and the elbow is flexed.

Probe: 25-mm linear probe oscillating at 13 MHz.

Probe Orientation: Transverse.

Needle: 22-gauge, 5-cm blunt needle.

Local Anesthetic: 3 to 5 mL of 0.5% ropivacaine or 0.5% bupivacaine with epinephrine.

Technique: Oxygen by face mask is initiated. Patient monitors are placed, and sedation is administered. A brief preprocedural "time out" is conducted at the bedside, and the anesthesiologist marks the surgical site. An antiseptic is utilized to prepare the skin of the block area.

After establishing an appropriate image of the ulnar or median nerve at the elbow or forearm, or the radial nerve just proximal to the elbow, the physician may choose either an in-plane or out-of-plane approach to nerve blockade. The in-plane technique allows closer observation of the tip of the needle and facilitates direct deposit of local anesthetic on the posterior side of the nerve. The skin is infiltrated with local anesthetic in the appropriate site for introduction of the block needle, depending on which technique is chosen.

Next, the block needle is introduced. Peripheral nerve stimulation may be elected to guide the block in concert with ultrasound imaging. After the needle approximates the nerve, with or without nerve stimulation, local anesthetic is injected in small aliquots to surround the nerve in question. Care must be taken when blocking nerves adjacent to small vessels, such as the ulnar artery, to avoid intravascular injection. Small arteries are difficult to visualize and may be compressed when subjected to pressure applied with the probe.

Summary of Evidence: Evidence supporting distal nerve block in the upper extremity with ultrasound guidance is relatively scant and primarily consists of observational studies or small case series. Gray described block of the ulnar nerve in the forearm utilizing this technique for surgery on the fifth finger.

References

1. Neal JM, Hebl JR, Gerancher JC, et al. Brachial plexus anesthesia: essentials of our current understanding. Reg Anesth Pain Med 2002;27:402–428.
2. Chelly JE. Blocks at the elbow. In: Chelly JE, ed. Peripheral Nerve Blocks-A color Atlas. 2nd ed. Philadelphia: Lippincott Williams Wilkins; 2004:58–60.
3. Gray AT, Schafhalter-Zoppoth I. Ultrasound guidance for ulnar nerve block in the forearm. Reg Anesth Pain Med 2003;28:335–339.
4. McCartney CJL, Xu D, Constantinescu C, Abbas S, Chan VWS. Ultrasound examination of peripheral nerves in the forearm. Reg Anesth Pain Med 2007;32:434–439.

Section III

Lower Extremity Blocks

12 Ultrasound-Guided Lumbar Plexus Block (Transverse Approach)

13 Ultrasound-Guided Inguinal Nerve Block

14 Ultrasound-Guided Transversus Abdominis Plane Block

15 Ultrasound-Guided Femoral Nerve Block

16 Ultrasound-Guided Lateral Femoral Cutaneous Block

17 Ultrasound-Guided Saphenous Nerve Block

18 Ultrasound-Guided Obturator Nerve Block

19 Ultrasound-Guided Parasacral Block

20 Ultrasound-Guided Anterior Sciatic Nerve Block

21 Subgluteal Sciatic Block

22 Ultrasound-Guided Popliteal Sciatic Block

23 Ultrasound-Guided Ankle Block

12

Ultrasound-Guided Lumbar Plexus Block (Transverse Approach)

SHINICHI SAKURA, KAORU HARA, JEAN-LOUIS HORN

 Introduction and Indications: The lumbar plexus consists of roots L1 through L4. In some patients, roots T12 and L5 contribute. The roots join together to form the subcostal, iliohypogastric, ilioinguinal, lateral femoral cutaneous, genital-femoral, and obturator nerves. The lumbar plexus usually lies within the posterior substance of the psoas muscle. The lateral femoral cutaneous and femoral nerves usually lie within the same fascial plane, but the obturator nerve often lies within a separate fold of the muscle. Lumbar plexus block is used to provide intraoperative and postoperative analgesia for lower extremity surgery, sometimes in combination with sciatic nerve block. It may also be used as a series of injections for patients suffering from chronic lower extremity pain.

 Anatomy: The spinous process, the articular process, and the transverse process are important landmarks. These bony structures are hyperechoic and create a shadow. When the transducer is moved slightly cephalad or caudad, a clear image of the psoas and quadratus lumborum muscles is obtained. The lumbar plexus generally is expected to lie within the posterior one third of the psoas major muscle and 2 to 3 cm deep to the anterior surface of the transverse process. The lumbar plexus is not always visualized under ultrasound but may be observed as a hyperechoic structure in a young population (Fig. 12-1).

 Patient Position: Lateral decubitus position with the side to be blocked uppermost.

 Transducer: 40- to 60-mm curved array oscillating at 2 to 5 MHz.

 Transducer Position: The transducer is positioned transversely in the midline of the back at the L4 level to capture the spinous process. The transducer is then moved laterally (approximately 3 cm) while scanning the paravertebral region until a clear image of the articular and transverse processes is obtained.

 Needle: A 100- to 150-mm long, short-bevel, 21-gauge insulated needle.

 Local Anesthetic: 20 to 35 mL of ropivacaine 0.5% to 0.75%.
a) Pain Therapy: 10 mL of ropivacaine 0.25%.

Approach and Technique: The skin is washed with sterile solution, and the transducer is covered with a sterile sheath. Ultrasound-guided lumbar plexus block requires advanced skill because of the depth of needle placement. After the optimal transducer position is found, the transducer is angled laterally or medially in the transverse plane depending on the needle insertion site while the target is kept in the middle of the ultrasound image. This allows the practitioner to view the needle more easily.

Lateral Insertion Approach: After skin infiltration with local anesthetic, the needle is inserted in-plane from the lateral edge of the transducer. The transducer is perpendicular to

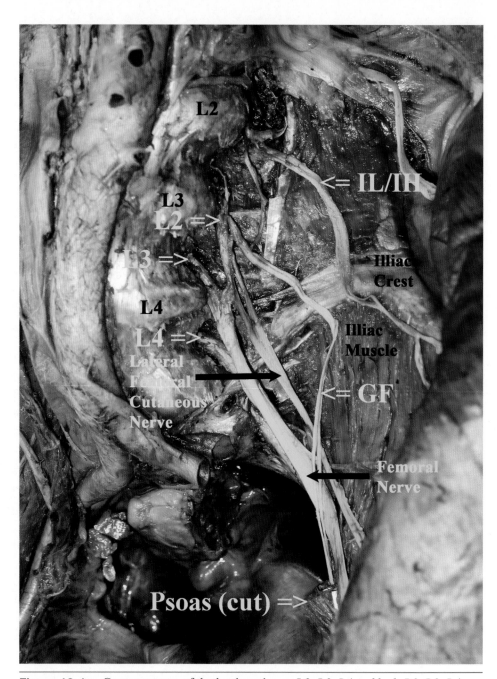

Figure 12-1a. Gross anatomy of the lumbar plexus. L2, L3, L4 *in black*; L2, L3, L4 *vertebrae*; L2, L3, L4 *in yellow*; *nerve roots* L2, L3, L4; *IL/IH,* ilioinguinal and iliohypogastric nerves; *GF,* genital-femoral nerve.

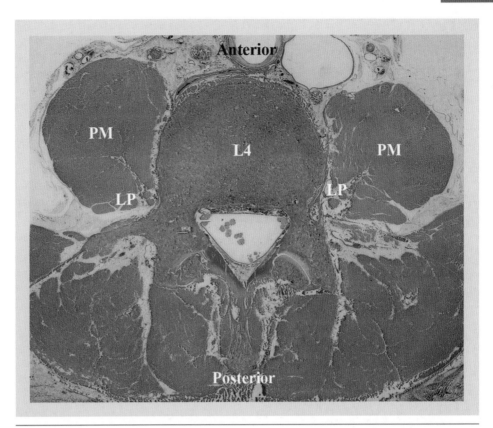

Figure 12-1b. Histological cross section showing lumbar plexus embedded in psoas muscle. *LP*, lumbar plexus; *PM*, psoas muscle.

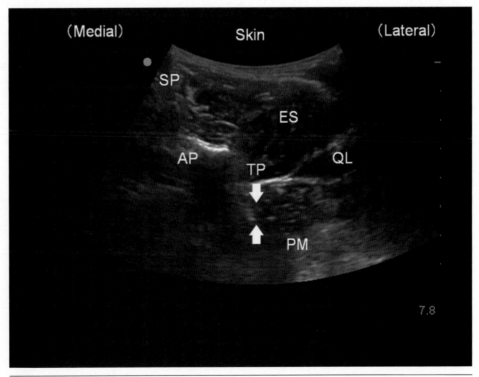

Figure 12-1c. Ultrasound image. *Arrows*, lumbar plexus; *SP*, spinous process; *AP*, articular process; *TP*, transverse process; *ES*, erector spinae muscle; *QL*, quadratus lumborum muscle; *PM*, psoas muscle.

the skin (Fig. 12-2). The needle insertion site should be around 5 cm lateral to the midline, and the needle direction should be perpendicular to the body plane or directed slightly toward the midline. When the lumbar plexus is visualized, the needle should be advanced directly to the plexus. If the lumbar plexus is not visualized, the location of the target can be estimated from the distance of the skin to the transverse process. In either case, electrical stimulation helps identify and confirm the target. When the needle tip is near the target, a nerve stimulator with pulse duration of 0.1 ms and stimulating frequency of 2 Hz is turned on to elicit twitches of the quadriceps muscle. After contractions are obtained by stimulation between 0.5 and 1.0 mA, local anesthetic is injected in small increments after negative aspiration. This allows the practitioner to test for an intravascular or intrathecal position of the needle. During injection, local anesthetic and tissue expansion are observed within the psoas muscle and may surround the lumbar plexus (Fig. 12-3).

Medial Approach: The needle can be inserted in-plane from the medial edge of the transducer. In this case, the transducer should be angled slightly toward the midline (Fig. 12-4). The needle insertion site should be 3 to 4 cm lateral to the midline with the needle direction perpendicular to the body. In some cases, it may be necessary to angle the needle slightly laterally (Fig. 12-5). The remainder of the procedure is the same as above.

Sagittal Approach: Some practitioners prefer to use a sagittal orientation of the probe. In this approach, the iliac crest and posterior superior iliac spine are identified and the

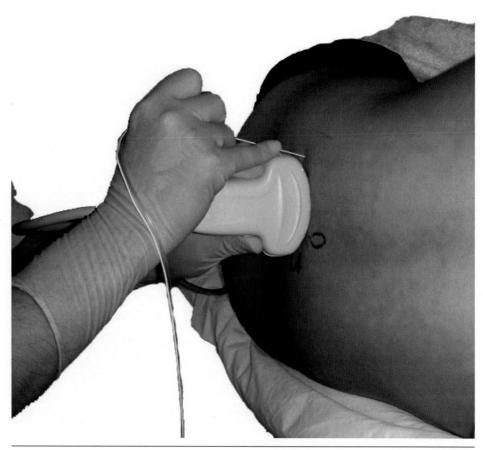

Figure 12-2a. Transducer position to obtain the ultrasound image as shown in Figure 12-1 and needle insertion from the lateral edge of the transducer.

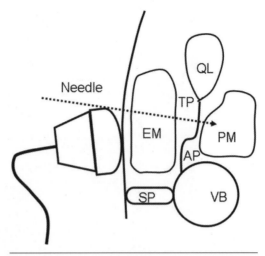

Figure 12-2b. A schematic diagram of the transverse view showing needle insertion from the lateral edge of the transducer. *SP*, spinous process; *AP*, articular process; *TP*, transverse process; *VB*, vertebral body; *ES*, erector spinae muscle; *QL*, quadratus lumborum muscle; *PM*, psoas muscle.

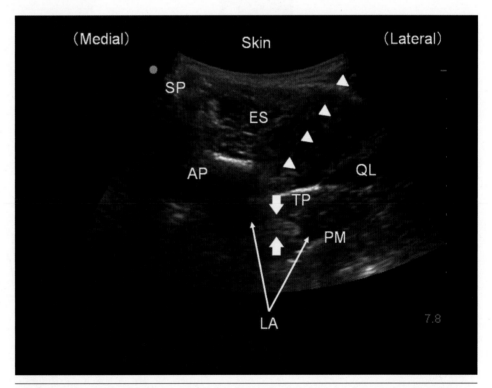

Figure 12-3. Ultrasound image after local anesthetic injection. *Arrows*, lumbar plexus; *SP*, spinous process; *AP*, articular process; *TP*, transverse process; *ES*, erector spinae muscle; *QL*, quadratus lumborum muscle; *PM*, psoas muscle; *LA*, local anesthetic; *triangles*, needle.

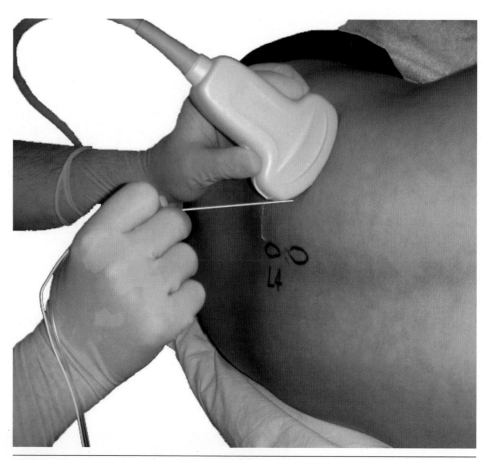

Figure 12-4a. Transducer position and needle insertion from the medial edge of the transducer.

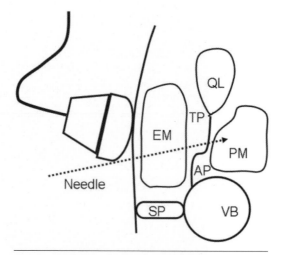

Figure 12-4b. A schematic diagram of the transverse view showing needle insertion from the medial edge of the transducer. *SP*, spinous process; *AP*, articular process; *TP*, transverse process; *VB*, vertebral body; *ES*, erector spinae muscle; *QL*, quadratus lumborum muscle; *PM*, psoas muscle.

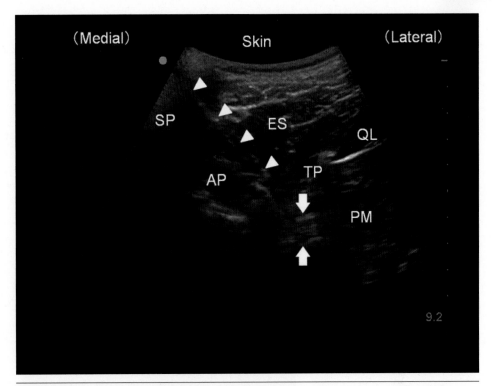

Figure 12-5. Ultrasound image showing the needle approaching the lumbar plexus from the medial edge of the transducer. *Arrows*, lumbar plexus; *SP*, spinous process; *AP*, articular process; *TP*, transverse process; *ES*, erector spinae muscle; *QL*, quadratus lumborum muscle; *PM*, psoas muscle; *triangles*, needle.

probe is sited in a sagittal plane at the level of L4 approximately 4 to 5 cm lateral to the midline (Fig. 12-6). The hyperechoic shadows of L3, L4, and L5 are identified (Fig. 12-6). A stimulating needle set at 1 mA is inserted either in-plane or out-of-plane in the space between L3 and L4. The needle is advanced between the spinous processes of L3 and L4 until a contraction is elicited in the quadriceps muscle. Fifteen to 25 mL of local anesthetic is then injected in aliquots of 3 to 5 mL. Because of the depth of the plexus in obese patients, some practitioners simply use ultrasound to determine the depth and location of the transverse processes, and then proceed with a blind technique using electrolocation, a paresthesia, or a loss of resistance technique.

Tips

1. Because of the depth of the target and the angle of the needle, it is difficult to observe the entire needle during the whole procedure. However, the needle tip should be observed, or at least the estimated tissue movement, when the needle is moved under real-time ultrasound imaging. The use of an echogenic tip needle is preferable.
2. To obtain a better needle image under ultrasound, the transducer should be angled medially or laterally, so that the angle of needle in the ultrasound beam is less steep. This will allow visualization of the needle tip and shaft more easily. Needle insertion should not be too lateral to avoid kidney puncture nor should it be too medial to avoid subarachnoid injection.

   Continuous lumbar plexus block is useful for the management of postoperative pain after major lower extremity surgery. The technique is similar to a single-shot injection, but the use of a Tuohy needle is recommended. A catheter is inserted approximately 5 to 10 cm beyond the needle tip after administration of local anesthetic.
3. In some patients, the iliac artery can be visualized anterior to the psoas muscle.

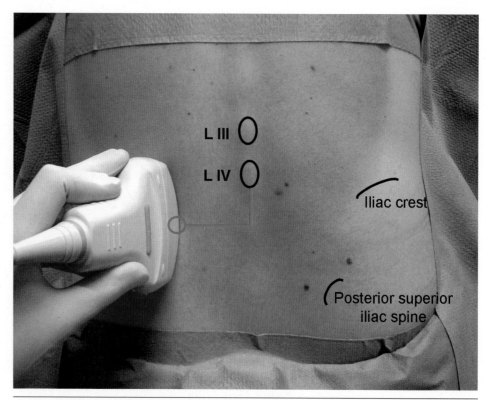

Figure 12-6a. Probe position for longitudinal scan.

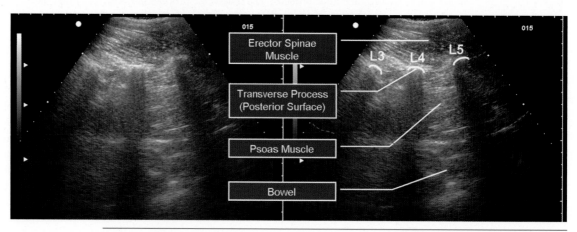

Figure 12-6b. Longitudinal scan showing transverse processes and psoas muscle.

Suggested Readings

Awad I, Dugan E. Posterior lumbar plexus block: anatomy, approaches, and techniques. Reg Anesth Pain Med 2005;30:143–149.

Karmakar MK, Ho AM, Li X, et al. Ultrasound-guided lumbar plexus block through the acoustic window of the lumbar ultrasound trident. Br J Anaesth 2008;100:533–537.

Kirchmair L, Enna B, Mitterschiffthaler G, et al. Lumbar plexus in children: a sonographic study and its relevance to pediatric regional anesthesia. Anesthesiology 2004;101:445–450.

Kirchmair L, Entner T, Kapral S, et al. Ultrasound guidance for the psoas compartment block: an imaging study. Anesth Analg 2002;94:706–710.

Robards C, Hadzic A. Lumbar plexus block. In: Hadzic A, ed. Textbook of regional anesthesia and acute pain management. New York: McGraw-Hill Medical: 2007:481–488.

13

Ultrasound-Guided Inguinal Nerve Block

URS EICHENBERGER

Background and Indication: The ilioinguinal and iliohypogastric nerves are part of the lumbar plexus and formed from roots T12 and L1. The nerves travel between the psoas and iliacus muscles as they emerge from the spine. More distally, they travel in the layer between the transversus abdominis muscle and the internal oblique muscle (Fig. 13-1). As the transversus abdominis muscle fuses with the internal oblique muscle, the nerves pierce the fascia between the internal and external oblique muscles. Branches of the nerves also subserve the skin over the lower quadrant of the abdomen. The ilioinguinal nerve also supplies innervation to the inguinal canal. Ilioinguinal/iliohypogastric block is used to provide intraoperative and postoperative analgesia for hernia repair. It may also be used for diagnostic nerve block or a therapeutic series of injections for patients suffering from chronic pain after hernia repair.

Anatomy: The three muscle layers of the abdominal wall, from superficial to deep, are the external oblique, the internal oblique, and the transverse abdominal muscle. More distally, you will usually only find one or two muscle layers—the external oblique and transversus abdominis muscles may present as only a thin aponeurosis. The nerves at this level can be found between the internal oblique and transverse abdominal muscles in more than 90% of cases. The nerves appear as oval hypoechoic areas with hyperechoic spots and are often accompanied by small vessels (Fig. 13-2). The ilioinguinal nerve can be found close to the iliac crest (4–10 mm) and the iliohypogastric nerve lies 8 to 15 mm more medial. The diameters of both nerves are between 2 to 4 mm. The lateral end of the transducer sits on the iliac crest with a bony shadow as an important landmark (Figs. 13-2 and 13-3).

Patient Position: Supine.

Transducer: 25-mm linear array oscillating at 13 MHz.

Transducer Position: 5 cm superior and slightly lateral to the anterior superior iliac spine. Transverse oblique plane, perpendicular to the course of both nerves (Fig. 13-3).

Needle: 5-cm, 22-gauge blunt needle.

Local Anesthetic: 5 to 10 mL of 0.5 % ropivacaine or bupivacaine with epinephrine.

Technique: The skin is washed with sterile solution and the probe is covered with a sterile sheath. The external, internal, and transversus abdominis muscles are imaged, and the two nerves are sought in the plane between the internal oblique and transversus abdominis

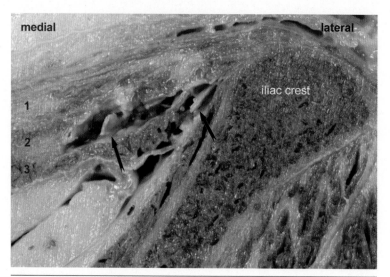

Figure 13-1. Corresponding anatomical cross section to Figure 13-2. Arrows, ilioinguinal nerve (the lateral one, close to the iliac crest) and iliohypogastric nerve (the medial one); *1*, external oblique; *2*, internal oblique; *3*, transverse abdominal muscle.

muscles. Occasionally, the nerves will be found between the external and internal oblique muscles. After the optimal probe position is found, the target nerve or nerves are brought into the middle of the ultrasound image. The needle is advanced out of plane (Fig. 13-4), medial to the ilioinguinal or lateral to the iliohypogastric nerve. At this point, local anesthetic is injected in small increments after negative aspiration to test for intravascular injection. A distension of tissue should occur with each injection, and the injected local anesthetic should surround the nerve be seen between the internal oblique and transversus abdominis muscles. The needle should be repositioned near to the second nerve after half of local anesthetic has been injected.

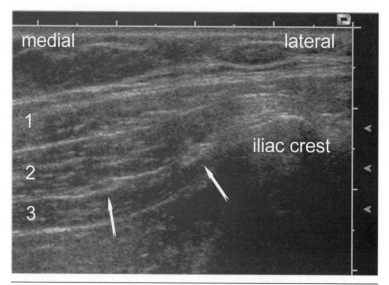

Figure 13-2. Ultrasound image. Arrows, ilioinguinal nerve (the lateral one, close to the iliac crest) and iliohypogastric nerve (the medial one); *1*, external oblique; *2*, internal oblique; *3*, transverse abdominal muscle.

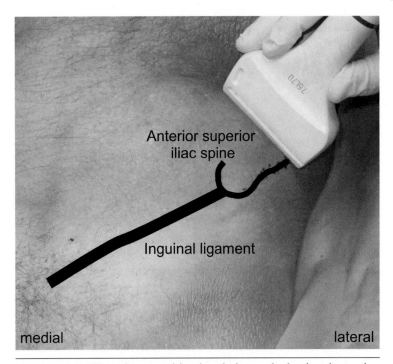

Anterior superior
iliac spine

Inguinal ligament

medial   lateral

Figure 13-3. Transducer position in relation to the landmarks to obtain the ultrasound image as shown in Figure 13-2.

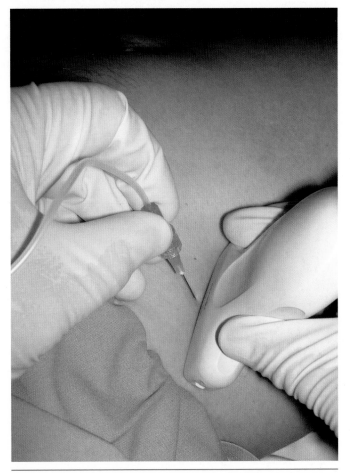

Figure 13-4. Needle position in relation to the transducer. Out-of-plane, short-axis approach.

For pain therapy, the practitioner's goal should be to target each nerve to provide a more accurate diagnosis. In this case, the needle should be placed lateral to the ilioinguinal nerve and then medial to the iliohypogastric nerve so that each nerve can be blocked separately. Unfortunately, this cannot be guaranteed in all cases.

 Tips

1. The in-line technique is difficult to perform in this region. At the lateral end of the probe, the iliac crest lies in the path of the needle.
2. If the nerves cannot be identified clearly (especially in obese patients), the local anesthetic can be injected between the internal oblique and transversus abdominis muscle.
3. In pain patients, two positive diagnostic blocks of the targeted nerve suggest that cryoanalgesia may be a good treatment. In these cases, the ice ball can be seen on an ultrasound.
4. A third nerve—the genitofemoral nerve—may play an important role, especially in chronic pain patients. This nerve lies anterior to the psoas muscle and cannot be visualized by ultrasound. Near the pubic symphysis, it becomes superficial but often divides into several branches. At this level, the femoral part of the nerve may sometimes be visualized on ultrasound, but the genital part of the nerve is usually too thin. The genital branches can be blocked using a subcutaneous field block near the symphysis.

Suggested Reading

Eichenberger U, Greher M, Kirchmair L, et al. Ultrasound-guided blocks of the ilioinguinal and iliohypogastric nerve: accuracy of a selective new technique confirmed by anatomical dissection. Br J Anaesth 2006;97:238–243.

Jamieson RW, Swigart LL, Anson BJ. Points of parietal perforation of the ilioinguinal and iliohypogastric nerves in relation to optimal sites for local anaesthesia. Q Bull Northwest Univ Med Sch 1952;26:22–26.

Willschke H, Bösenberg A, Marhofer P, et al. Ultrasonographic-guided ilioinguinal/iliohypogastric nerve block in pediatric anesthesia: what is the optimal volume? Anesth Analg 2006;102:1680–1684.

Ultrasound-Guided Transversus Abdominis Plane Block

KIM RUSSON, RAFAEL BLANCO

 Background and Indications: The transversus abdominis plane, more commonly referred to as the TAP block, places local anesthetic in the lateral abdominal wall in a plane between the internal oblique and the transversus abdominis muscles. Here, the local anesthetic block can block many of the abdominal nerves as they pass to the abdominal structures. The TAP block was first described by McDonnell et al[1] in 2006. Their original technique was a blind technique using a blunt regional anesthesia needle and relied on feeling a double pop as the needle passed through the layers in an area known as the triangle of Petit. Since then, the technique has been modified to utilize ultrasound to confirm placement of the local anesthetic. Studies (although numbers remain small) have shown bilateral TAP blocks to provide effective postoperative analgesia after prostatectomy,[1] large and small bowel resection,[2] and cesarean section[3] compared with morphine. Intuition suggests that if the nerves to the abdominal wall and peritoneum can be numbed with this block, then it is likely to be useful in providing pain relief following many other abdominal surgical, gynecological, and urological procedures.

 Anatomy: The abdominal wall between the iliac crest and the subcostal margin consists of three layers of muscle (external oblique, internal oblique, transversus abdominis) covered by connective tissue and skin (Fig. 14-1). The transversus abdominis is the deepest layer, and below is the peritoneum. The skin, muscles, and peritoneum of the anterior abdominal wall are innervated by the lower 6 thoracic nerves and the first intercostals nerve. At the costal margin, thoracic nerves 7 to 11 leave their intercostals spaces and enter the neurovascular plane of the abdominal wall between transversus abdominis and internal oblique (Fig. 14-1). Running across the surface of the transversus abdominis muscle and aponeurosis are the lower intercostals, subcostal, and iliohypogastric nerves.

 Patient Position: Supine.

 Probe: 40- or 60-mm curved array oscillating at 3 to 8 MHz.

 Probe Position: Transverse or transverse oblique between the margin of the 12th rib and superior iliac spine.

 Needle: 22-gauge blunt needle (5–10 cm) for single injection. 18-gauge Tuohy needle (5–10 cm) for continuous infusions.

 Local Anesthetic: Bupivaciane 0.25% (20–30 mL), ropivacaine 0.2% (20–30 mL).

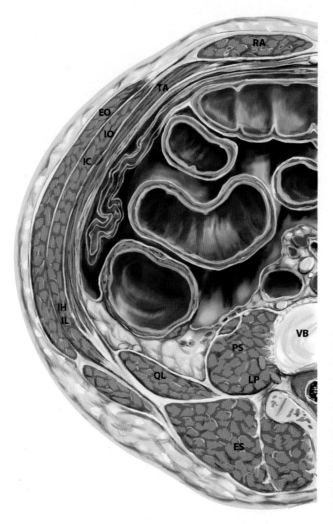

Figure 14-1. Cross section through the abdomen. *EO*, external oblique muscle; *IO*, internal oblique muscle; *TA*, transversus abdominus muscle; *IC*, intercostal nerves; *IL*, ilioinguinal nerve; *IH*, iliohypogastric nerve; *PS*, psoas; *ES*, erector spinae; *VB*, vertebral body; *QB*, quadratus lumborum.

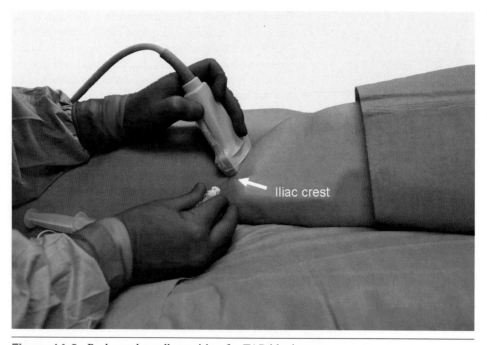

Figure 14-2. Probe and needle position for TAP block.

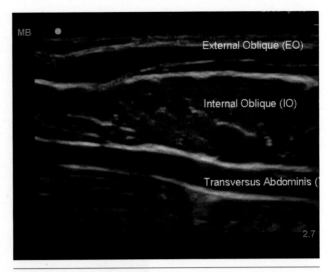

Figure 14-3. Ultrasound scan through the abdomen.

Technique: This block may be performed before or following induction of general or spinal anesthesia. The patient needs to be lying supine. An aseptic technique is advocated using a no-touch technique, an appropriate cleaning solution, and a sterile cover for the ultrasound probe. The ultrasound probe is positioned horizontally on the skin just above the iliac crest in the midaxillary line (Fig. 14-2). The muscle layers are identified (Fig. 14-3). We prefer to use a peripheral nerve block needle because it allows "distant" injection by your assistant while you remain in control of ultrasound probe and needle. A 50-mm needle is usually sufficient. We use an in-plane approach inserting the needle posteriorly and directing anteriorly. The needle is followed under direct vision as it passes through the muscle layers until the tip lies between the internal oblique and transversus abdomenus muscles (Fig. 14-4).

Injection of the local anesthetic must be seen to ensure correct placement. It is very characteristic to see the layer expanding in an ellipsoid way (Fig. 14-5). We use 20 mL of 0.25% levobupivacaine in each side as do McDonnell et al.[2] Use of 20 mL of 0.5% ropivacaine[4] has also been described resulting in a block from T8 to the symphysis pubis.

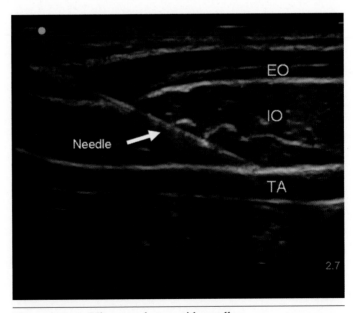

Figure 14-4. Ultrasound scan with needle.

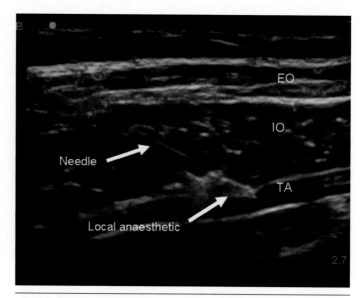

Figure 14-5. Ultrasound scan after local anesthetic injection.

References

1. O'Donnell BD, McDonnell JG, McShane AJ. The transversus abdominis plane (TAP) block in open retropubic prostatectomy. Reg Anesth Pain Med. 2006;31(1):91. PMID: 16418039.
2. McDonnell JG, O'Donnell B, Curley G, et al. The analgesic efficacy of transversus abdominis plane block after abdominal surgery: a prospective randomized controlled trial. Anesth Analg 2007; 104(1):193–197. PMID: 17179269.
3. McDonnell JG, Curley G, Carney J, et al. The analgesic efficacy of transversus abdominis plane block after cesarean delivery: a randomized controlled trial. Anesth Analg 2008;106(1):186–191. PMID: 18165577.
4. Hebbard P, Fujiwara Y, Shibata Y, et al. Ultrasound-guided transversus abdominis plane (TAP) block. Anaesth Intensive Care 2007;35(4):616–617. PMID: 18020088.

Ultrasound-Guided Femoral Nerve Block

STEPHEN M. BRENEMAN

 Background and Indications: Femoral nerve block has traditionally been used in conjunction with block of the sciatic nerve for surgery of the knee, leg, foot, or saphenous vein stripping. In the past, practitioners used a blind approach (fascia iliaca) which relied on palpating the iliac crest and the pubic ramus. Other practitioners used electrolocation, paresthesia, or simply infiltrated around the femoral artery after palpating a pulse. Because of the variable distribution and location of the femoral nerve, ultrasound has made the procedure more reliable.

 Anatomy: The femoral nerve is formed from roots L2, L3, and L4. These roots combine to form the femoral nerve that travels in the space between the psoas and iliacus muscles (Fig. 15-1A). In most cases, the nerve actually travels within the substance of the psoas muscle (Fig. 15-1B). The nerve emerges below the inguinal ligament, lateral to the femoral artery, and deep to the fascia iliaca. Many textbooks portray the nerve as a single round or oval structure. In fact, the nerve is often flat, giving rise to its many branches that subserve the thigh.

 Patient Position: Supine or recumbent with groin exposed.

 Transducer: 8- to 12-MHz linear array or 5- to 8-MHz curved array.

 Transducer Position: The transducer is placed axially anywhere between the inguinal crease to the inguinal ligament (Fig. 15-2A).

 Needle: 5-cm, 22-gauge nerve block needle.

 Local Anesthetic: 10 mL (saphenous), 20 mL (femoral), 20 to 40 mL (fascia iliaca).

 Technique: The groin is exposed and examined for skin breakdown or infection. The skin is washed with sterile solution. The inguinal crease, anterior superior iliac spine, and lateral superior pubic ramus are identified. The transducer is placed axially anywhere between the inguinal crease to the inguinal ligament. The femoral artery and vein are identified as the curved surface of the iliopsoas muscle and the hyperechoic triangle formed between the muscle and the artery that are covered by the fascia iliaca (Fig. 15-2A,B). This triangle can have a mirror image on the medial aspect of the femoral vein (Fig. 15-2C).

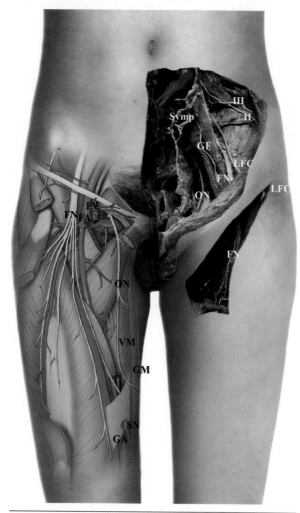

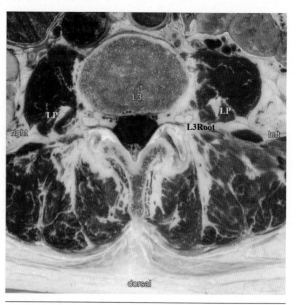

Figure 15-1b. *L3*, third lumbar verteba; *LP*, lumbar plexus in psoas muscle.

Figure 15-1a. *FN*, femoral nerve; *LFC*, lateral femoral cutaneous nerve; *IH*, iliohypogastric nerve; *IL*, ilioinguinal nerve; *ON*, obturator nerve; *GF*, genital-femoral nerve; *SYM*, sympathetic chain.

The needle entry is lateral to the probe using an in-line approach. A 30- to 45-degree needle trajectory should pierce the surface of the iliopsoas muscle until a distinct "pop" of the fascia iliaca is seen as the triangle is entered. (The fascia lata pop is often missed visually on ultrasound.) The triangle is filled, and most of the time the hyperechoic nerve will show more clearly once it has been surrounded with local anesthetic.

Tips

1. When using a nerve stimulator, set the current to 0.8 to 1.0 mA, which is used for verification rather than localization. This lower amperage is especially important in young patients with significant muscle development.
2. The most common initial contraction is the sartorius muscle over the medial thigh. This represents the anterior branch of the femoral nerve (Fig. 15-3), which is deep to the fascia lata but superficial to the fascia iliaca. Thus, an injection in this superficial plane will not lead to adequate anesthesia of the thigh and knee. Usually, moving the needle more

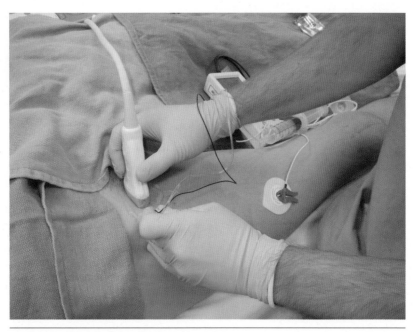

Figure 15-2a. Probe and needle position.

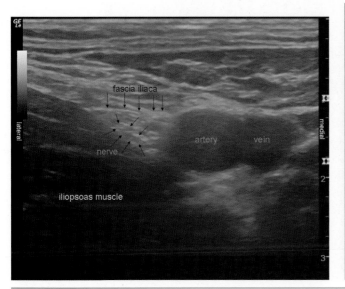
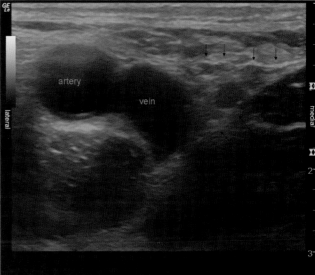

Figure 15-2b,c. Ultrasound scan showing false femoral nerve.

laterally and deeper (and pop) will lead to a contraction of the quadriceps muscle and anterior movement of the patella (Fig. 15-4). With very small needle movements, the contraction may move back and forth from the medial thigh to the anterior and lateral thigh. If the stimulating needle is too deep, there will be a local twitch of the iliopsoas muscle that does not extend to the patella.

3. Unlike nerves of the brachial plexus or the sciatic nerve, the femoral nerve is not always apparent prior to injection (Fig. 15-5). In addition, hyperechoic areas do not always indicate the nerve (Fig. 15-6). Because of the difficulty in visualization, often the injection is intraneural (Fig. 15-7), thus keep injection pressures low.

4. For obese patients, one may need to tape the pannus up and away from the groin. Beware of yeast infections in this location. Also, use a longer needle and start fur-

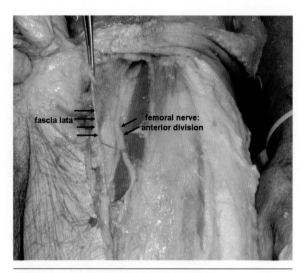

Figure 15-3. Dissection showing nerve to sartorius muscle.

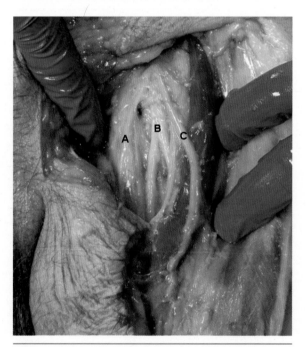

Figure 15-4. Deep dissection showing nerve to quadratus femoris. A, nerve to vastus medialis; B, nerve to quadriceps femoris; C, nerve to sartorius.

ther ateral from the probe, so that the needle angle does not become too steep. A needle angle great than 30 to 45 degrees can make the block needle even harder to visualize.

5. This block has other names including *3-in-1* and *fascia iliaca* block. The 3-in-1 described by Winnie included coverage for the obturator nerve. His results have not been replicated. Thus, the femoral block could be considered a 2-in-1 block that includes the lateral femoral cutaneous nerve when higher volumes of local anesthetic are administered. The fascia iliaca block was a "block by feel." The practitioner placed a finger on

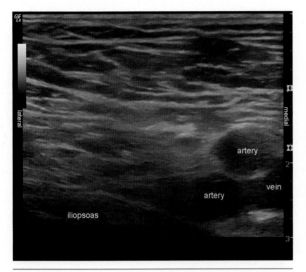

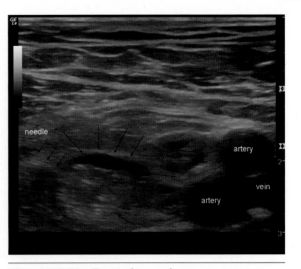

Figure 15-5a. Femoral nerve is not apparent before injection.

Figure 15-5b. Femoral nerve becomes apparent after injection.

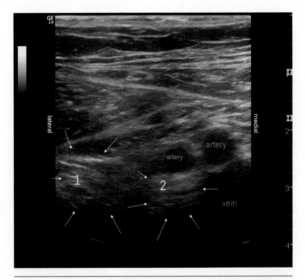

Figure 15-6a. *1*, femoral nerve; *2*, false femoral nerve.

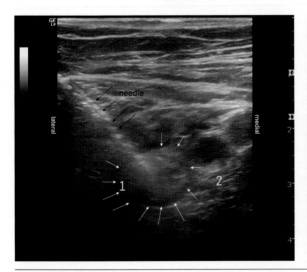

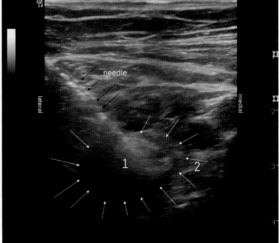

Figure 15-6b,c. *1*, femoral nerve after injection; *2*, false femoral nerve.

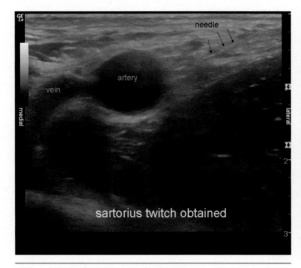

Figure 15-7a. Nerve and needle.

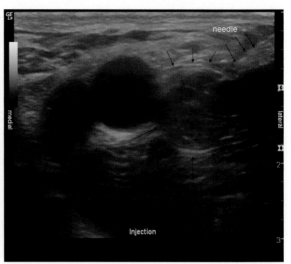

Figure 15-7b. Intraneural injection.

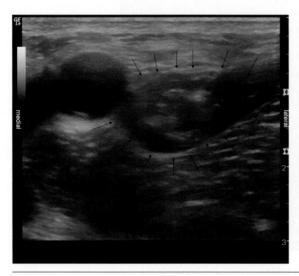

Figure 15-7c,d. Rupture of the epineurium and spread of local anesthetic around the femoral nerve.

the artery. A blunt bevel needle was sited several centimeters lateral to the pulse, with the needle oriented perpendicular to the skin. The needle was inserted through the skin, and then the practitioner advanced the needle until two additional pops were felt. After this, 20 to 40 mL of local anesthetic was injected.

6. For ultrasound-guided catheter placement next to the femoral nerve, use the same lateral approach with an 18-gauge Tuohy needle. Once the tip of the needle is properly sited, inject local anesthetic through the needle to dilate the area around the nerve. This also allows visualization of the Tuohy needle tip adjacent to the nerve. Next, direct the bevel cranially and pass the catheter. An out-of-plane method can be used as well with the subsequent injection of local via the catheter. When using a stimulating catheter, D5W can be used to expand the space to allow easier passage of the stimulating catheter while maintaining a contraction in the muscle. The catheter can be threaded cranially to the lumbar plexus region.

Suggested Readings

Casati A, Baciarello M, Di Cianni S, et al. Effects of ultrasound guidance on the minimum effective anaesthetic volume required to block the femoral nerve. Br J Anaesth 2007;98(6):823–827.

Marhofer P, Schrögendorfer K, Wallner T, et al. Ultrasonographic guidance reduces the amount of local anesthetic for 3-in-1 blocks. Reg Anesth Pain Med 1998;23(6):584–588.

Sites BD, Beach M, Gallagher JD, et al. A single injection ultrasound-assisted femoral nerve block provides side effect-sparing analgesia when compared with intrathecal morphine in patients undergoing total knee arthroplasty. Anesth Analg 2004;99(5):1539–1543.

Tsui BC, Dillane D, Pillay J, Ramji AK, Walji AH. Cadaveric ultrasound imaging for training in ultrasound-guided peripheral nerve blocks: lower extremity. Can J Anaesth 2007;54(6):475–480.

16

Ultrasound-Guided Lateral Femoral Cutaneous Block

PAUL E. BIGELEISEN, MILENA MORENO, STEVEN L. OREBAUGH

 Background and Indications: Lateral femoral cutaneous nerve block is useful when sensory anesthesia of the lateral thigh is necessary. In most cases, this block is used in conjunction with femoral nerve block, or when a "three-in-one" block does not provide adequate anesthesia of the lateral thigh. The block is also useful in the diagnosis and treatment of meralgia paresthetica.

 Anatomy: The lateral femoral cutaneous nerve is a branch of the brachial plexus. The nerve arises from the L2 and L3 nerve roots. After exiting the intervertebral foramina at these levels, the roots join the plexus and branches combine to form the nerve, which travels in the space between the quadratus lumborum and psoas major muscles (Fig. 16-1). It then passes under the inguinal ligament and over the sartorius muscle into the thigh where it divides into an anterior and posterior branch. The anterior branch becomes superficial about 10 cm below the inguinal ligament and supplies the skin of the anterior and lateral parts of the thigh as far as the knee. The posterior branch pierces the fascia lata and passes backward across the lateral and posterior surfaces of the thigh. After the nerve passes medial to the sartorius muscle and distal to the inguinal ligament, it can usually be imaged 2 cm medial and 5 cm inferior to the anterior-superior iliac spine (Fig. 16-2). The nerve appears as a hyperechoic linear streak deep to the fascia iliaca (Fig. 16-3) at a depth of 1 to 3 cm. If the nerve is imaged lateral to the femoral artery and nerve, it can be found deep to the fascia iliaca or in the layer between the fascia iliaca and the fascia lata (Fig. 16-4).

 Patient position: The patient lies in a supine position for this block.

 Transducer: A linear transducer, such as 5 to 10 MHz or 6 to 13 MHz.

 Transducer Orientation: Transverse or axial oblique position (Fig. 16-2).

 Needle: 50-mm, 22-gauge, short-bevel needle.

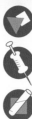 **Local Anesthetic:** 5 mL of ropivacaine (0.2%) or 5 mL of bupivacaine (0.25%).

 Technique: Patient monitors are attached, and sedation is administered. Oxygen by face mask is initiated. Appropriate markings are placed on the indicated extremity for confirmation, and a brief preprocedural "time out" is conducted at the bedside. An antiseptic is utilized to prepare the skin over the block area.

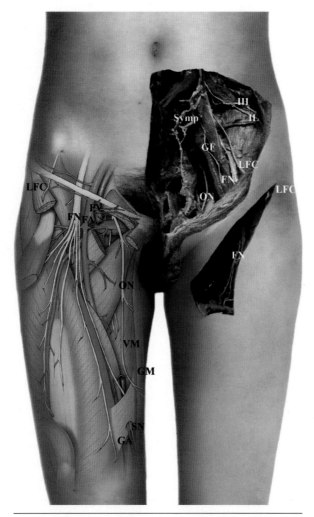

Figure 16-1. *FN*, femoral nerve; *LFC*, lateral femoral cutaneous nerve; *IH*, iliohypogastric nerve; *IL*, ilioinguinal nerve; *ON*, obturator nerve; *GF*, genital femoral nerve; *Symp*, sympathetic chain.

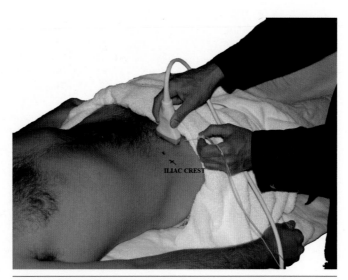

Figure 16-2. Needle and probe position for lateral femoral cutaneous nerve block.

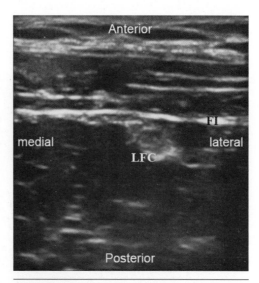

Figure 16-3. Ultrasound scan of the lateral femoral cutaneous nerve. *FI*, fascia iliaca; *LFC*, lateral femoral cutaneous nerve.

The probe is placed on the skin medial and inferior to the anterior-superior iliac spine. The sartorius muscle is seen along the lateral aspect of the probe in this position, and the fascia lata and iliaca are identified (Fig. 16-3). Using an in-plane approach, the needle can be placed either medial or lateral to the transducer. After anesthetizing the skin, the needle is advanced through the fascia iliaca until it is adjacent to the nerve. Five to ten milliliters of local anesthetic solution are injected in incremental doses. Injection of large volumes of local anesthetic in this location will also anesthetize the femoral nerve.

Some practitioners prefer to place the probe in a transverse orientation in the inguinal crease over the femoral artery. The fascial iliaca is identified, and then the probe is moved laterally. The lateral femoral cutaneous nerve is identified medial to the iliac crest. In this location, the nerve or its anterior and posterior branches are usually found in the layer

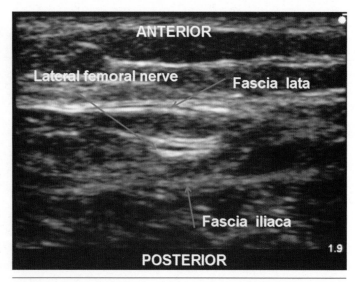

Figure 16-4. Ultrasound scan of the lateral femoral cutaneous nerve.

between the fascia lata and fascia iliaca. Once the nerve is identified, anesthesia of the nerve is accomplished by infiltrating deep to the fascia lata.

Summary of Evidence: Ng et al have shown that the nerve lies approximately 2 cm medial and 5 cm distal to the anterior-superior iliac spine. In a comparative study carried out by Shannon et al, use of ultrasound resulted in a 100% success rate for lateral femoral cutaneous nerve block in volunteers compared with a 40% success rate using a blind technique.

Suggested Reading

Ng I, Vaghadia H, Choi PT, et al. Ultrasound imaging accurately identifies the lateral femoral cutaneous nerve. Anesth Analg 2008;107:1070–1074.

Shannon J, Lang SA, Yip RW, et al. Lateral femoral cutaneous nerve block revisited. A nerve stimulator technique. Reg Anesth 1995;20:100–104.

17

Ultrasound-Guided Saphenous Nerve Block

STEVEN L. OREBAUGH, MILENA MORENO, STEPHEN M. BRENEMAN, PAUL E. BIGELEISEN

Background and Indications: Saphenous nerve block has been described using different approaches. Techniques for guiding the block have included sensory nerve stimulation, motor nerve stimulation (of adjacent femoral nerve branches), and surface landmarks alone. Described approaches include the perifemoral, condylar, infrapatellar/subcutaneous, medial malleolar/cutaneous, and subsartorial. Although the subsartorial has been found in one study to be superior to the others, none have consistently high success rates. Ultrasonography may allow increased precision for this block. Block of the saphenous nerve is useful for anesthesia and postoperative analgesia for foot and ankle procedures involving the medial dermatomes, as well as surgery involving the medial aspect of the leg.

Anatomy: The saphenous nerve may be approached with ultrasound guidance at several different levels. The nerve may be difficult to locate because of its small size, and therefore, the block relies on identification of nearby anatomy. An additional approach is to perform a femoral block, although this may have safety implications with regard to patients' inability to ambulate after same-day discharge.

The first approach requires identification of the saphenous vein of the leg, either distally, near the medial malleolus, or at the midcalf, if it is readily found (Fig. 17-1). A tourniquet on the distal thigh enhances its size. The depth of this vein is seldom more than 1 cm, even in the largest patients at the malleolus. At more proximal levels, the nerve may be more than 2 cm deep to the skin. This approach takes advantage of the proximity of the saphenous nerve to the vein for which it is named in the leg. After the vein is located, it is traced proximally to the level of the tibial tuberosity. Local anesthetic is then placed around the vein at this level.

A more proximal approach relies on the juxtaposition of the saphenous nerve to the femoral artery and vein in the thigh. After the arborization of the femoral nerve at the femoral crease, the saphenous nerve runs distally with the femoral artery and vein (Fig. 17-2). At approximately the junction of the proximal two thirds and distal one third of the thigh, the artery and vein dive deep through the adductor canal. The nerve may be blocked by placing local anesthetic perivascularly (Fig. 17-2A). Distal to the adductor canal, the saphenous nerve passes through the vastoadductor membrane, the fascial plane just deep to the sartorius muscle and adjacent to the vastus medialis (Fig. 17-3). At this point, the nerve is ensconced in the connective tissue septum and runs with a small artery and vein, which may be visible on ultrasound with the color Doppler feature. The nerve, artery, and vein within this plane have been described as a "string of beads." However, the individual structures are small and may require a very high-resolution transducer to distinguish. Local anesthetic may also be injected at this level to block the saphenous nerve.

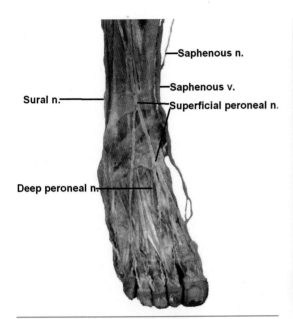

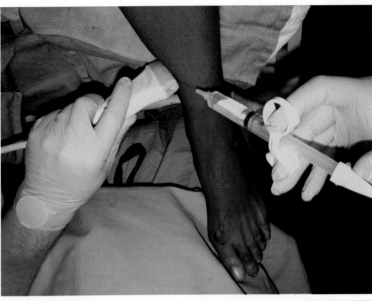

Figure 17-1a. Gross anatomy of the leg. *SV*, saphenous vein; *SN*, saphenous nerve; *SPN*, superficial peroneal nerve; *DPN*, deep peroneal nerve.

Figure 17-1b. Probe and needle position.

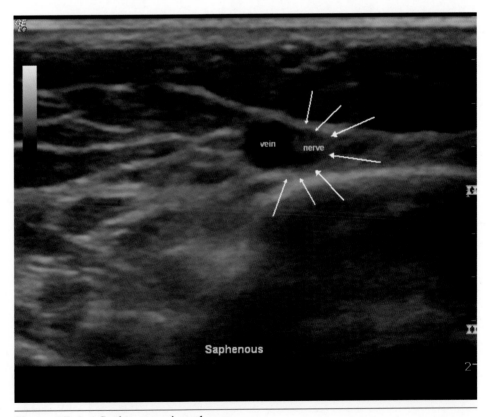

Figure 17-1c. Saphenous vein and nerve.

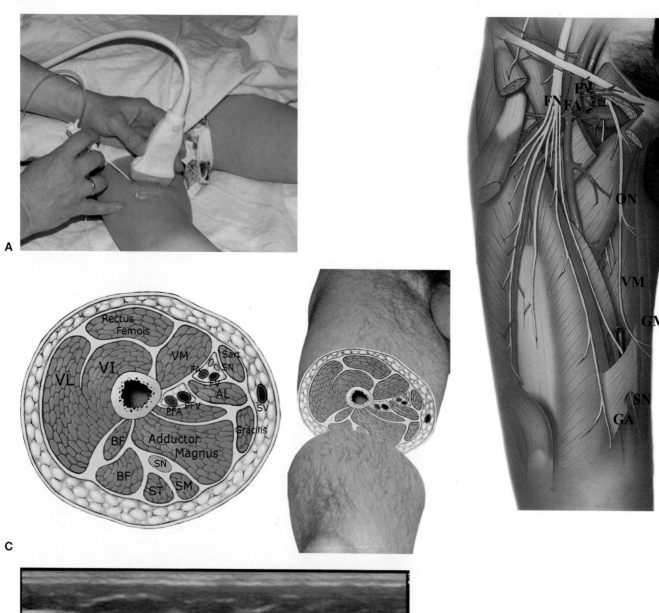

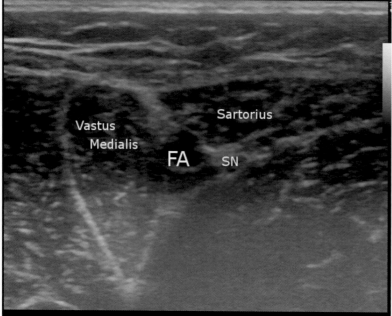

Figure 17-2a–d. *FA*, femoral artery; *FV*, femoral vein; *PFA*, profunda femoris artery; *PFV*, profunda femoris vein; *SN*, saphenous nerve; *Sart*, sartorius muscle; *Gracilis*, gracilis muscle; *Adductor magnus*, adductor magnus muscle; *AL*, adductor longus, *SM*, semimembranosis; *ST*, semitendonosis; *BF*, biceps femoris; *VM*, vastus medialis; *VI*, vastus intermedius; *VL*, vastus lateralis; *SV*, saphenous vein.

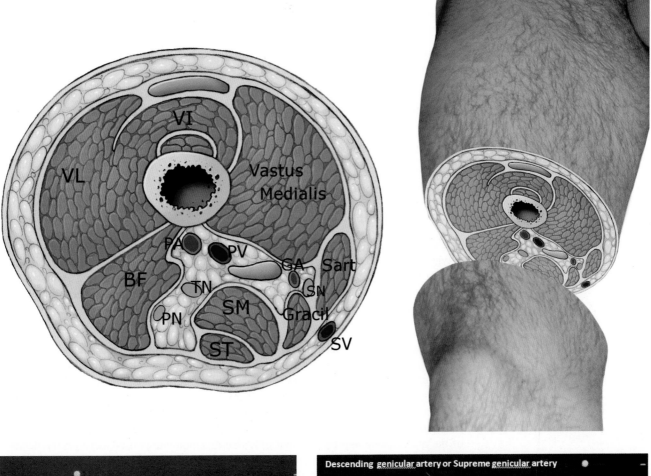

A

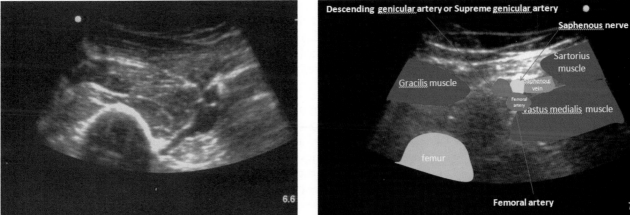

B   C

Figure 17-3a–c. *PA*, popliteal artery; *PV*, popliteal vein; *FV*, femoral vein; *SN*, saphenous nerve; *Sart*, sartorius muscle; *Gracil*, gracilis muscle; *vastus medialis*, vastus medialis muscle; *VI*, vastus intermedius; *VL* vastus lateralis; *GA*, geniculate artery; *SV*, saphenous vein; *BF*, biceps femoris; *SM*, semimembranosis; *ST*, semitendonosis; *TN*, tibial nerve; *PN*, peroneal nerve.

Patient Position: Supine with the thigh and leg externally rotated.

Transducer: 25-mm linear transducer oscillating at 13 MHz (ankle or tibia) 11-mm curved transducer oscillating at 6 to 10 MHz (thigh).

Transducer Position: Transverse.

Needle: 22-gauge, 5-cm blunt needle; 18-gauge, 5-cm Tuohy needle (continuous blocks).

Local Anesthetic: 5 to 10 mL of 0.2% ropivacaine or 0.25% bupivacaine with epinephrine.

Technique: The patient monitors are placed, and judicious sedation is introduced. Oxygen by face mask is initiated. Appropriate markings are placed on the indicated extremity for confirmation, and a brief preprocedural "time out" is conducted at the bedside. An antiseptic is utilized to prepare the skin of the block area. Peripheral nerve stimulation is not typically used for this block, because there is no motor component.

For the perivenous approach to the saphenous nerve in the upper calf, one should identify the saphenous vein and trace it to the level of the tibial tubercle. Lower approaches may allow branching to occur above the level of the block, resulting in incomplete anesthesia of the nerve. Once the vein is identified, the skin is anesthetized with 0.5 to 1 mL of lidocaine 1%, and the block needle is inserted through this site. Either an in-plane or out-of-plane technique is possible for any of the saphenous nerve block techniques. One advantage of the out-of-plane approach is that only one injection site is used, because the needle's angle of insertion can be changed, using the same entry point. In either case, ultrasound guidance is used to guide the tip of the needle to a perivenous position (Fig. 17-1), and 2 to 3 mL of local anesthetic are injected on each side. Completely surrounding the vein with local anesthetic is desirable, because the nerve is frequently not well distinguished. Two injections may be required to accomplish this.

In the distal thigh approach, the ultrasound probe is placed over the femoral artery at the mid-thigh, and the vessels are followed distally toward the adductor canal. Just distal to the entry of the femoral vessels into the adductor canal, the vastoadductor membrane is visible as a fascial plane deep to the sartorius and along the medial edge of the vastus medialis (Fig. 17-2). More distally, this membrane contains both the saphenous nerve and an accompanying small vein and artery, giving the appearance of a string of beads. Injecting the membrane with 6 to 8 mL of local anesthetic at this point results in anesthesia of the saphenous nerve. It should be noted that the needle may traverse the sartorius muscle or the vastus medialis via this approach (in-plane approach), depending on whether the needle is inserted medial or lateral to the transducer. Other practitioners prefer to search for the nerve itself (Fig. 17-3) that may have a variable position relative to the artery. Some practitioners have used this site for continuous catheter infusions. Other practitioners prefer to place a catheter next to the femoral nerve. If the nerve is not visible, infiltration around the artery is an acceptable alternative.

Summary of Evidence: Gray and Collins in 2003 described the approach to perivenous block of the saphenous nerve in the calf. The authors at that time described the utility of the block as "uniformly successful." However, 4 years later, Krombach and Gray noted that the small size of the nerve at this level frustrates attempts at imaging, as does the presence of multiple veins in many patients. In addition, they pointed out that significant branching of the nerve may have occurred proximal to this point, rendering the block less effective. Instead, the authors described the block in the distal thigh, usually 5 to 7 cm proximal to the flexion crease of the knee, to be more reliable because of the more consistent course of the saphenous nerve in the thigh, and its larger size, rendering it more amenable to imaging at least with the 14-MHz linear transducer that they used. The authors had, by this time, evaluated the blocks effect in 20 patients with success.

Suggested Reading

Benzon HT, Sharma S, Calimaran A. Comparison of the different approaches to the saphenous nerve block. Anesthesiology 2005;102:633–638.

Krombach J, Gray AT. Sonography for saphenous nerve block near the adductor canal (letter). Reg Anesth Pain Med 2007;32:369–370.

Gray AT, Collins AB. Ultrasound-guided saphenous nerve block. Reg Anesth Pain Med 2003;28:148.

De May JC, Deruyck LJ, Cammu G, et al. A paravenous approach for the saphenous nerve block. Reg Anesth Pain Med 2001;26:504–506.

Dunaway DJ, Steensen RN, Wiand W, et al. The sartorial branch of the saphenous nerve: its anatomy at the joint line of the knee. Arthroscopy 2005;21:547–551.

18

Ultrasound-Guided Obturator Nerve Block

YOSHIHIRO FUJIWARA, TORU KOMATSU

 Background and Indication: The obturator nerve emerges from the medial border of the iliopsoas muscle, posterior to the psoas muscle and anterior to the obturator internus muscle. The nerve lies approximately 2 cm lateral and 2 cm distal to the pubic tubercle (Fig. 18-1). It carries a mixed population of sensory and motor fibers from roots L2, L3, and L4. As it enters the obturator canal, it divides into an anterior and posterior branch. The anterior branch supplies the adductor longus, adductor brevis, and gracilis muscles as well as the skin over the medial thigh or posterior knee and a branch to the hip joint. The posterior branch supplies the obturator externus muscle, the quadratus femoris and adductor magnus muscles as well as the knee joint. Ten percent of patients have an accessory branch from the lumbar plexus.

Obturator nerve block is used to prevent adductor contraction evoked by electrocautery near the bladder wall and to supplement analgesia for major knee surgery. Obturator nerve block can also be used to treat spasticity of the adductor thigh muscles, obturator neuralgia, or pain in the hip joint.

 Anatomy: The femoral neurovascular bundle and pectineus muscle medial to the femoral vein serve as major landmarks. More medially, the three muscle layers of the adductor muscles, from superficial to deep: adductor longus muscle, adductor brevis muscle, and adductor magnus muscle, must also be identified. The anterior branches of the obturator nerve at this level can be found between adductor longus muscle and adductor brevis muscle. The posterior branch is found between the adductor brevis muscle and adductor magnus muscle. The nerves appear as oval hypoechoic structures within the hyperechoic fascia (Fig. 18-2).

 Patient Position: Supine. The leg is externally rotated with the hip and knee flexed.

 Transducer Type: 25-mm linear probe oscillating at 10 to 13 MHz. 11-mm curved array oscillating at 6 to 10 MHz (obese patients).

 Transducer Position: The probe is positioned parallel to the inguinal crease and medial to the femoral artery (Fig. 18-3).

 Needle: Short-beveled, insulated, 70-mm, 22-gauge needle. Whenever possible, a nerve stimulator should be used in combination.

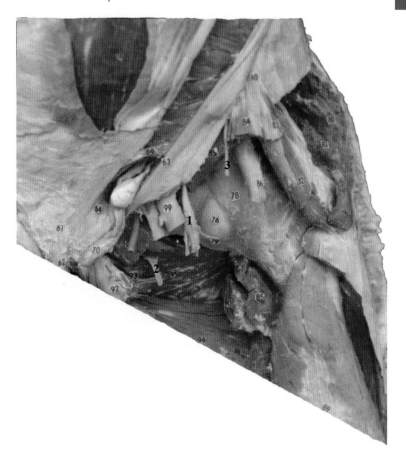

Figure 18-1a. Gross anatomy of the obturator nerve. *1*, femoral nerve; *2*, obturator nerve; *3*, lateral femoral cutaneous nerve; *95*, obturator externus muscle; *90*, pectineus; *85*, iliopsoas; *92*, adductor longus; *93*, adductor brevis; *94*, adductor magnus; *99*, femoral artery.

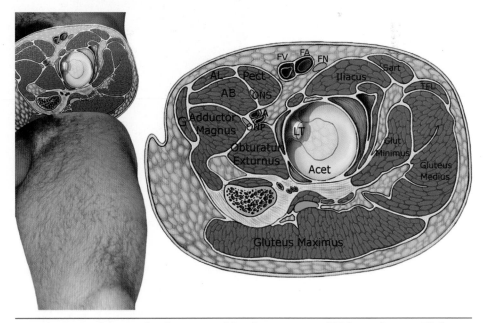

Figure 18-1b. Cross sectional anatomy of the obturator nerve. *FV*, femoral nerve; *FA*, femoral artery; *FN*, femoral nerve; *AI*, adductor longus; *AB*, adductor brevis; *Pect*, pectineus; *Sart*, sartprius; *TFL*, tensor fascia lata; *IG*, inferior gamellus; *G*, gracilis, *LT*, ligamentum teres; *Acet*, acetabulum; *PM*, psoas major; *ONS*, superficial obturator nerve; *ONP*, deep obturator nerve.

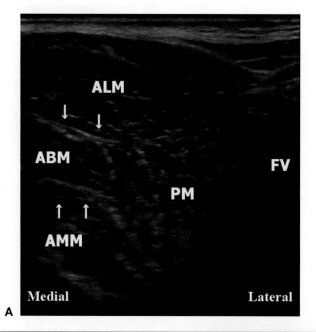

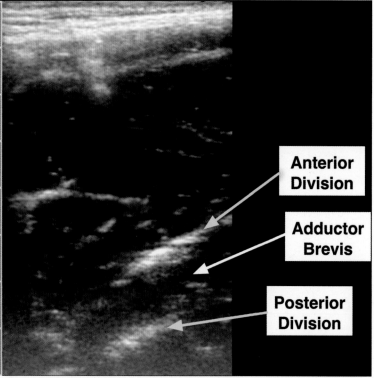

Figure 18-2a,b. Ultrasound scan of the obturator nerve. *ALM,* adductor longus muscle; *ABM,* adductor brevis muscle; *AMM,* adductor magnus muscle; *PM,* pectineus muscle; *FV,* femoral vein; *arrows between ALM and ABM,* anterior branch of obturator nerve; *arrows between ABM and AMM,* posterior branch of obturator nerve.

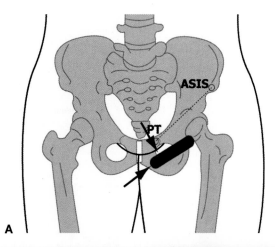

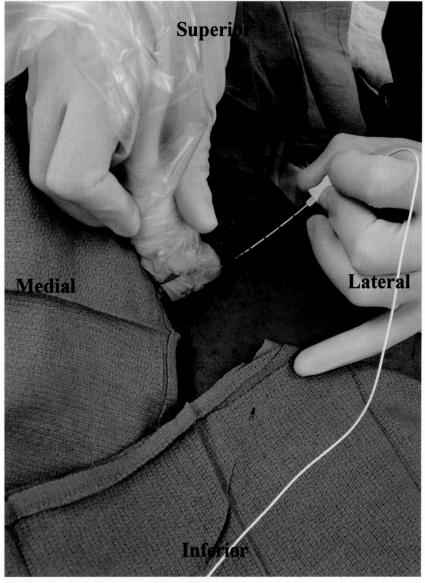

Figure 18-3a,b. Probe and needle position.

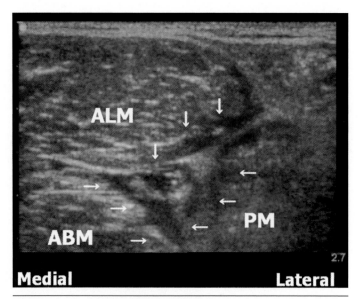

Figure 18-4. Ultrasound image after injection of local anesthetics. Arrows, local anesthetics; *ALM*, adductor longus muscle; *ABM*, adductor brevis muscle; *PM*, pectineus muscle. Adapted from Fujiwara Y, Sato Y, Kitayama M, et al. Anesth Analg 2008;106:350–351.

Local Anesthetic: 10 to 15 mL of 0.2% ropivacaine or 0.25% bupivacaine with epinephrine. 5 mL of 6% phenol in glycerin (neuroablation for pain patients).

Technique: After sterile skin preparation, a short-beveled stimulating needle is advanced via an out-of-plane or an in-plane technique (Fig. 18-3). The needle is placed at the lateral border of the probe and under ultrasound guidance and is advanced toward the fascia between the adductor longus and adductor brevis muscles (Fig. 18-2). Then the nerve stimulator is turned on. The intensity of the stimulating current is initially set to deliver 1 mA and gradually decreased. If a stimulating current less than 0.6 mA evokes a motor response, 3 to 5 mL of local anesthetic is injected after negative aspiration (Fig. 18-4). This procedure is repeated along the fascia until the motor response is eliminated. The needle is then advanced until it contacts with the posterior branch between the adductor brevis and adductor magnus muscles. After the nerve is identified by stimulation, 3 to 5 mL of local anesthetic is injected. The same approach and technique are used as for surgical block. After a prognostic block with 1% lidocaine, neurolytic agents (alcohol or phenol) are injected.

Tips

1. We usually block the anterior branch first. In some patients, a motor response to the posterior branch cannot be obtained. This is presumably because of posterior or proximal spread of local anesthetic injected around the anterior branch.
2. Even complete block of both branches may not guarantee the complete inactivation of adductor muscle of lower limb. In some patients, an accessory obturator nerve, which may not be blocked with this technique, innervates the adductor muscles.
3. When you provide this block for patients without general or spinal anesthesia, subcutaneous infiltration of local anesthetic is needed. If you infiltrate too deep, you may lose the motor response to nerve stimulation as a result of unintentional block of the anterior branch.

4. At this site of injection, both branches of the obturator nerve may consist of several small fibers. Thus, we search for an adductor response along the fascia and inject small amounts of local anesthetic to each adductor response, rather than give a large single injection.

5. Puncture of the obturator artery has led intraperitoneal and retroperitoneal hemorrhage.

Suggested Reading

Fujiwara Y, Sato Y, Kitayama M, et al. Obturator nerve block: from anatomy to ultrasound guidance. Anesth Analg 2008;106:350–351.

Fujiwara Y, Sato Y, Kitayama S, et al. Obturator nerve block using ultrasound guidance. Anesth Analg 2007;105:888–889.

Helayel PE, da Conceição DB, Pavei P, et al. Ultrasound-guided obturator nerve block: a preliminary report of a case series. Reg Anesth Pain Med 2007;32:221–226.

Saranteas T, Paraskeuopoulos T, Alevizou A, et al. Identification of the obturator nerve divisions and subdivisions in the inguinal region: a study with ultrasound. Acta Anaesthesiol Scand 2007;51:404–1406.

Soong J, Schafhalter-Zoppoth I, Gray AT. Sonographic imaging of the obturator nerve for regional block. Reg Anesth Pain Med 2007;32:146–151.

19

Ultrasound-Guided Parasacral Block

ALON BEN-ARI, BRUCE BEN-DAVID

 Background and Indications: Parasacral block was first described by Masour using a blind approach and electrolocation. Success rates ranging from 60% to 90% have been described with this approach. Ultrasound may enable the practitioner to improve on this success rate. The sacral plexus takes origin form roots L4, L5, and S1, S2, and S3. The roots emerge from the deep surface of the sacrum where they fuse to form the sciatic nerve and its tributaries. Here, the nerve is covered by the gluteus maximus and the piriformis muscles. Once the sciatic nerve is formed from its roots, it traverses the greater sciatic foramen and then courses down the posterior aspect of the leg. After the nerve passes underneath the piriformis muscle, it overlies the superior and inferior gemelli muscles and the obturator internus muscles (Fig. 19-1). This approach caries some risk of bowel or rectum perforation if it is performed incorrectly. Ultrasound-guided parasacral block is useful for total hip surgery and more distal parts of the lower extremity, when it is accompanied by a lumbar plexus block.

 Anatomy: The posterior superior iliac spine and ischial tuberosity are identified by palpation. A line is drawn connecting these two points, and the transducer is placed in the transverse position at level of the coccyx. The sacral plexus is a flat hyperechoic structure at the same depth as the ischium and sacrum.

 Patient Position: Lateral decubitus with the operative side up. The hip and knee are flexed.

 Transducer: 60-mm curved array oscillating at 2 to 5 MHz.

 Transducer Position: Transverse.

 Needle: 10- to 15-cm, 21-gauge blunt needle or 18-gauge Tuohy needle.

 Local Anesthetic: 10 to 20 mL of 0.5% ropivacaine or 0.5% bupivacaine with epinephrine.

 Technique: The patient is placed in the lateral decubitus position with the operative side up. The hip and knee are flexed whenever possible. Standard monitors are applied, sedation is administered, and the skin over the lower back and buttock is washed. The posterior superior iliac spine and the ischial tuberosity are identified. A line connecting these two points is drawn, and the transducer is placed lateral to this line at the level of the

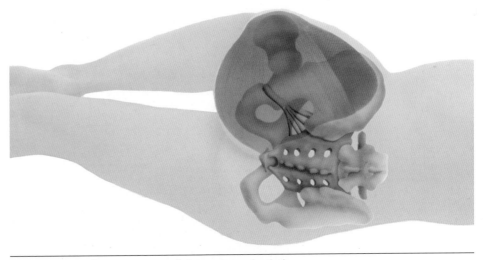

Figure 19-1. Gross anatomy of the parasacral sciatic nerve.

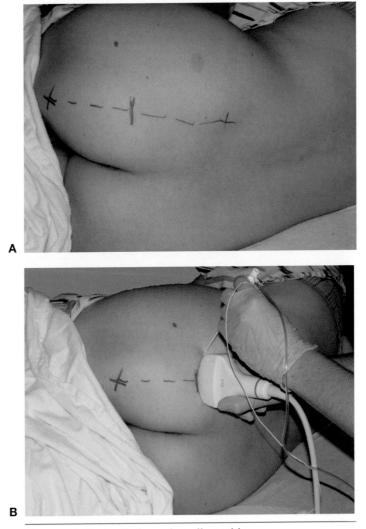

A

B

Figure 19-2a,b. Probe and needle position.

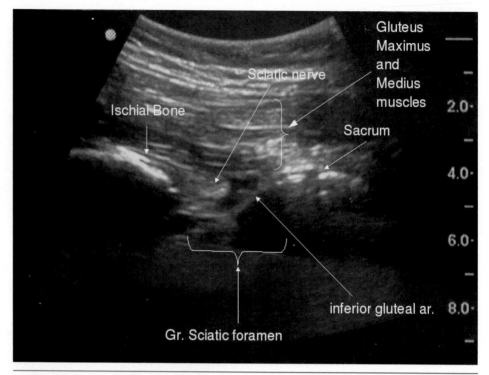

Figure 19-3. Ultrasound scan of the parasacral sciatic nerve.

coccyx in the transverse position (Fig. 19-2). The sacrum and the ischium are identified on ultrasound. The sciatic nerve or the sacral plexus are identified on ultrasound as a flat, hyperechoic structure at the same depth as the ischium and sacrum (Fig. 19-3). The needle is inserted medial or lateral to the probe, using an in-plane approach. Most practitioners prefer to use a stimulating needle for this block with a current amplitude of 1 to 1.5 mA. Once the nerve has been identified, 10 to 20 mL of local anesthetic is injected around the nerve. Because of the large size of the nerve, there is a long latency until surgical anesthesia is achieved. Care should be taken not to puncture the nerve roots themselves or the deeper visceral structure of the pelvis.

Suggested Reading

Ben-Ari AY, Joshi R, Uskova A, et al. Ultrasound localization of the sacral plexus using a parasacral approach. Anesth Analg 2009;108:1977–1980.

Ultrasound-Guided Anterior Sciatic Nerve Block

YASUYUKI SHIBATA, TORU KOMATSU, LAURENT DELAUNAY

 Background and Indications: Ultrasound-guided block of the sciatic nerve can be conducted from the anterior aspect of the patient as well as from the lateral or posterior positions. When the block is conducted from the anterior approach (at the level of the lesser trochanter), it is too distal to be of use in hip surgery. However, the anterior approach allows the patient to remain supine. This is especially advantageous in patients who have fractures of the lower extremity. Anterior sciatic block is used for surgery of the distal thigh, knee, leg, or foot.

 Anatomy: From the anterior approach, the sciatic nerve lies deep and medial to the femur (Fig. 20-1). The nerve is bounded laterally by the gluteus maximus muscle and medially by the biceps femoris and semimembranosus/semitendinosus muscles (which are frequently referred to as the *hamstring muscles*). Just anterior to the nerve lies the adductor magnus muscle. Medial to the nerve, and quite superficial in the thigh at these levels, the femoral vessels and nerve can be seen (Fig. 20-1). On ultrasound, the sciatic nerve will appear as a hyperechoic oval or round structure (Fig. 20-2). In some patients, the obturator artery and nerves can also be seen lying deep to the adductor longus and between the adductor brevis and adductor magnus muscles (Fig. 20-3).

 Patient Position: The patient remains supine. The thigh is externally rotated, and the knee is flexed. The leg should be externally rotated, so that the sciatic nerve is rotated to a position medial to the femur.

 Transducer: 60-mm curved array oscillating at 2 to 5 MHz.

 Transducer Orientation: The transducer is placed transversely on the anterior thigh (Fig. 20-2).

 Needle: 10- to 15-cm, 21-gauge (single injection) or 18-gauge Tuohy (continuous block) insulated needle.

 Local Anesthetic: 10 to 20 mL of ropivacaine 0.5% or bupivacaine 0.5% with epinephrine.

 Technique: Patient monitors are attached, and sedation is administered. Oxygen by face mask is initiated. Appropriate markings are placed on the indicated extremity for confirmation, and a brief preprocedural "time out" is conducted at the bedside. An antiseptic is utilized to prepare the skin over the block area.

ANTERIOR

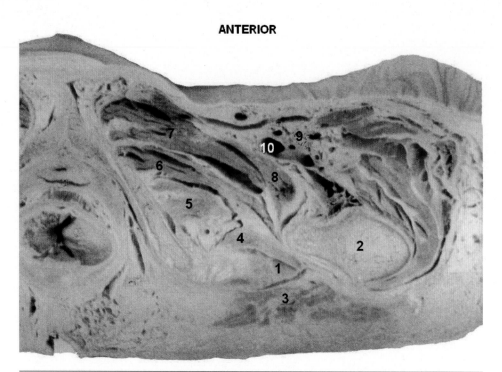

Figure 20-1. Cross section through the lesser trochanter. *1*, sciatic nerve; *2*, femur; *3*, gluteus maximus muscle; *4*, quadratus femoris muscles; *5*, obturator externus muscle; *6*, adductor magnus muscle; *7*, adductor brevis muscle; *8*, adductor longus muscle; *9* femoral nerve; *10* femoral vessels.

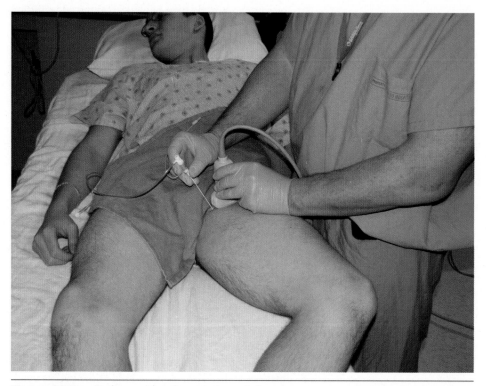

Figure 20-2a. Probe position for anterior sciatic scan.

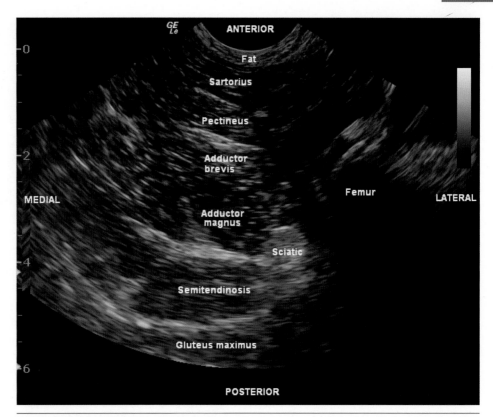

Figure 20-2b. Anterior sciatic scan.

The lesser trochanter is imaged, and the probe is moved proximally or distally along the thigh, until the nerve is imaged medial and posterior (deep) to the femur (Fig. 20-2). Toggling of the probe is usually necessary to create the optimum image of the nerve, usually at a depth of 6 to 10 cm. Some practitioners also use the femoral artery as a landmark. In many patients, the sciatic nerve lies along a line drawn perpendicular through the femoral artery. The needle is placed in-line, medial to the probe and advanced in a posterolateral direction, until the nerve is contacted or penetrated. Most practitioners prefer to utilize nerve stimulation in conjunction with ultrasound imaging with this approach

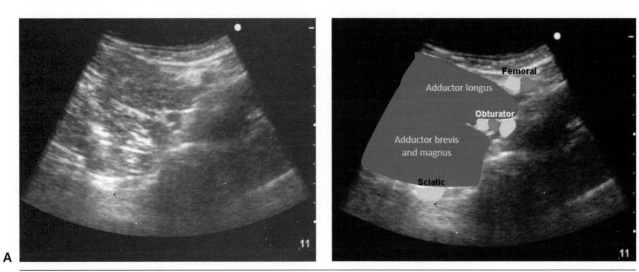

Figure 20-3a,b. Anterior sciatic scan with femoral and obturator nerves.

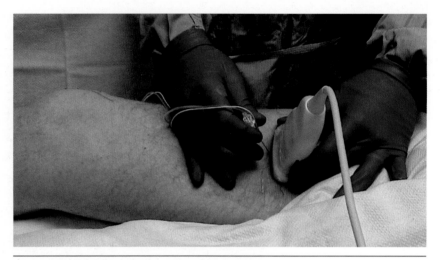

Figure 20-4. Probe position for out-of-plane approach.

because of the depth of the nerve. A stimulation threshold of 1 mA or more is utilized to identify the nerve. Even at this setting, puncture of the nerve is commonly required to elicit stimulation. Once the nerve is identified, local anesthetic is injected in 3 to 5 mL aliquots. If the needle is within the nerve sheath, or mesoneurium, 5 to 10 mL of local anesthetic solution is sufficient for a profound block. If the local anesthetic solution is deposited outside the nerve, a "halo" should be created around the nerve, utilizing 10 to 20 mL of solution. Because of the size of the nerve and the dual covering (epineurium and mesoneurium), long latencies are common when local anesthetic is deposited outside the nerve.

Some practitioners prefer to image the nerve in short axis and use an out-of-plane approach for the needle (Fig. 20-4). Other practitioners image the nerve in the short axis and then rotate the probe into a long-axis view. In this case, the nerve appears as a hyperechoic streak between the adductor magnus muscle and the gluteus maximus muscle. When this approach is used, the needle is inserted in-line with the probe.

Summary of Evidence: Chan et al (2006) evaluated 15 volunteers with ultrasound at different approaches to establish optimal visualization of the sciatic nerve. For the anterior approach, the authors utilized a 2 to 5 MHz curved probe. Overall, the nerve was easily visualized in 87% of patients, and the authors were able to stimulate the nerve within two attempts in all patients. Chantzi et al (2007) described the anterior approach to sciatic block in 18 obese subjects utilizing ultrasound guidance. The authors were able to identify the nerve in 17 out of 18 patients and provided successful nerve stimulation in all of these within four attempts. They noted that because of the depth of the nerve and the angle of needle insertion, it is quite difficult to simultaneously image both needle and nerve during this technique.

Suggested Readings

Chan VW, Nova H, Abbas S, et al. Ultrasound examination and localization of the sciatic nerve: a volunteer study. Anesthesiology 2006;104:309–314.

Chantzi C, Saranteas T, Zogogiannis J, et al. Ultrasound examination of the sciatic nerve at the anterior thigh in obese patients. Acta Anaesthesiol Scand 2007;51(1):132.

Tsui BC, Ozelsel TJ. Ultrasound-guided anterior sciatic nerve block using a longitudinal approach: expanding the view (letter). Reg Anesth Pain Med 2008;33:275–276.

21

Subgluteal Sciatic Block

STEVEN L. OREBAUGH, PAUL E. BIGELEISEN

 Background and Indications: Sciatic nerve block has been in use by anesthesiologists for more than 90 years. The traditional approach has been to create landmarks over the gluteus and traverse this large muscle en route to the nerve. However, di Benedetto et al[1] described a somewhat more distal approach, in which the nerve is blocked in the proximal thigh, just as it leaves the pelvis. In his original description, the subgluteus block, which will hereafter be referred to as the "infragluteal" approach to avoid confusion with the subgluteal space. When compared to the transgluteal approach, the infragluteal approach resulted in less patient discomfort and required less time with fewer needle punctures than the time-honored approach through the gluteus. Ultrasound has the potential to make the infragluteal sciatic block even more efficient with less discomfort for the patient. Sciatic block is provided for surgical procedures involving the distal femur, knee joint, leg, ankle, and foot.

 Anatomy: Infragluteal sciatic block guided by landmarks and nerve stimulation relies on palpation of the greater trochanter and ischial tuberosity because the nerve lies approximately midway between them. The "groove" that lies between the hamstring muscles, which originate from the ischial tuberosity, and the lateral edge of the vastus lateralis muscle are then palpated. The nerve typically lies deep to this groove and is sought 4 cm below the line connecting the two boney landmarks (Figs. 21-1 and 21-2).

With ultrasound, the same landmarks may be located. The ischial tuberosity and greater trochanter are readily imaged just proximal to the gluteal fold (Fig. 21-1), and below this fold, the overlying gluteus maximus muscle is seen to thin out considerably. Deep to the gluteus, and superficial to the quadratus femoris muscle, lies the sciatic nerve, at a depth of approximately 3 to 12 cm, depending on the patient's habitus. The nerve itself has a fusiform or wedge-shaped appearance and is hyperechoic (Fig. 21-2). As one proceeds distally, the quadratus femoris disappears, the nerve becomes more round or oval shape, and lies on the belly of the adductor magnus. Deeper, and lying somewhat more lateral than the nerve, the hyperechoic arc of the femur is evident. There are usually no significant vessels evident adjacent to the nerve at this level.

 Patient Position: Lateral decubitus position, with the affected side up, or prone.

 Transducer: 40- to 60-mm curved array oscillating at 2 to 5 MHz; 11-mm curved array oscillating at 6 to 10 MHz (smaller patients and children).

 Transducer Orientation: Transverse below the gluteal cleft. Significant pressure on the transducer may be necessary in larger subjects.

 Needle: 10-cm, 21-gauge blunt needle (single injection) or 18-gauge Tuohy needle (continuous infusion).

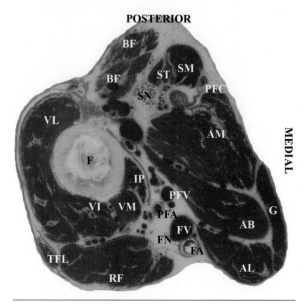

Figure 21-1. Gross anatomy of the upper thigh. *F*, femur; *BF*, biceps femoris; *ST*, semitendinosus; *SM*, semimembranosus; *FA*, femoral artery; *FV*, femoral vein; *TFL*, tensor fascia lata; *VI*, vastus intermedius; *RF*, rectus femoris; *PFA*, profunda femoris artery; *PFV*, profunda femoris vein; *S*, sartorius; *AL*, adductor longus; *G*, gracilis; *AB*, adductor brevis; *AM*, adductor magnus; *PFC*, posterior femoral cutaneous; *SM*, semimembranosus; *ST*, semitendinosus; *SN*, sciatic nerve; *FN*, femoral nerve; *VL*, vastus lateralis; *IP*, iliopsoas.

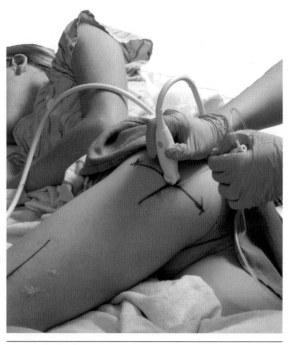

Figure 21-2a. Needle and probe position for subgluteal block.

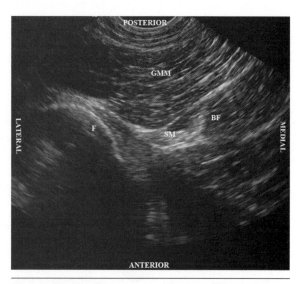

Figure 21-2b. *F*, greater trochanter; *SN*, sciatic nerve; *GMM*, gluteus maximus muscle; *BF*, biceps femoris.

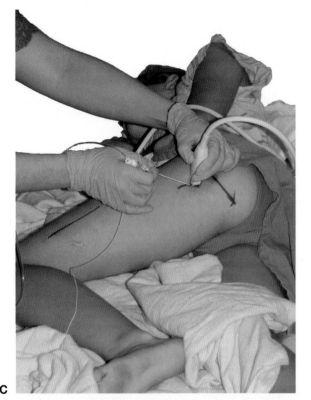

C

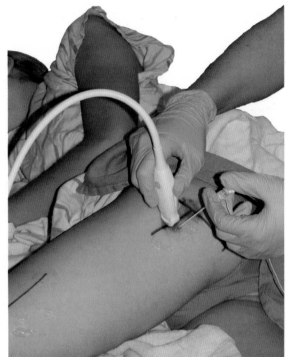

D

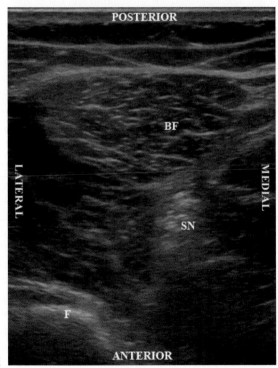

E

Figure 21-2c–e. More distal needle and probe position for subgluteal block. *BF*, biceps femoris; *SN*, sciatic nerve; *F*, femur.

Local Anesthetic: 10 to 20 mL of ropivacaine 0.5% or 0.5% bupivacaine with epinephrine.

Technique: The patient monitors are placed and judicious sedation introduced. Oxygen by face mask is initiated. Appropriate markings are placed on the indicated extremity for confirmation, and a brief preprocedural time-out is conducted at the bedside. An antiseptic is utilized to prepare the skin of the block area.

Infragluteal block with real-time ultrasound guidance may be conducted with or without nerve stimulator confirmation. In addition, the needle may be inserted using an out-of-plane (superior or inferior to the axis of the transducer, or in-plane approach at the medial or lateral end of the transducer.

After establishing an appropriate image of the nerve, the skin over the area of needle insertion is anesthetized, along with the subcutaneous tissues. The block needle is then introduced along the predicted pathway, with subtle transducer adjustments to maintain an image of both the nerve and needle. However, it is frequently difficult to maintain an image of the needle because of the steep insertion angle, and careful observation of tissue distortion caused by the advancing needle is necessary. If doubt exists as to the position of the tip, a small amount of dextrose may be injected to help localize the needle.

The nerve stimulator, if utilized, is turned on before needle introduction, or later, as the needle approaches the nerves. The threshold for stimulation has not been found to be of importance in this technique. Local anesthetic solution, typically 20 to 25 mL, is then injected under ultrasound guidance, ensuring that the nerve is surrounded by the solution. This frequently requires two or more needle positions to accomplish successfully. It is common to find that the needle, even though placed against the suspected nerve, does not elicit motor stimulation at typical currents (0.8–1.0 mA). As the needle is advanced further, stimulation frequently ensues, and may be vigorous. This may be a result of intraneural placement of the needle. To avoid intraneural injection, the needle should then be pulled back, and a 1-mL volume of local anesthetic solution injected to help localize the needle tip before the full dose is injected.

For indwelling catheter placement, either an in-plane or an out-of plane technique is possible. A sterile sheath should be utilized for placement of an indwelling device, along with sterile gloves, cap, mask, and drapes. After establishing an optimal view of the nerve, similar to that for the single-injection block, the skin is anesthetized with a subcutaneous wheal of local anesthetic. The needle is then guided to the nerve, and nerve stimulation is utilized for confirmation if desired. For nonstimulating catheters, a bolus of local anesthetic, saline, or dextrose solution is used to confirm accurate needle-tip placement and the catheter is then inserted. If a stimulating catheter is desired, then the stimulator is attached to the catheter after needle localization, and placement is confirmed by continued stimulation as the catheter is inserted (ultrasound will not be particularly useful during this step). By either technique, after catheter placement, ultrasound imaging can be used to confirm that solution injected through the catheter is deposited in juxtaposition to the nerve. Color flow Doppler may improve the ability to image in this situation, as the injection occurs.

Summary of Clinical Evidence: Chan et al[2] described the ultrasound-guided sciatic nerve block via several different routes, including the transgluteal, infragluteal, and anterior approach. The authors reviewed the relevant anatomy in 15 volunteers and were able to easily visualize the nerve in 87% of them. Although blocks were not performed, nerve stimulation was conducted successfully in all patients within two attempts.

In an evaluation of the subgluteal space with ultrasound, Karmakar et al[3] emphasized the importance of the ischial tuberosity, greater trochanter, and space between the fascia lining the deep aspect of the gluteus muscle and that lining the superficial aspect of the quadratus femoris muscle in which the sciatic nerve lies. The subgluteal space, while somewhat proximal to the true infragluteal block, is distal to the site of traditional transgluteal blocks. The authors evaluated five patients undergoing ultrasound-guided blocks with deposition of local anesthetic in the subgluteal space and noted successful anesthesia in all of them within 20 minutes.

Van Geffen et al[5] described placement of subgluteal catheters in 10 children receiving lower limb surgery, utilizing the ultrasound guidance as well as nerve stimulation for the placement of the stimulating catheters. Spread of injectate on ultrasound predicted successful catheter placement, and all 10 children received excellent postoperative analgesia. In a randomized trial of ultrasound guidance versus nerve stimulation for placement of sciatic blocks, Oberndorfer et al[6] found that the success rate in 46 children was similar, but that sensory block was prolonged in the ultrasound group.

References

1. di Benedetto P, Bertini L, Casati A, et al. A new posterior approach to the sciatic nerve block: a prospective, randomized comparison with the classic posterior approach. Anesth Analg 2001;93:1040–1044.
2. Chan VW, Nova H, Abbas S, et al. Ultrasound examination and localization of the sciatic nerve: a volunteer study. Anesthesiology 2006;104:309–314.
3. Karmakar MK, Kwok WH, Ho AM, et al. Ultrasound guided sciatic nerve block: description of a new approach at the subgluteal space. Br J Anaesth 2007;98:390–395.
4. Perlas A, Niazi A, McCartney C, et al. The sensitivity of motor response to nerve stimulation and paresthesia for nerve localization as evaluated by ultrasound. Reg Anesth Pain Med 2006;31:445–450.
5. van Geffen GJ, Gielen M. Ultrasound guided subgluteal sciatic nerve blocks with stimulating catheters in children: a descriptive study. Ped Anesth 2006;103:328–333.
6. Oberndorfer U, Marhofer P, Bösenberg A, et al. Ultrasonographic guidance for sciatic and femoral nerve block in children. Br J Anaesth 2007;98:797–801.
7. Sinha SK, Abrams JH, Weller RS. Ultrasound-guided interscalene needle placement produces successful anesthesia regardless of motor stimulation above or below 0.5 mA. Anesth Analg 2007;105:848–852.

22

Ultrasound-Guided Popliteal Sciatic Block

STEVEN L. OREBAUGH, PAUL E. BIGELEISEN

Background and Indications: Block of the sciatic nerve at the popliteal fossa is the most distal of the many approaches to the sciatic nerve. When ultrasound is used for imaging, local anesthetic is readily deposited around the sciatic nerve or around the tibial and common peroneal nerves when the block is done distal to the bifurcation of the sciatic nerve. Historically, the block was done with patient prone (posterior approach). With the advent of ultrasound, the patient is usually placed in the lateral decubitus position with the operative side up or in the supine position.

Block of the sciatic nerve at the popliteal fossa is indicated for surgical procedures involving the toes, foot, or subtalar joint. It may not be suitable as a primary anesthetic for major ankle procedures, because surgeons often choose a thigh (rather than calf) tourniquet for control of bleeding during the procedure.

Anatomy: It is useful to identify the arteries and veins in the area because of their position relative to the nerve. In the popliteal region, the popliteal artery and vein can be located at the flexor crease (Fig. 22-1). The tibial nerve is usually visible at this level, just lateral and/or superficial to the vein.[1] Lateral to the nerve lies the biceps femoris muscle. Medial to the nerve lie the semimembranosis and semitendonosis muscles (Fig. 22-1). Once the tibial nerve is identified at the flexor crease, the probe can be moved slowly proximally, keeping the nerve in the center of the image. The tibial nerve is joined by the common peroneal nerve as the hamstring muscle bellies in the surrounding area enlarge and more subcutaneous adipose tissue becomes evident (Fig. 22-2). Between 5 and 10 cm above the flexor crease, the smaller peroneal nerve will be seen to approximate the tibial nerve, and above this level, one round, large nerve structure is apparent (Fig. 22-3). The peroneal nerve is frequently more difficult to locate than the tibial, because it is smaller and often appears to be made up of one or more large fascicles with little surrounding connective tissue.

At the level at which the sciatic nerve bifurcates, the popliteal vessels are usually considerably deeper than the nerve (Fig. 22-2). Because significant pressure is usually required to optimize the nerve image, it is important to "press up and down" with the transducer periodically, revealing the vein, which otherwise may remain compressed and invisible. Deep to the vessels, the hyperechoic, arcuate form of the cortex is evident.

Patient Position: Lateral decubitus with the operative side up. Supine with the hip slightly rotated away from the operator.

Transducer: 11-mm curved array oscillating at 6 to 10 MHz (small patients). 40- to 60-mm curved array oscillating 2 to 5 MHz.

 Transducer Orientation: Transverse.

 Needle: 10-cm, 21-gauge (single injection) or 18-gauge Tuohy needle (continuous infusion).

 Local Anesthetic: 10 to 20 mL of 0.5% ropivacaine or 0.5% bupivacaine with epinephrine. Patients should be positioned in the lateral decubitus position with the operative side up. A linear, 5- to 10-MHz transducer is ideal for this application. Only in the heaviest patients would a lower frequency, curvilinear transducer be necessary. For small or thin subjects, a higher frequency linear transducer, such as 10 to 13 MHz, will provide excellent

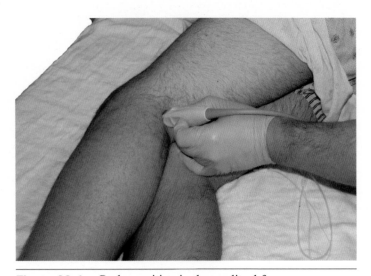

Figure 22-1a. Probe position in the popliteal fossa.

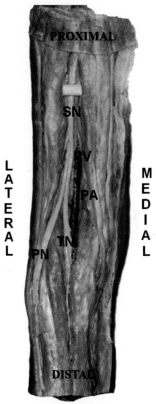

Figure 22-1b. Sciatic nerve and popliteal artery and vein. *PA*, popliteal artery; *PN*, peroneal nerve; *PV*, popliteal vein; *SN*, sciatic nerve; *TN*, tibial nerve.

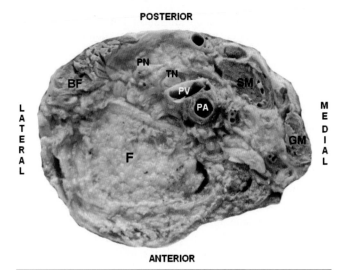

Figure 22-1c. *BF*, biceps femoris muscle; *F*, femur; *GM*, gracilis muscle; *PA*, popliteal artery; *PN*, common peroneal nerve; *PV*, popliteal vein; *SM*, sartorius muscle; *TN*, tibial nerve.

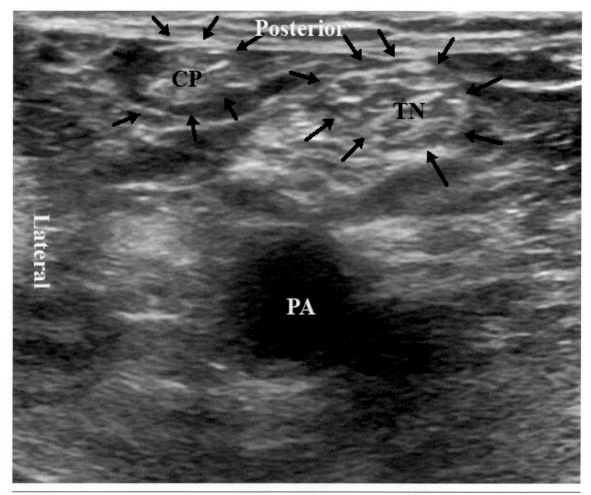

Figure 22-1d. Ultrasound scan at the knee crease.

images. The transducer is held in the transverse position, directly over the flexor crease and is moved proximally (Fig. 22-3). Very commonly, the image is optimized with a significant degree of caudad tilt of the transducer. For the supine approach, a 40- to 60-mm curved array oscillating at 3 to 5 MHz is required. For thin patients, a small curved array oscillating at 6 to 10 MHz will suffice.

 Technique: Patient monitors are attached, and sedation is administered. Oxygen by face mask is initiated. Appropriate markings are placed on the indicated extremity for confirmation, and a brief preprocedural "time out" is conducted at the bedside. An antiseptic is utilized to prepare the skin over the block area.

Posterior Popliteal Approach

Sciatic block at the popliteal level with ultrasound guidance may be conducted with or without nerve stimulator confirmation. The needle is inserted lateral to the transducer using an in-plane approach (Fig. 22-3). One may also utilize an out-of-plane approach, in which the transducer position is identical, but the needle is introduced from a position superior or inferior to the midpoint of the transducer.

The tibial nerve is located with scanning (Fig. 22-1), and traced to the level of its union with the peroneal nerve, or just proximal to this level. The skin is anesthetized along with the subcutaneous tissues, at the site of block needle entry. The block needle is then introduced

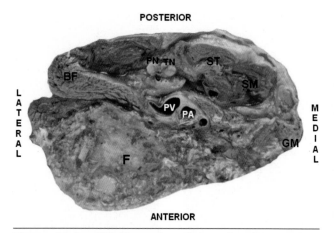

POSTERIOR

LATERAL

MEDIAL

ANTERIOR

Figure 22-2a. *BF*, biceps femoris muscle; *CP*, common peroneal nerve; *F*, femur; *PA*, popliteal artery; *PV*, popliteal vein; *SM*, semimembranosus muscle; *ST*, semitendonosis muscle; *TN*, tibial nerve.

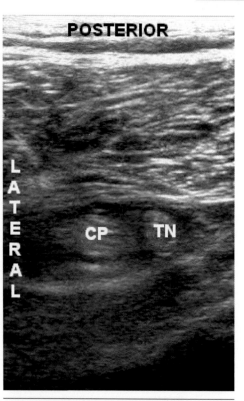

Figure 22-2b. *CP*, common peroneal nerve; *TN*, tibial nerve.

along the predicted path to the nerve, with subtle adjustments made to the needle and/or transducer to maintain the image. The nerve stimulator, if utilized, is switched on as the needle is introduced, or as the needle-tip approaches the nerve. The threshold for stimulation has not been found to be of importance. The authors prefer to start with a threshold of 5 mA. After the needle is positioned next to the nerve, and the desired motor response is elicited, local anesthetic solution in a volume sufficient to surround the nerve is injected (typically 20–25 mL) (Fig. 22-3). If necessary, the needle is repositioned during intermittent injection to completely surround the nerve. When nerve stimulation is used to assist with ultrasound-guided sciatic block, intraneural placement of needle is common when thresholds less than 1 mA are used. Injection within the nerve will be readily apparent if this occurs (Fig. 22-3). Some practitioners prefer to perform the block at the midthigh. In this case, the nerve is still located at the popliteal crease and then traced more proximally (Fig. 22-4).

For indwelling catheter placement, either an in-plane or out-of-plane technique may be utilized. A sterile sheath is placed on the transducer, and sterile gloves, gown, and drapes are utilized, along with a face mask. After establishing an optimal image of the tibial and peroneal nerves as they come together, or of the sciatic nerve just above this level, the skin is anesthetized. For an out-of-plane technique, the needle should be inserted distal to the midpoint of the transducer at a distance equal to the depth of the nerve on ultrasound imaging. The needle is inserted at a 45-degree angle. This should bring the needle tip to the nerve in the imaging plane of the transducer. The needle is then guided to the nerve, and stimulation is used for confirmation if desired. For nonstimulating catheters, a bolus of local anesthetic, saline, or dextrose solution may be utilized to confirm accurate needle tip placement as well as catheter tip placement. When the needle has been accurately placed, the catheter is inserted. If a stimulating catheter is utilized, the nerve stimulator is attached to the catheter after needle placement, and the catheter is placed using stimulation as a guide. Once catheter insertion is begun, the transducer may be put aside. When the catheter

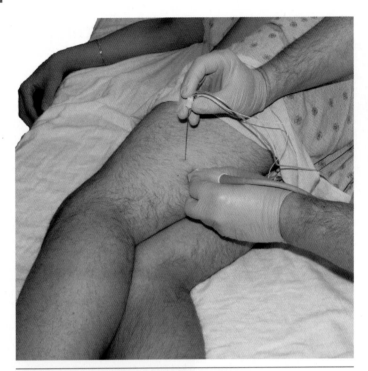

Figure 22-3a. Needle and probe position.

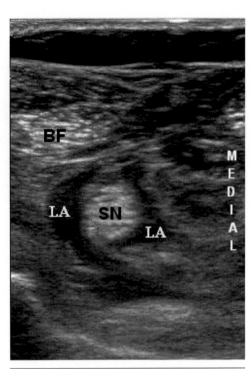

Figure 22-3b. Sciatic nerve surrounded by local anesthetic. *BF*, biceps femoris; *LA*, local anesthetic; *SN*, sciatic nerve.

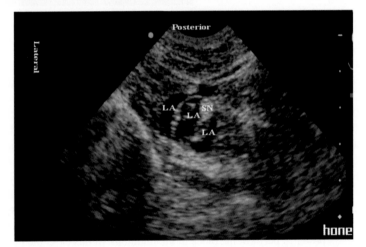

Figure 22-3c. Intraneural sciatic injection. *LA*, local anesthetic around and in the sciatic nerve; *SN*, sciatic nerve.

is in its desired position, it may be imaged by injecting local anesthetic, saline, or dextrose through it. Color flow Doppler may improve the ability to image in this situation.

Supine Lateral Approach

The lateral approach to sciatic block is convenient for patients who cannot turn over, who have fractures, or who have immobilization devices in place. Some practitioners use this approach exclusively. Ultrasound-guided lateral block of the sciatic nerve can be performed at a level 5 to 10 cm above the patella or at the mid-thigh (Figs. 22-5 and 22-6). At the mid-thigh, the sciatic nerve lies anterior to the semimembranosis and semitendonosis muscles. It is bounded laterally by the long and short heads of the biceps femoris muscles and medially by the adductor brevis muscle (Fig. 22-6).

At this level, the sciatic nerve is encased by a thick mesoneurial sheath. Within the nerve, both the peroneal and tibial nerves are incased by their own epineurial sheath. Within the epineurium of each nerve lie the fascicles, which are bounded by their own perineurium.

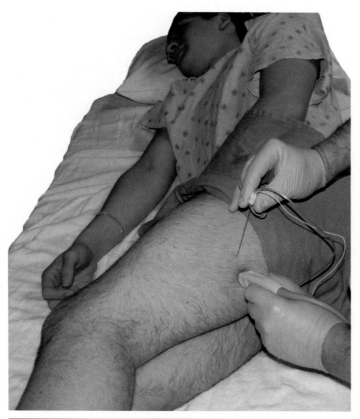

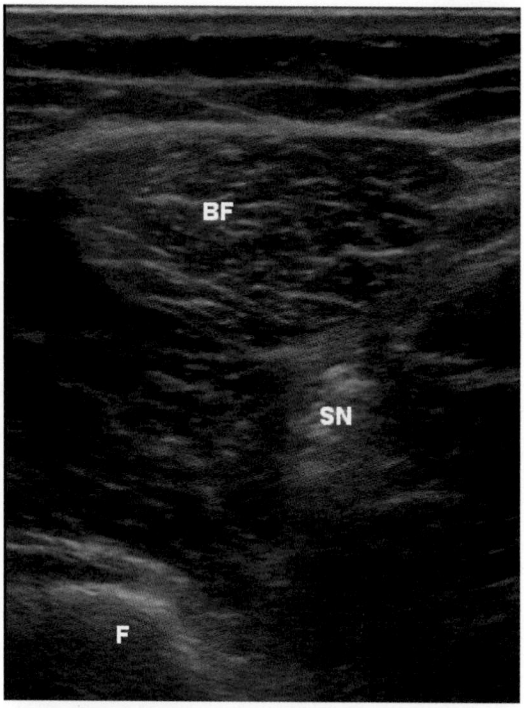

Figure 22-4b. *BF*, biceps femoris; *F*, femur; *N*, sciatic nerve.

Figure 22-4a. Upper thigh posterior approach. Needle and probe position.

With the patient supine, the thigh and leg are internally rotated 30 degrees if this is not painful to the patient. Standard monitors are applied, sedation is administered as needed and the skin is cleansed. In slim patients, the sciatic nerve can be easily found at the lateral suprapatellar level or at the mid-thigh. In heavier patients, the nerve is difficult to see at the mid-thigh level. For this reason, some practitioners prefer to start the scan just proximal to the head of the fibula and trace the common peroneal and tibial nerves (Fig. 22-5) proximally where they join to form the sciatic nerve (Fig. 22-6). A 60-mm curved array oscillating at 2 to 5 MHz is placed in transverse orientation just above the patella. The common peroneal and tibial nerves are imaged several centimeters deep to the bone. Here, the nerves usually appear as round or oval hyperechoic structures. Toggling the transducer is often necessary to bring the nerves into focus. Once the proper level of block is imaged, the needle is inserted in line, superior to the probe. The needle is directed posteriorly and medially at a 30- to 45-degree angle until the nerve is contacted or penetrated. Some practitioners prefer to use a stimulating needle to help localize the nerve. When thresholds less than 1 mA are used, the needle invariably penetrates the mesoneurium. Injection of local should proceed slowly in aliquots of 3 to 5 mL. If the needle appears within the nerve, 5 to 10 mL of local anesthetic is sufficient. The needle should be withdrawn from the nerve if pain or resistance occurs during injection. If the needle lies outside the nerve, the entire nerve must be surrounded with 10 to 20 mL of local anesthetic. Because of the size of the nerve and its dual sheath, a long latency is expected when the local anesthetic is injected around the nerve.

Summary of Clinical Evidence: Sinha and Chan[1] described use of ultrasound guidance for posterior popliteal block in 10 patients. In eight patients with circumferential spread of local anesthetic solution around the nerve, complete foot anesthesia ensued in the sciatic territory. In patients with spread of solution around only part of the nerve, only a partial block

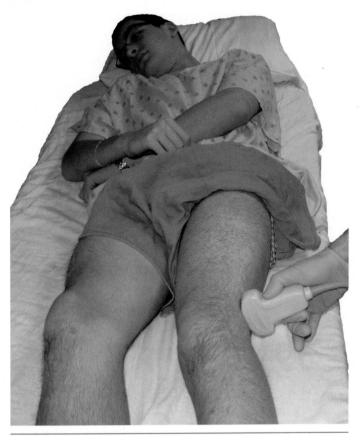

Figure 22-5a. Probe position.

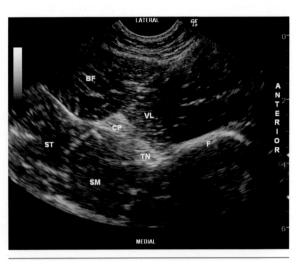

Figure 22-5b. *BF*, biceps femoris; *CP*, common peroneal nerve; *F*, femur; *SM*, semimembranosus muscle; *ST*, semitendinosus muscle; *TN*, tibial nerve; *VL*, vastus lateralis muscle.

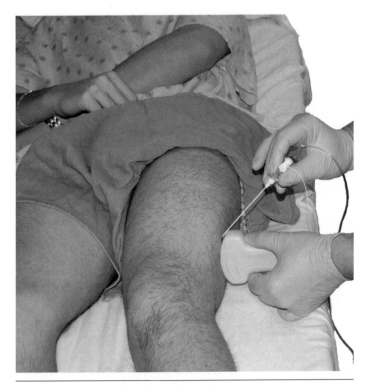

Figure 22-6a. Probe and needle position.

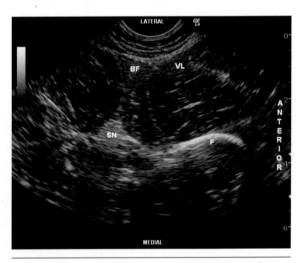

Figure 22-6b. *BF*, biceps femoris muscle; *F*, femur; *SN*, sciatic nerve; *VL*, vastus lateralis muscle.

occurred. More recently, Perlas et al[2] conducted a randomized, controlled trial of posterior sciatic block. Seventy four patients were randomized to receive the popliteal block conducted by either peripheral nerve stimulation/landmark technique, or ultrasound-guided technique, including nerve stimulation for confirmation. The authors reported a greater degree of successful block with ultrasound guidance (89% versus 61%) as well as enhanced onset of the block. In a randomized, prospective evaluation of ultrasound guidance (with nerve stimulation for confirmation) compared with landmark-nerve stimulation technique, Dufuour[3] found a much higher degree of complete anesthesia of the sciatic territory at 30 minutes in the ultrasound guidance group (65% versus 16%), though block times were similar for both groups.

Sites et al[4] described a case series in which two diabetic patients, one with a history of peripheral neuropathy, underwent posterior sciatic block. The authors noted significant difficulty in stimulating the nerves, despite apparent contact of needle with nerve during ultrasound imaging. They report stimulation thresholds considerably higher than those usually considered optimal for needle localization (2.6 and 2.4 mA), and relied on local anesthetic placement by ultrasound guidance instead of persisting in establishing a lower stimulation threshold. Both patients developed successful sciatic nerve block by this technique. The authors concluded that diabetic patients may not have normal nerve stimulation characteristics or thresholds, and suggest that ultrasound is an effective way to guide blocks in such circumstances.

Domingo-Triadó et al[5] compared ultrasound-guided midfemoral sciatic block with that localized by nerve stimulation alone. With 31 patients in each group, the authors found that localizing the nerve on the first attempt was significantly more successful with ultrasound guidance, and that the quality of sensory block was improved when ultrasound was utilized. Block success, and latency times for both sensory and motor anesthesia, did not differ between the two groups. These authors utilized a linear transducer, placed on the posterior aspect of the mid-thigh, necessitating hip and knee flexion to carry out the block. In a clinical–anatomical study, Barrington[6] utilized ultrasound-guided mid-thigh sciatic block, successfully identifying the nerve in 38 of 40 patients. The authors noted that nerve stimulation was required in 37.5% of cases because of suboptimal imaging of the nerve.

Although no randomized trials exist, lateral suprapatellar approach to catheter insertion for block of the sciatic nerve has been described by McCartney et al[7] for postoperative analgesia after repair of a foot fracture. Gray et al[8] describe the technique as successful in a 30-patient series.

References

1. Sinha A, Chan VW. Ultrasound imaging for popliteal sciatic nerve block. Reg Anesth Pain Med 2004;29:130–134.
2. Perlas A, Brull R, Chan VW, et al. Ultrasound guidance improves the success of sciatic nerve block at the popliteal fossa. Reg Anesth Pain Med 2008;33:259–265.
3. Dufour E, Quennesson P, Van Robais AL, et al. Combined ultrasound and neurostimulation guidance for popliteal sciatic nerve block: a prospective, randomized comparison with neurostimulation alone. Anesth Analg 2008;106:1553–1558.
4. Sites BD, Gallagher J, Sparks M. Ultrasound-guided popliteal block demonstrates an atypical motor response to nerve stimulation in 2 patients with diabetes mellitus. Reg Anesth Pain Med 2003;28:479–482.
5. Domingo-Triadó V, Selfa S, et al. Ultrasound guidance for lateral midfemoral sciatic nerve block: a prospective, comparative, randomized study. Anesth Analg 2007;104:1270–1274.
6. Barrington MJ, Lai SL, Briggs CA, et al. Ultrasound-guided midthigh sciatic nerve block-A clinical and anatomic study. Reg Anesth Pain Med 2008;33:369–376.
7. McCartney CJ, Brauner I, Chan VW. Ultrasound guidance for a lateral approach to the sciatic nerve in the popliteal fossa. Anaesthesia 2004;59:1023–1025.
8. Gray AT, Huczko EL, Schafhalter-Zoppoth I. Lateral popliteal nerve block with ultrasound guidance. Reg Anesth Pain Med 2004;29:507–509.

23

Ultrasound-Guided Ankle Block

STEPHEN M. BRENEMAN

Background and Indications: The sciatic nerve gives off four branches below the knee that must be blocked for surgery of the ankle or the foot. These are the sural nerve, superficial and deep peroneal nerves and posterior tibial nerve. In addition, the saphenous nerve, a branch of the femoral nerve must also be anesthetized when surgery on the ankle or foot is planned. The superficial peroneal and sural nerves are very small and difficult to image on ultrasound. Because they are superficial, most practitioners prefer to block these with skin infiltration. The deep peroneal nerve runs along the anterior surface of the tibia, deep to the extensor retinaculum (Fig. 23-1). The posterior tibial nerve can be found posterior to the medial malleolus near the posterior tibial artery (Fig. 23-2). The saphenous nerve can be found next to the saphenous vein usually posterior to the vein (Fig. 23-3). Ankle block is indicated for surgery on the foot below the ankle.

Anatomy: The deep peroneal nerve can often be found lateral to the anterior tibial artery. The nerve has a round or oval hyperechoic appearance (Fig. 23-1). The posterior tibial nerve can be found posterior to the posterior tibial artery where it has a round hyperechoic appearance (Fig. 23-2). The saphenous nerve is located inferolateral to the saphenous vein. The nerve has a hyperechoic appearance (Fig. 23-3).

Patient Position: Supine or recumbent with foot and ankle exposed.

Transducer: A 25-mm linear array oscillating at 10 to 13 MHz provides an excellent image. The small transducer size makes it easy to control the probe.

Transducer Position: Deep Peroneal: axially superior to the anterior ankle (Fig. 23-1A).

Tibial: Axially posterosuperior to the medial malleolus (Fig. 23-2A).

Saphenous: Axially anterosuperior to medial malleolus (Fig. 23-3A).

Needle: 3-cm, 25-gauge nerve block needle.

Local Anesthetic: 2 to 5 mL/nerve of 0.5 % ropivacaine or 0.5% bupivacaine.

Technique: The skin is washed and sterile ultrasound gel is applied to the skin. A sterilized or covered probe is used for the procedure. The foot is stabilized, the probe is applied, and the hand is anchored to hold the probe steady. Use a lateral approach for the deep peroneal nerve to place the needle by the nerve. For the tibial nerve, use a posterior

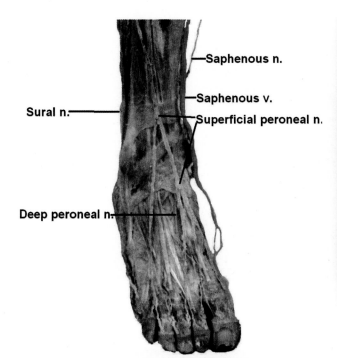

Figure 23-1a. Nerves of the ankle.

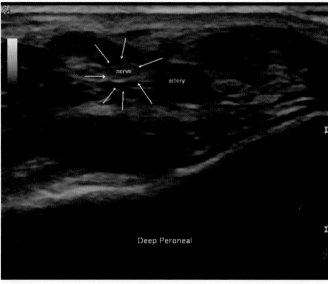

Figure 23-1c. Deep peroneal nerve.

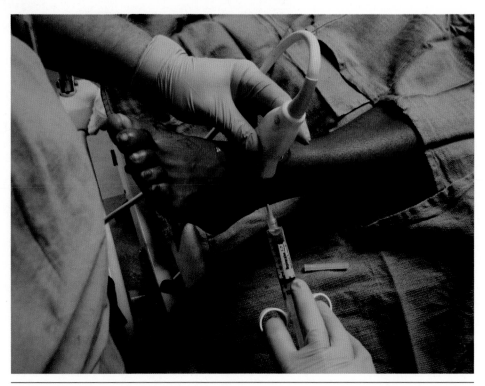

Figure 23-1b. Injection of the deep peroneal nerve.

approach and infiltrate around the nerve and artery. An anterior or posterior approach may be used for the saphenous. Very little volume is necessary to create circumferential spread. To cover the remaining superficial peroneal and sural nerve, perform an infiltration field block from the lateral aspect of the Achilles tendon to medial malleolus superior to the malleoli.

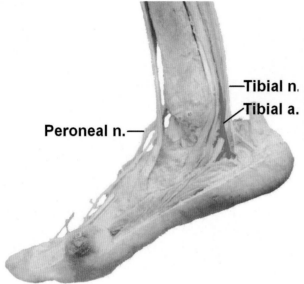

Peroneal n.

Tibial n.
Tibial a.

Figure 23-2a. Posterior tibial nerve.

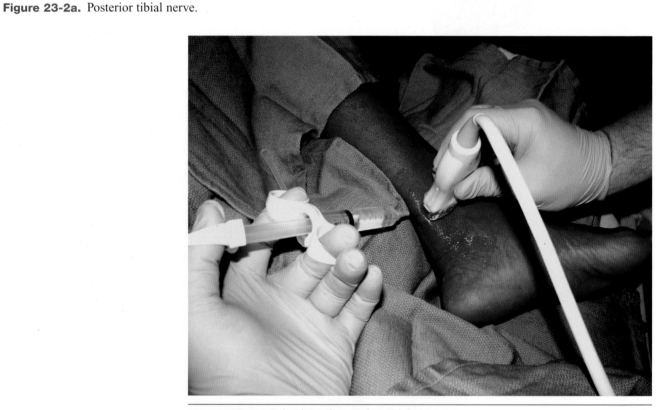

Figure 23-2c. Posterior tibial nerve and vein.

Figure 23-2b. Injection of posterior tibial nerve.

 Tips

1. Use a control-top syringe to place block when working alone.
2. This is a very shallow block on a curved surface, so a smaller ultrasound probe makes the block easier to perform.
3. Typically, only the two deep nerves associated with the arteries (deep peroneal and tibial) are targeted directly with ultrasound, whereas the infiltration field block covers the highly arborized superficial nerves (i.e., saphenous, superficial peroneal, and sural).

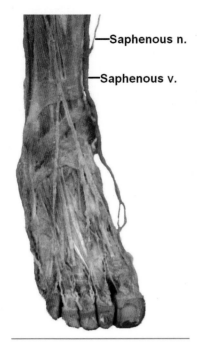

Figure 23-3a. Nerves of the ankle.

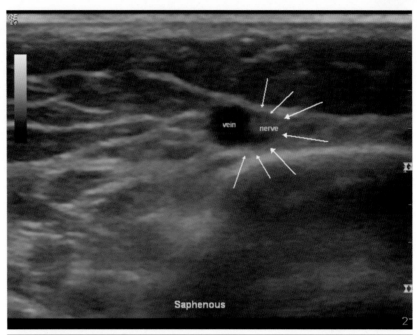

Figure 23-3c. Saphenous nerve and artery.

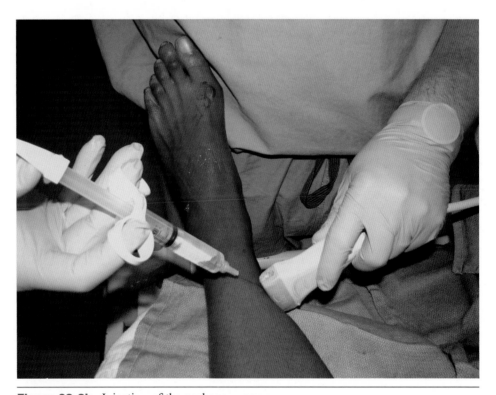

Figure 23-3b. Injection of the saphenous nerve.

Suggested Reading

Sites B, Spence B, Beach M, et al. Ultrasound guidance in regional anesthesia: techniques for lower-extremity nerve blocks. Pocket guide. New York: McMahon Publishing Group; 2006.

Section *IV*

Central Blocks

24   Ultrasound for Labor Epidural Placement

25   Ultrasound-Guided Thoracic Paravertebral Block

26   Ultrasound-Guided Thoracic Paravertebral Block: Classic Approach

Ultrasound for Labor Epidural Placement

MANUEL C. VALLEJO

 Background and Indications: The first stage of labor begins with maternal perception of regular, painful uterine contractions and ends with complete cervical dilatation. Analgesia for the first stage of labor can be achieved by blocking segments from the 10th thoracic dermatome to the 5th lumbar dermatome (T10-L5). The second stage of labor begins with complete cervical dilatation and ends with delivery of the neonate. Analgesia for the second stage of labor can be achieved by blocking the pudendal nerve distribution; sacral nerves 1 through 5 (S1-S5).

Accidental dural puncture is a common complication of epidural insertion for labor analgesia, with a reported incidence of 1% to 5%. Resultant postdural puncture headache (PDPH), following accidental dural puncture, can be very distressing and extremely disabling. A failed labor epidural is also challenging, because the parturient has inadequate analgesia, requires another neuraxial block for analgesia, or a potentially emergent general anesthetic with its inherent complications consisting of respiratory obstruction, difficult ventilation and intubation, aspiration, and increased morbidity and mortality.

Ultrasound assistance for epidural placement can be used to calculate the distance from the skin to the epidural space, to provide an estimation of the proper insertion angle, to determine the best epidural insertion point, especially in patients with difficult or altered anatomy (e.g., scoliosis, obesity, decompressive neuraxial surgery, surgical rods), and ultimately to decrease the failed epidural placement rate. Epidural analgesia is used for the first and second stage of labor. Epidural anesthesia is used for cesarean section.

 Anatomy: Epidural needle insertion traverses the skin, followed by the supraspinous ligament, then the interspinous ligament, and then the ligamentum flavum. Entering the epidural space is confirmed with a loss of resistance to air or saline, and the epidural catheter is inserted 3 to 5 cm into the epidural space and then secured with adhesive dressing and tape. Identifiable anatomy using the longitudinal approach includes the sacrum, articular process, ligamentum flavum, and posterior dura mater, anterior dura mater, posterior longitudinal ligament, and vertebral body (Fig. 24-1). Identifiable anatomy using the transverse approach include spinous process, articular process, transverse process, ligamentum flavum, and posterior dura mater, anterior dura mater, posterior longitudinal ligament, and vertebral body (Fig. 24-2).

 Patient Position: Sitting or lateral position, flexed forward, and curled inward.

 Transducer: 40- to 60-mm curved array oscillating at 2 to 5 MHz.

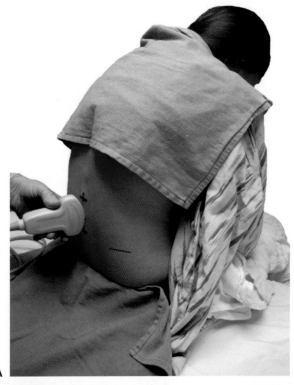

A

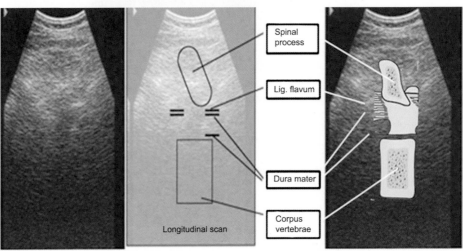

Spinal
process

Lig. flavum

Dura mater

Corpus
vertebrae

Longitudinal scan

B

Figure 24-1a,b. Longitudinal scan.

Transducer Orientation: Longitudinal and then transverse.

Needle Size: 18-gauge or 17-gauge epidural Tuohy needle.

Local Anesthetic: 5 to 15 mL of 0.2% ropivacaine or 0.25% bupivacaine. Fentanyl, 2 mcg/mL is frequently added to the local anesthetic solution.

Technique: For the longitudinal approach, the ultrasound scan is performed by positioning the ultrasound probe vertically, perpendicular to the long axis of the spine. A "saw" sign will be visually seen (Fig. 24-3). The "saw" represents the spinous processes (saw teeth),

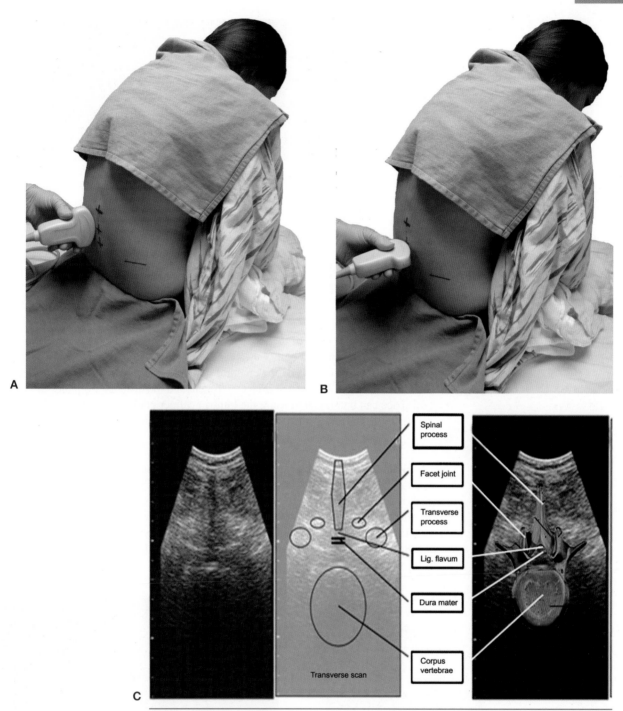

Figure 24-2a–c. Transverse scan.

and the interspinous spaces (groves of the saw) represent the ligamentum flavum, dura, and vertebral body (Fig. 24-3). For the transverse approach, the probe is placed horizontally, perpendicular to the long axis of the spine in the intervertebral space. In the midline, the spinous process is identified as a small hyperechoic signal immediately underneath the skin, which continues as a long triangular hypoechoic (dark) acoustic shadow (Fig. 24-2). The probe is then moved slightly cephalad or caudad to capture a view of an acoustic window that represents the vertebral interspace. On the midline and within the vertebral interspace, an equal sign "=" or a "flying bat" sign may be seen (Fig. 24-2). A hyperechoic band corresponding

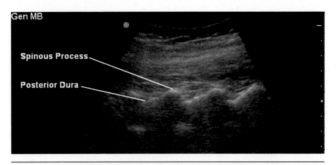

Figure 24-3. Longitudinal scan.

to the ligamentum flavum and the dorsal dura is visualized, which corresponds to the upper most part of the = sign. A second hyperechoic band, parallel and beneath the first part of the = sign, corresponds to the anterior dura, the posterior longitudinal ligament, and the vertebral body (Fig. 24-4). In thin patients, the ligamentum flavum anterior and posterior epidural spaces transverse processes, and facet joints can be seen clearly (Fig. 24-5).

The exact level of each of the interspaces (L3-S1) can be marked on the skin to facilitate epidural placement, and both views can be used as points of reference to determine the optimal vertebral interspace for epidural puncture and insertion. Once the clear image of the interspace is obtained, the image is frozen, and the distance from the skin to the epidural space can be measured using the built-in caliper equipped on the ultrasound machine.

 Tips

1. Both the longitudinal and transverse approaches should be used to visualize the epidural space because both views provide two points of reference.
2. Of the two approaches, the transverse approach provides the most reliable distance to the epidural space.
3. The ultrasound probe angle that produced the best visualization of the epidural space is the angle that should be used for epidural needle placement.

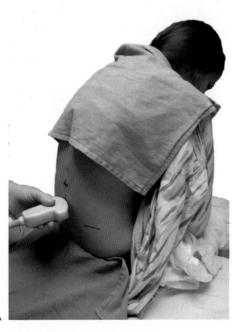

A

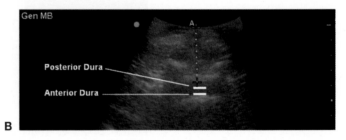

B

Figure 24-4a,b. Transverse scan.

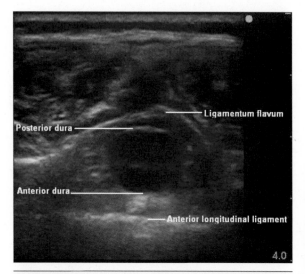

Figure 24-5a. Transverse scan in a thin patient.

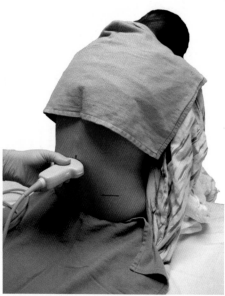

Figure 24-5b. Transverse scan at intervertebral level.

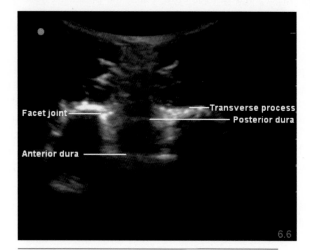

Figure 24-5c. Transverse scan at vertebral level.

4. Because of excessive adipose tissue, extreme obesity can present difficulty in visualization of the epidural space. Aids to visualization include increasing the ultrasound depth on the ultrasound machine and increasing the penetrance of the ultrasound machine.

Suggested Reading

Baraz R, Collis RE. The management of accidental dural puncture during labour epidural analgesia: a survey of UK practice. Anesthesia 2005;60:673–679.

Carvalho JC. Ultrasound-facilitated epidurals and spinals in obstetrics. Anesthesiol Clin 2008 Mar;26(1): 145–158.

Grau T, Leipold RW, Horter J, et al. The lumbar epidural space in pregnancy: visualization by ultrasonography. Br J Anaesth 2001 Jun;86(6):798–804.

Vallejo MC. Anesthetic management of the morbidly obese parturient. Curr Opin Anaesthesiol 2007;20: 175–180.

25

Ultrasound-Guided Thoracic Paravertebral Block

PAUL E. BIGELEISEN, ALON BEN-ARI

Background and Indications: Ultrasound-guided thoracic paravertebral block is indicated for procedures on the thorax that are lateral to the paravertebral muscles, such as breast surgery and thoracotomy. When the pleura is entered surgically, intubation is required. Breast surgery can be done without intubation. Superficial surgery of the upper abdominal wall can be done with bilateral thoracic paravertebral block.

The thoracic spinal nerve roots and sympathetic chain emerge from the lateral vertebral foramina and course anterior to the transverse processes close to the parietal pleura (Fig. 25-1). Medially, the nerve root is bounded by the vertebral body. As the nerve root travels laterally, it is bounded anteriorly by the endothoracic fascia and superiorly by the inferior margin of the rib. The nerve becomes the intercostal nerve as it enters the plane between the innermost and inner intercostal muscles (Fig. 25-1). Posteriorly, the nerve is bounded by the transverse process and the costotransverse ligament.

Historically, thoracic paravertebral block was performed 2 to 3 cm lateral to the midline using a blind approach. In this space, there is a fascial plane, so that local anesthetic can spread from two to six dermatomes with a single injection. When this technique is used, there is occasional spread to the epidural space.

Anatomy: Ultrasound has some benefit when performing thoracic paravertebral block close to the midline. The transverse spinous process and rib can often be visualized, and measuring their approximate depth from the skin can be helpful. This is particularly true in obese patients where the posterior spinous process may be difficult to palpate. Unfortunately, it is difficult to visualize the costotransverse ligament in all but the thinnest of patients. For this reason, we prefer to use a lateral subcostal approach at the angle of the rib. Here, the space between the external and internal intercostal muscles and the space between the internal and inner intercostal muscles can be identified. Local anesthesia injected into either of these potential spaces can track back to the paravertebral space where it can ascend or descend several dermatomes, depending on the volume of local anesthetic injected. When this technique is used, the thick paraspinous muscles are avoided so that the block is usually less painful to perform.

Patient Position: Supine.

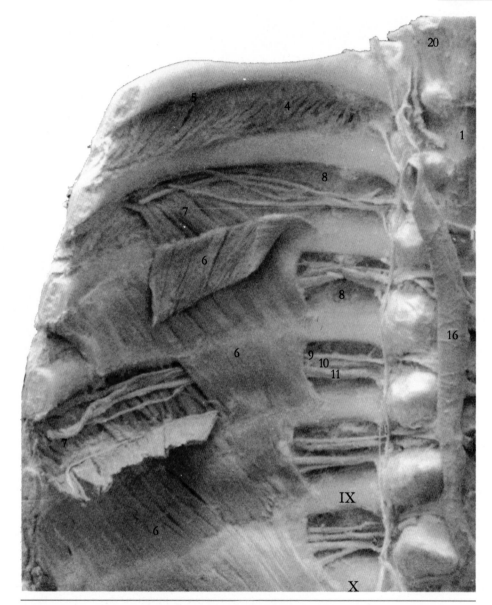

Figure 25-1. Gross and sonoanatomy of the intercostal space. *4*, external intercostal muscles; *5*, costal groove; *6*, innermost intercostal muscles; *7*, internal intercostal muscle; *8*, internal intercostal membrane; *9*, intercostal vein; *10*, intercostal artery; *11*, intercostal nerve; *IX*, 9th rib; *X*, 10th rib; *16*, azygous vein.

 Transducer: 11-cm curved array oscillating at 5 to 8 MHz or 25-mm linear array oscillating at 10 to 13 MHz.

 Transducer Orientation: Initially sagittal to identify the rib and pleura. The transducer is then rotated 90 degrees to an oblique axial position. Here, the rib, intercostal muscles, and pleura are identified.

 Needle: 5- to 10-cm, 22-gauge blunt needle or 18-gauge Tuohy needle.

 Local Anesthetic: 10 to 15 mL of 0.5% ropivacaine.

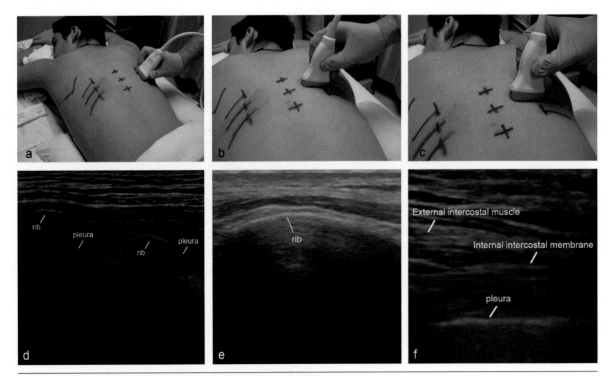

Figure 25-2. A, D: Probe position and longitudinal scan or ribs and pleura. **B, E**: Probe position and transverse scan of rib. **C, F**: Probe position and transverse scan of intercostal space.

Technique: The patient is placed prone with the arms at the side or under the chest. The desired thoracic level is identified, and the rib is palpated at its angle lateral to the paraspinous muscles (Fig. 25-2). The transducer is originally oriented sagitally and the rib and pleura are identified. The transducer is then rotated so that it is along the long axis of the rib. In this orientation, toggling the transducer allows the practitioner to identify the rib and pleura. By asking the patient to breathe deeply, the visceral and parietal pleura can usually be identified as they slide past each other (Fig. 25-2). In thin patients, the fascia between the intercostal muscles can also be identified. The needle is introduced at the lateral border of the transducer using an in-plane approach (Fig. 25-3). As the needle passes below the depth of the rib, 2 to 3 mL of local anesthetic is injected. If a plane appears between muscles, this is likely the plane between the external and internal intercostal muscles. The needle is then advanced until it lies approximately 2 mm superficial to the pleura. Another 3 mL of local anesthetic is injected. If a second tissue plane appears, this is the plane between the internal and inner intercostal muscles (Fig. 25-3). Once this plane has been identified, an additional 10 to 15 mL of local anesthetic can be injected in aliquots of 5 mL. At the conclusion of this injection, a catheter may be inserted 5 to 10 cm beyond the end of the needle if a continuous block is desired (Fig. 25-4). If radio-opaque dye is injected through the catheter, and a chest x-ray is obtained, then the dye usually spreads in a spindle-like pattern in the paravertebral space (Fig. 25-5).

Tips

1. The block usually takes 20 to 30 minutes to set up.
2. Sympathetic block is common. When bilateral block is performed, hypotension is possible.
3. Pneumothorax can occur.
4. If the space between the pleura is entered by mistake, a catheter may be inserted into the intrapleural space, and local anesthetic can be infused to provide analgesia if a chest tube is not present.

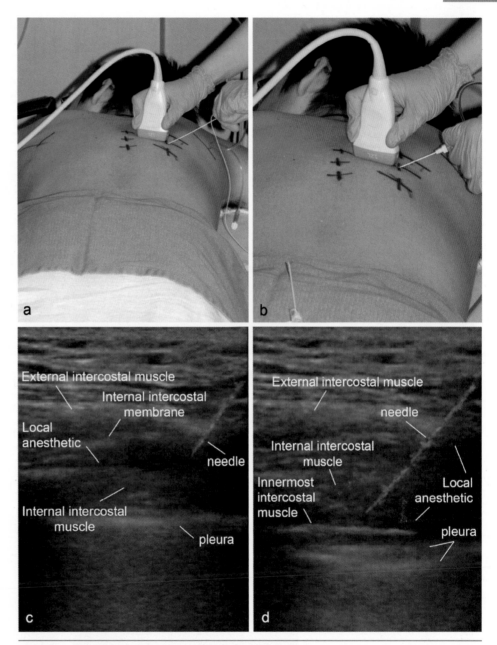

Figure 25-3. Probe and needle position: probe. **A, C**: Superficial needle position and injection. **B, D**: Deep needle position with injection between internal and innermost intercostal muscles.

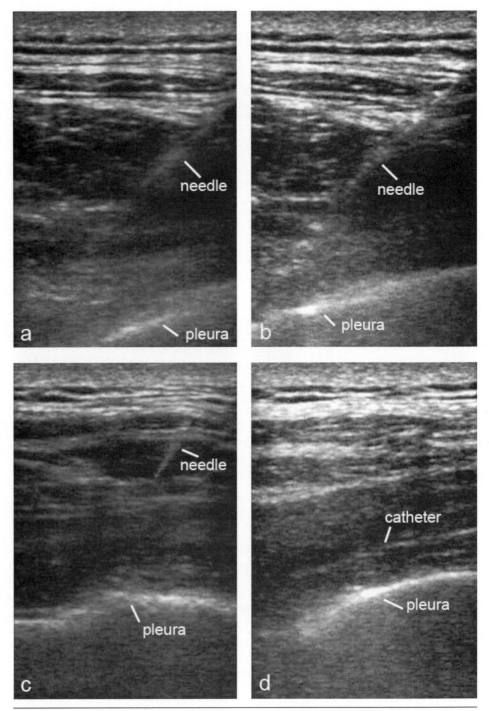

Figure 25-4. A, B: Positioning the needle in the intercostal space. **C**: Injection of local anesthetic in the intercostal space displacing the pleura posteriorly. **D**: Catheter in the intercostal space.

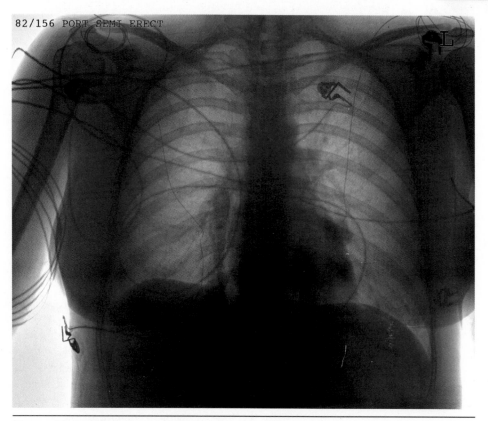

Figure 25-5. Bilateral pravertebral catheters at T9 (note spindle pattern on right and cloud pattern on left).

26

Ultrasound-Guided Thoracic Paravertebral Block: Classic Approach

ANDREA FANELLI, MARIO I. MONTOYA, DANIELA ELENA FRANCESCA GHISI

 Background and Indications: Thoracic paravertebral blocks have been shown to provide anesthesia and postoperative analgesia, which is comparable with thoracic epidural anesthesia and analgesia.[1,2] In addition, paravertebral blocks have decreased the recurrence of cancer in a retrospective study.[3] Their indications include anesthesia and postoperative analgesia for breast surgery, video-assisted thoracoscopies, inguinal and ventral hernia repairs, and postoperative analgesia of major and minor thoracic and abdominal procedures.[4] In our practice, the use of paravertebral block has nearly eliminated the need for thoracic epidural analgesia.

The classic technique of paravertebral block uses a blind approach in which the needle is inserted 2.5 to 4 cm lateral to the posterior spinous process in search of the transverse process. When the transverse process is contacted, the needle is withdrawn and directed caudad to the transverse process and approximately 1 cm deep to the transverse process.[5,6] Once the costotransverse ligament is pierced, local anesthetic is injected. Recent advances in ultrasonography have made it possible to place the needle in the paravertebral space under direct ultrasound guidance in some patients.

 Anatomy: The thoracic paravertebral space, in transverse cross section, is triangular. Its boundaries include posteriorly the superior costotransverse ligament, the vertebral body and vertebral foramen medially, and the endothoracic fascia that forms the deep border of the space and separates the nerve root from the sympathetic ganglia (Fig. 26-1 and 26-2). In most cases, the endothoracic fascia cannot be visualized on ultrasound, and the pleura, which lies immediately deep to the endothoracic fascia, is used as a landmark to prevent the needle from being inserted too far. In thin patients, the epidural space, the transverse process, the costotransverse ligament, and the pleura can be imaged in longitudinal view by placing the transducer lateral to the posterior spinous process and toggling from medial to lateral.

 Transducer: 40- to 60-cm curved array oscillating at 2 to 5 MHz. An 11-mm curved array oscillating at 5 to 8 MHz may be used in small patients.

 Needle: 18-gauge, 10-cm, Tuohy needle.

 Local Anesthetic: Ropivacaine 0.5%, 5 to 15 mL.

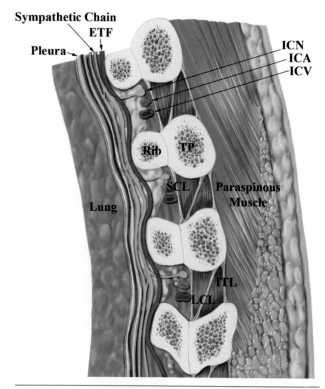

Figure 26-1. Anatomy of the paravertebral space. *ETF*, endothoracic fascia; *SCL*, superior costotransverse ligament; *LCL*, lateral costotransverse ligament; *ITL*, interspinous costotransverse ligament.

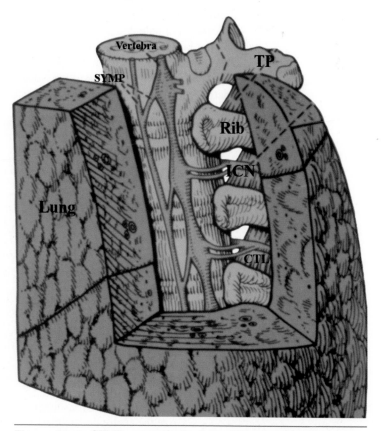

Figure 26-2. *SYMP*, sympathetic chain; *TP*, transverse process; *ICN*, intercostal nerve; *CTL*, superior costotransverse ligament.

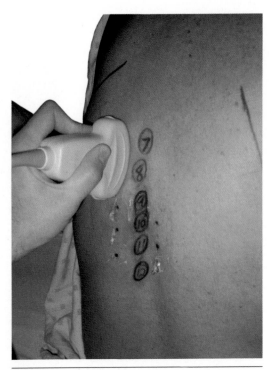

Figure 26-3. The skin landmarks are identified and marked. The spinous processes of T7 to T12 are identified and marked. The site of insertion of the needle is located 2.5 cm lateral from the tip of each spinal process.

Technique: The patient is placed in a sitting position. The relevant thoracic spinous processes are palpated and marked on the skin. A point 2.5 cm lateral to the tip of the spinous process is marked (Fig. 26-3). The region is scanned using a 2- to 5-MHz curved array transducer placed parallel to the spinous processes (longitudinal) in search of the transverse processes, the costotransverse ligament and the pleura (Fig. 26-4). Once the anatomical structures are clearly identified, the skin is disinfected and anesthetized with

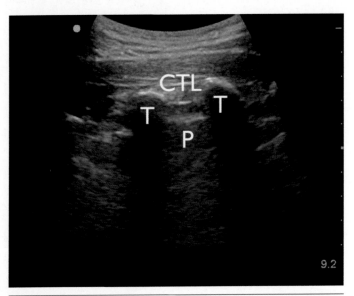

Figure 26-4. Ultrasonographic scanning performed to visualize the anatomic landmarks. *CTL*, costotransverse ligament; *T*, transverse process; *P*, pleura.

1% lidocaine, using a 25-gauge, 3.75-cm needle at the site of introduction of the block needle. The probe is covered by a sterile cover and repositioned longitudinally in search of the initial anatomic landmarks (Fig. 26-5). An 18-gauge Tuohy needle, connected to an extension tube, is inserted at the cephalad end of the transducer using an in-plane technique (Fig. 26-6). The needle is directed deep to the costotransverse ligament and superficial to the endothoracic fascia (Fig. 26-7). If the needle is placed deep to the endothoracic fascia, then the local anesthetic may spread anteriorly into the space containing the sympathetic ganglia. After negative aspiration for blood, 5 mL of ropivacaine 0.5% is injected slowly into the paravertebral space. This results in a slight anterior displacement of the pleura. Multiple levels may need to be injected if the local anesthetic volume is limited to 5 mL. Some practitioners prefer to inject an additional 10 to 15 mL at the same site, with the assumption that it will spread to both caudal and cephalad levels. Once the injection is complete, a 20-gauge multiport catheter is introduced through the needle and placed 4 to 5 cm beyond the tip of the needle. The needle is removed, and the catheter is fixed in place using Steri-Strips and then covered with a transparent dressing. An additional 5 to 10 mL of ropivacaine 0.5% is slowly injected through the catheter after negative aspiration for blood.

 Tips

1. The paravertebral space is bisected by the endothoracic fascia, which creates two compartments. The anterior compartment contains the sympathetic chain, and the posterior compartment contains the intercostal nerve, dorsal ramus, intercostal blood vessels, and rami communicantes (Fig. 26-1).

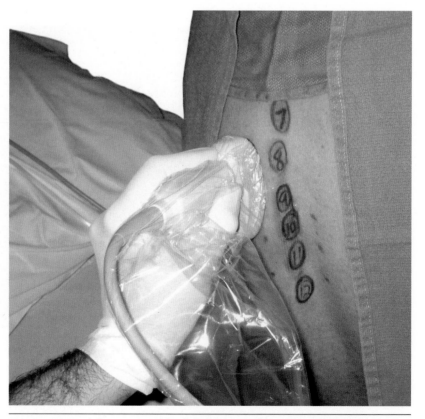

Figure 26-5. After proper skin disinfection and local anesthetic injection, the transducer cover with a sterile cover is positioned longitudinally.

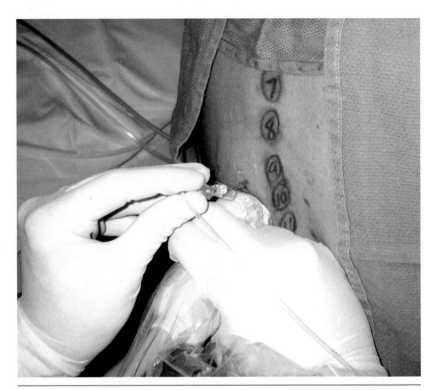

Figure 26-6. The transducer is positioned with a 22-gauge needle introduced in plane.

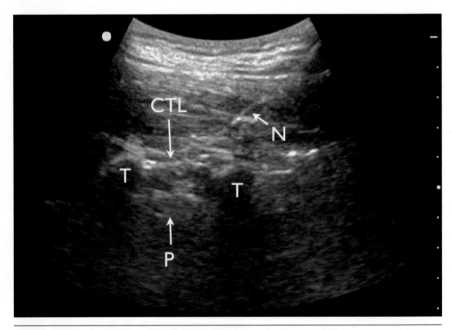

Figure 26-7. *N*, needle; *T*, transverse process; *P*, pleura; *CTL*, costotransverse ligament.

2. The paravertebral catheter can also be placed using an ultrasound-guided intercostal approach.
3. To decrease the risk of epidural spread, the needle should not be introduced in a latero-medial direction.
4. The use of a Tuohy needle is recommended to minimize the risk of nerve or pleural puncture.

For higher thoracic levels, a 5- to 10-MHz linear array can be used, because the paravertebral space is more superficial at these levels.

References

1. Joshi GP, Bonnet F, Shah R, et al. A systematic review of randomized trials evaluating regional techniques for postthoracotomy analgesia. Anesth Analg 2008 Sep;107:1026–1040.
2. Davies RG, Myles PS, Graham JM. A comparison of the analgesic efficacy and side effects of paravertebral vs. epidural blockade for thoracotomy–a systematic review and meta-analysis of randomized trials. Br J Anaesth 2006 Apr;96:418–426.
3. Exadaktylos AK, Buggy DJ, Moriarty DC, et al. Can anesthetic technique for primary breast cancer surgery affect recurrence or metastasis? Anesthesiology 2006 Oct;105:660–664.
4. Karmakar MK. Thoracic paravertebral block. Anesthesiology 2001;95:771–780.
5. Chelly JE. Peropheral Nervs Blocks: A Color Atlas. Philadelphia: Lippincott Williams & Wilkins; 1999.
6. Chelly JE, Uskova A, Merman R, et al. A multifactorial approach to the factors influencing determination of paravertebral depth. Can J Aneasth 2008;55:587–594.

Section *V*

Pediatric Anesthesia

27   Fundamentals of Ultrasound-Guided Pediatric Regional Anesthesia

28   Ultrasound-Guided Brachial Plexus Blockade in Infants and Children

29   Ultrasound-Guided Regional Anesthesia of the Thorax, Trunk, and Abdomen in Infants and Children

30   Ultrasound-Guided Lower Extremity Block in Children

27

Fundamentals of Ultrasound-Guided Pediatric Regional Anesthesia

JOSEPH D. TOBIAS

In the pediatric-aged patient, there has been increasing use of regional anesthesia in the perioperative period. In this age group, regional anesthetic techniques are used most commonly as an adjunct to general anesthesia, either to supplement general anesthesia or to provide postoperative analgesia. However, many of these regional anesthetic techniques can also be used instead of general anesthesia in circumstances where anatomic or physiologic alterations may make the conduct of general anesthesia more difficult or dangerous. Regional anesthetic techniques may also be used during painful or invasive procedures in situations where the conduct of general anesthesia may not be readily possible or as a therapeutic modality to provide sympathetic blockade in patients with vascular insufficiency and in the treatment of chronic pain. Regardless of the situation, accurate placement is mandatory to ensure the success and safety of the technique.

In pediatric-aged patients, caudal epidural anesthesia remains the most frequently performed regional anesthetic technique.[1] Although this technique is effective for lower abdominal and lower extremity procedures, other approaches are obviously necessary when the operative procedure involves the upper extremity. Additionally, for unilateral extremity procedures, there has been an increased use of peripheral nerve block to allow for unilateral anesthesia and avoid the potential complications of neuraxial techniques such as caudal epidural anesthesia. The potential advantages of peripheral block are illustrated by Giaufre et al[2] in their survey of regional anesthetic techniques employed by the French-Language Society of Pediatric Anesthesiologists. Central neuraxial block (mostly caudal epidural block) accounted for 60% of the 24,409 regional anesthetic techniques. There were 4090 peripheral nerve blocks, 997 of which were placed in the upper extremity. No complications were noted related to the peripheral nerve blocks, whereas the complication rate related to caudal epidural block was 1.5%. These results prompted the authors to suggest that "the extremely low incidence of complications (zero in the study) after peripheral nerve blocks should encourage anesthesiologists to use them more often, when they are appropriate, in the place of a central block."

Ongoing advancements in technique and refinement of the available equipment have improved the applicability of regional anesthetic techniques in the pediatric population. The use of ultrasound-guided block has gained widespread applicability in the adult population. Given its ease of use, noninvasive modality, and potential to improve the success rate and decrease the incidence of adverse effects, it is likely that the use of ultrasound-guided regional anesthesia will increase in the pediatric population.[3,4] Of the many differences between the practices of adult and pediatric regional anesthesia, the major one is that in the pediatric-aged patient, these techniques are performed in the anesthetized or deeply sedated patient.[5] This practice is well within the standard of care for infants and children,

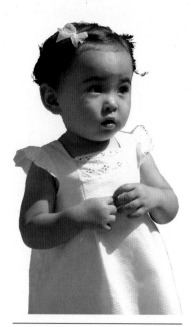

Figure 27-1. Image of a child.

and as such a means of ensuring correct placement of the needle is mandatory. This chapter reviews basic information regarding the use of ultrasound to guide regional anesthesia procedures in infants and children, discusses some of the appropriate equipment needed for such a practice, and reviews issues related to the use of local anesthetic agents in pediatric patients, including dosing regimens and the issue of test dosing to identify inadvertent intravascular injection.

Equipment for Regional Anesthesia in Infants and Children

Ultrasound

The use of ultrasound to guide peripheral and caudal epidural block in children has great utility because the nerves are superficial and easily imaged. Regional anesthetic techniques in children are often performed under deep sedation or general anesthesia. In this setting, the ability to identify the nerve and the needle tip may prevent adverse effects of these techniques, including damage to or injection within nerves, puncture of vascular structures, or pneumothorax. In smaller patients, the safe dose of local anesthetic is often a limiting factor in the successful performance of peripheral nerve block. Ultrasound-guided block is an asset in this setting because it has been shown to speed the onset of the block, improve its efficacy, and, most importantly, diminish the dose of local anesthetic agent that is necessary to provide a successful block.[6-8] With such accuracy and efficacy, ultrasound-guided peripheral nerve block in children can now be used instead of caudal epidural block, which was previously used for surgery of the lower extremities and abdomen. Although neuraxial block (caudal and lumbar epidural analgesia) in children is efficacious, adverse effects, including urinary retention, as well as bilateral sensory block and motor weakness may occur. If hydrophilic opioids such as morphine or hydromorphone are added to neuraxial block, additional adverse effects, including nausea, vomiting, pruritus, and respiratory depression may occur. Greater experience with the use of ultrasound-guided lower extremity blocks, transversus abdominis block, paravertebral or intercostal block, and rectus sheath block may replace many of the neuraxial techniques previously used in pediatric patients.

The true echogenicity of a nerve is visualized only when the ultrasound beam is directed perpendicular to the nerve axis. Consequently, linear probes with parallel sound beam emission are used for ultrasound-guided regional anesthesia. Using a transverse scanning technique, peripheral nerves may appear as dark (hypoechoic) structures surrounded by white/bright (hyperechoic) structures or a single hyperechoic structure. These differences in the appearance of the nerves on ultrasound depend on the size of the nerve, the frequency of the ultrasound, and the angle at which the ultrasound beam contacts the nerve. Given these issues, the nerves may appear as round or oval hypoechoic structures or as a single hyperechoic structure. With some techniques (transversus abdominis, rectus sheath, or fascia iliaca block), the nerves are not individually identified, but rather ultrasound is used to identify the appropriate fascial plane for the deposition of the local anesthetic agent. Needles (see below) can be inserted in-line with the transducer so that the needle and its tip can be visualized or at an angle of 90 degrees (cross-sectional technique) to the transducer. With the latter technique, only the tip of the needle can be seen and so the course of the needle is identified by tissue displacement.

Just like in adults, various probes and transducers can be used for the performance of regional anesthesia in infants and children; the choice being based on the patient's weight and the type of block that is being performed.[9,10] There is an inverse relationship between frequency and depth of penetration, so higher frequency probes provide better resolution of superficial structures and can generally be used in smaller pediatric patients given the proximity of the structures to the skin. In general, three types of probes provide most of what is needed for ultrasound-guided regional anesthesia in infants and children.

1. A 25-mm (hockey-stick), high-frequency (10–14 MHz) linear transducer is suitable for the performance of most regional blocks in children who weigh less than 20 to 30 kg.
2. A curved (11 mm), intermediate-frequency (5–10 MHz) probe may be useful for the performance of blocks where there is limited space for the placement of the probe such as the supraclavicular area. This probe can also be used in larger children and adolescents to survey surrounding anatomical structures such as muscles, bones, and the vasculature to identify deep-lying structures such as the sciatic nerve.
3. A 35-mm linear probe with a frequency range of 8 to13 MHz is useful in children who weigh more than 40 kg.

Needles

As children come in all sizes, ages, and shapes, various needles of different gauges and lengths are necessary for the successful use of regional anesthesia in the pediatric patient. When selecting the appropriate needle, an additional advantage of ultrasound is that the depth of the structures to be anesthetized from the skin surface can be estimated and thereby help in the choice of the length of the needle to be used. In our practice, we have access to various lengths and gauges of insulated needles, which include 20- (6 in), 21- (4 in), 22- (2 in), and 24-gauge (1 in) needles for single-shot techniques. Additional equipment for placement of catheters for continuous postoperative infusions may be also considered in the pediatric patient. Most of these catheters, which are 20 gauge, are placed through an insulated 18-gauge Tuohy needle. Various lengths of insulated 18-gauge Tuohy needles are available including 4-, 2-, and 1.5-in varieties.

Nerve Stimulator

Although ultrasound-guided blockade provides the greatest likelihood of safety and success with regional anesthesia, the use of surface landmarks and a nerve stimulator is still practiced in many centers especially during the transition to using ultrasound. Although some argue that the fusion of nerve stimulation and ultrasound guidance is unnecessary, until our expertise with ultrasound has been established, nerve stimulation provides additional assurance that the needle is in the correct location. The author's practice is to set the nerve stimulator at 1.5 to 2 mA to initially identify the nerve and then fine tune the position to achieve adequate nerve stimulation at ≤1 mA. The most recent information from the pediatric population demonstrates that the success of a block is no different when twitches are attained with the nerve stimulator at 0 to 0.5 mA versus 0.5 to 1.0 mA.[11] Additionally, it has been suggested that use of lower thresholds (<0.5 mA) may increase the risk of intraneural injection. The addition of neurostimulation for peripheral nerve blocks is largely a matter of preference rather than practice based on outcome studies. For those practitioners who choose to add neurostimulation to ultrasound in children, stimulation thresholds between 0.5 to 1 mA are appropriate. The use of the nerve stimulator requires avoidance or reversal of neuromuscular blocking agents. Ilioinguinal/iliohypogastric, transversus abdominis, paravertebral, and intercostal blockade are essentially field blocks, and the addition of neurostimulation to ultrasound guidance serves no purpose in these blocks.

Local Anesthetic Dosing Guidelines: In the pediatric-aged patient, most experience with regional anesthesia has included the use of either 0.25% bupivacaine or 0.2% ropivacaine. As most of these patients are already anesthetized, the decreased degree of motor block with the lower concentration of local anesthetic is not generally an issue. If the limited motor blockade becomes a problem, the administration of a neuromuscular blocking agent and controlled ventilation can be provided. When used solely for the purpose of postoperative analgesia, several studies have demonstrated, at least when used for caudal epidural blockade, that 0.125% bupivacaine is as effective as 0.25% bupivacaine.[12–14] However, concentrations of ropivacaine less than 0.2% have been shown to be ineffective.[15] An additional advantage of the more dilute concentrations of local anesthetic agent is the limitation of motor blockade and the ability to ambulate postoperatively if outpatient surgery is planned. When catheters are placed for continuous infusions, ropivacaine or bupivacaine at concentrations of 1 to 1.25 mg/mL (0.1%–0.125%) are generally effective. In some circumstances, the regional anesthetic technique is used instead of general anesthesia. Depending on the size of the patient, higher concentrations of bupivacaine or ropivacaine (0.5%) may be used to provide surgical anesthesia and a greater degree of motor blockade. As the concentration of the local anesthetic is increased, the total volume used should be decreased to limit the total dose of bupivacaine to ≤3 mg/kg. This would amount to 1.2 mL/kg of 0.25% bupivacaine or 0.6 mL/kg of 0.5% bupivacaine.

With regional anesthetic techniques in children, the greatest risk of morbidity and mortality lies in local anesthetic toxicity making calculation of the appropriate dose of great importance. Although blood levels achieved after plexus anesthesia or peripheral nerve block are less than those with neural block in more vascular areas (i.e., interpleural, intercostal, and caudal/lumbar/thoracic epidural), the total amount of bupivacaine administered during a single bolus injection should be limited to ≤3 mg/kg. Various studies have investigated plasma bupivacaine levels after regional blockade in infants and children. Following axillary block in children with either 2 mg/kg (n = 21) or 3 mg/kg (n = 20) of bupivacaine, Campbell et al[16] reported a rapid absorption with a mean time to peak concentration of 0.37 hours for either dose and mean peak plasma concentrations of 1.35 µg/mL with 2 mg/kg and 1.84 µg/mL after 3 mg/kg. The authors suggested that even after a 30% allowance for anticipated higher arterial levels, the plasma levels were well below what the authors considered to be the toxic concentration of bupivacaine (4 µg/mL). Sfez et al[17] evaluated plasma bupivacaine concentrations following penile block with either 0.1 mL/kg of 0.5% bupivacaine (0.5 mg/kg bupivacaine) or 0.1 mL/kg of 0.25% bupivacaine plus lidocaine 1% (0.25 mg/kg bupivacaine). The time to peak plasma concentration was similar between the two groups (27 ± 19 minutes versus 27 ± 18 minutes) as was the duration of analgesia (6.7 ± 1.7 hours versus 7.4 ± 1 hours).

Although the peak plasma concentrations were well below the toxic range in both groups (0.25 μg/mL and <0.1 μg/mL), the authors noted that the addition of lidocaine somehow altered the absorption of bupivacaine. Although the dose of bupivacaine used with lidocaine was one half of the dose used without lidocaine, the peak plasma concentration was less than one half.

As noted previously, one of the factors that may affect the plasma concentration achieved with any local anesthetic agent is the site of injection. The intercostal space is one of the most vascular areas into which local anesthetic agents are injected, and hence high plasma concentrations may occur following intercostal blockade. Bricker et al[18] evaluated bupivacaine plasma levels and pharmacokinetics following single-shot intercostal injections with a dose of bupivacaine (1.5 mg/kg) in 11 neonates (<1 month of age) and 11 infants (1–6 months of age). Peak plasma concentrations of bupivacaine occurred within 10 minutes in most patients and were 0.82 ± 0.56 μg/mL in neonates and 0.91 ± 0.27 μg/mL in infants. They noted no difference between the two age groups in regard to clearance or elimination half-life. Likewise, no difference was noted when comparing cyanotic and acyanotic patients. Plasma concentrations have also been shown to be well within acceptable ranges following the administration of 2 to 3 mg/kg of bupivacaine or ropivacaine for caudal epidural blockade.[19–21] More recently, other investigators have demonstrated low free plasma concentrations following the use of 1.25 mg/kg of either bupivacaine or ropivacaine for caudal epidural block.[22]

When ongoing continuous infusions are administered via an indwelling catheter, it has been suggested that the dose of bupivacaine should be less than 0.3 to 0.4 mg/kg/h in children and less than 0.2 to 0.25 mg/kg/h in neonates and infants.[23,24] More recently, concerns have been expressed regarding the potential for bupivacaine plasma concentrations to continue to escalate when continuous infusions are used in younger patients. To date, these data have been derived from studies with bupivacaine administered via a continuous epidural infusion. In eight infants, varying in age from 3 to 13 months, bupivacaine was administered via an epidural catheter as a bolus dose of 1.2 mg/kg followed by an infusion of 0.36 to 0.39 mg/kg/h for up to 44 hours.[25] Although the maximum bupivacaine plasma concentration was 2.02 μg/mL, there was evidence of the potential for accumulation with more prolonged infusions as three of eight patients had increasing levels at the time of discontinuation of the infusion. Similar results were reported by Larsson et al,[26] who noted increasing bupivacaine levels in five of eight patients at 48 hours after an initial bolus dose of 1.8 mg/kg and an infusion of 0.2 mg/kg/h.

The potential for bupivacaine toxicity with continuous infusions appears to be magnified in the youngest pediatric-aged patients. Luz et al[27,28] reported higher plasma bupivacaine concentrations in infants less than 4 months of age compared to those who were more than 9 months of age and higher free bupivacaine concentrations in infants compared to older children during continuous epidural infusions. The potential for an increased free fraction of plasma bupivacaine in young infants has been noted in other studies.[29] Decreased clearance and an increased free fraction has also been reported in neonates and young infants with a continuous epidural infusion of ropivacaine; however, these studies have demonstrated a stable plasma concentration over time without an increasing plasma concentration as has been demonstrated with bupivacaine.[30,31] These studies used ropivacaine in doses of 0.2 mg/kg/h in neonates and infants and up to 0.4 mg/kg/h in older children.

The risk of local anesthetic toxicity is greatest during the injection of the initial bolus dose. To limit the risks of toxicity, the lowest effective volume and concentration should be used.

As demonstrated by Willschke et al,[7] ultrasound guidance may be beneficial in this regard as visualization of local anesthetic deposition, which may allow lower volumes to be used without affecting efficacy. In addition, many practitioners still recommend the addition of epinephrine in a concentration of 1:200,000 (5 μg/mL) to the anesthetic solution to act as a test dose to identify inadvertent intravascular injection. Although the addition of low-dose epinephrine (1:200,000) is a time-honored practice as a means of inducing tachycardia and thereby alerting the clinician should inadvertent intravascular injection occur, there is debate regarding this practice. The accuracy of the hemodynamic response to the epinephrine "test dose" during halothane or sevoflurane has been questioned.[32,33] The criteria to identify inadvertent intravascular injection had been a heart rate increase $\geq$20 beats per minute. However, the sensitivity of this response has been shown to be altered by the inhalational anesthetic agent that is used as well as whether atropine has been administered. Although the blunting of the heart rate response is less with sevoflurane than with halothane, further studies have demonstrated that changes in the T wave (increase in amplitude $\geq$25%) or an increase in systolic blood pressure is more sensitive indicators of inadvertent intravascular injection than changes in heart rate.[34,35] In fact, in children anesthetized with sevoflurane, the positive response rate to the injection of the epinephrine test dose was shown to be 100% for a T wave amplitude increase $\geq$25%, 95% for a systolic blood pressure increase $\geq$15 mm Hg, and 71% for a heart rate increase $\geq$10 beats per minute. More recently, use of peripheral indicators of perfusion have been suggested as a sensitive tool for the identification of an inadvertent intravascular injection. The newest generation of pulse oximeters provides what is termed the plethysmographic pulse wave amplitude (PPWA), an indicator of peripheral perfusion. Mowafi et al[36] have demonstrated that a decrease in the PPWA is a sensitive means of identifying intravascular injection. In their study of 80 infants and children anesthetized with either 0.5 or 1 minimum alveolar concentration (MAC) of sevoflurane, they reported that the sensitivity, specificity, positive predictive value, and negative predictive value of the PPWA was 100% with either 0.5 or 1 MAC of sevoflurane. Although the use of the epinephrine test dose is not embraced by all practitioners of regional anesthesia, there may be other potential benefits to the addition of epinephrine. In addition to providing the potential to alert the clinician should inadvertent intravascular injection, the addition of epinephrine may also slow vascular absorption of the local anesthetic agent, thereby decreasing peak plasma concentrations. Doyle et al[37] demonstrated that the addition of epinephrine to the solution used for fascia iliaca compartment blocks resulted in a lower peak plasma concentration (0.35 μg/mL with epinephrine versus 1.1 μg/mL without epinephrine) as well as a delay in the time to reach the peak plasma concentration (45 minutes versus 20 minutes).

Summary: Given its many benefits, the use of peripheral regional blockade continues to increase in infants and children. Over the past 10 years, there have been improvements in the equipment available for this practice. Although initially used in the practice of adult regional anesthesia, there is growing interest in the applicability of ultrasound-guided techniques in infants and children. Along with this interest has come evidence-based medicine that supports the benefits of this practice. Major benefits include not only improved accuracy but also potentially decreased morbidity. Although the practice of peripheral blockade in infants and children has included primarily single-shot techniques, the refinement of the equipment and improvements in technique, including the use of ultrasound imaging, has led to interest in the use of continuous infusions to provide prolonged analgesia following major surgical procedures.[38]

References

1. Yaster M, Maxwell LG. Pediatric regional anesthesia. Anesthesiology 1989;70:324–338.
2. Giaufré E, Dalens B, Gombert A. Epidemiology and morbidity of regional anesthesia in children: a one-year prospective survey of the French-Language Society of Pediatric Anesthesiologists. Anesth Analg 1996;83:904–912.

3. Oberndorfer U, Marhofer P, Bösenberg A, et al. Ultrasonographic guidance for sciatic and femoral nerve blocks in children. Br J Anaesth 2007;98:797–801.
4. Schwemmer U, Markus CK, Greim CA, et al. Sonographic imaging of the sciatic nerve and its division the popliteal fossa in children. Paediatr Anaesth 2004:14:1005–1008.
5. Bernards CM, Hadzic A, Suresh S, et al. Regional anesthesia in anesthetized or heavily sedated patients. Reg Anesth Pain Med 2008;33:449–460.
6. Marhofer P, Sitzwohl C, Greher M, et al. Ultrasound guidance for infraclavicular brachial plexus anaesthesia in children. Anaesthesia 2004;59:642–646.
7. Willschke H, Bösenberg A, Marhofer P, et al. Ultrasonographic-guided ilioinguinal/iliohypogastric nerve block in pediatric anesthesia: what is the optimal volume? Anesth Analg 2006;102:1680–1684.
8. Willschke H, Marhofer P, Bösenberg A, et al. Ultrasonography for ilioinguinal/iliohypogastric nerve blocks in children. Br J Anaesth 2005;95:226–230.
9. Marhofer P, Frickey N. Ultrasonographic guidance in pediatric regional anesthesia Part 1: Theoretical background. Paediatr Anaesth 2006;16:1008–1018.
10. Marhofer P, Chan VW. Ultrasound-guided regional anesthesia: current concepts and future trends. Anesth Analg 2007;104:1265–1269.
11. Gurnaney H, Ganest A, Cucchiaro G. The relationship between intensity for nerve stimulation and success of peripheral nerve blocks performed in pediatric patients under general anesthesia. Anesth Analg 2007;105:1605–1609.
12. Tobias JD. Caudal epidural block with 0.125% bupivacaine for postoperative analgesia in children following lower extremity orthopedic procedures. Am J Pain Manage 1997;7:89–91.
13. Malviya S, Fear DW, Roy WL, et al. Adequacy of caudal analgesia in children after penoscrotal and inguinal surgery using 0.5 or 1.0 mL/kg-1 bupivacaine 0.125%. Can J Anaesth 1992;39:449–453.
14. Wolf AR, Valley RD, Fear DW, et al. Bupivacaine for caudal analgesia in infants and children: the optimal effective concentration. Anesthesiology 1988;69:102–106.
15. Luz G, Innerhofer P, Häussler B, et al. Comparison of ropivacaine 0.1% and 0.2% with bupivacaine 0.2% for single-shot caudal anaesthesia in children. Paediatr Anaesth 2000;10:499–504.
16. Campbell RJ, Ilett KF, Dusci L. Plasma bupivacaine concentrations after axillary block in children. Anaesth Intensive Care 1986;14:343–346.
17. Sfez M, Le Mapihan Y, Mazoit X, et al. Local anesthetic serum concentrations after penile nerve block in children. Anesth Analg 1990;71:423–426.
18. Bricker SR, Telford RJ, Booker PD. Pharmacokinetics of bupivacaine following intraoperative intercostal nerve block in neonates and in infants aged less than 6 months. Anesthesiology 1989;70:942–947.
19. Ala-Kokko TI, Partanen A, Karinen J, et al. Pharmacokinetics of 0.2% ropivacaine and 0.2% bupivacaine following caudal blocks in children. Acta Anaesthesiol Scand 2000;44:1099–1102.
20. Eyres RL, Bishop W, Oppenheim RC, et al. Plasma bupivacaine concentrations in children during caudal epidural analgesia. Anaesth Intensive Care 1983;11:20–22.
21. Bösenberg AT, Thomas J, Lopez T, et al. Plasma concentrations of ropivacaine following a single-shot caudal block of 1, 2 or 3 mg/kg in children. Acta Anaesthesiol Scand 2001;45:1276–1280.
22. Bozkurt P, Arslan I, Bakan M, et al. Free plasma levels of bupivacaine and ropivacaine when used for caudal blocks in children. Eur J Anaesthesiol 2005;22:640–641.
23. Berde CB. Convulsions associated with pediatric regional anesthesia. Anesth Analg 1992;75:164–166.
24. Berde CB. Toxicity of local anesthetics in infants and children. J Pediatr 1993;122:S14–S20.
25. Peutrell JM, Holder K, Gregory M. Plasma bupivacaine concentrations associated with continuous extradural infusions in babies. Br J Anaesth 1997;78:160–162.
26. Larsson BA, Lönnqvist PA, Olsson GL. Plasma concentrations of bupivacaine in neonates after continuous epidural infusion. Anesth Analg 1997;84:501–505.
27. Luz G, Wieser C, Innerhofer P, et al. Free and total bupivacaine plasma concentrations after continuous epidural anaesthesia in infants and children. Paediatr Anaesth 1998;8:473–478.
28. Luz G, Innerhofer P, Bachmann B, et al. Bupivacaine plasma concentrations during continuous epidural anesthesia in infants and children. Anesth Analg 1996;82:231–234.
29. Mazoit JX, Denson DD, Samii K. Pharmacokinetics of bupivacaine following caudal anesthesia in infants. Anesthesiology 1988;68:387–391.
30. Bösenberg AT, Thomas J, Cronje L, et al. Pharmacokinetics and efficacy of ropivacaine for continuous epidural infusion in neonates and infants. Paediatr Anaesth 2005;15:739–749.
31. Berde CB, Yaster M, Meretoja O, et al. Stable plasma concentrations of unbound ropivacaine during postoperative epidural infusions for 24–72 hours in children. Eur J Anaesthesiol 2008;25:410–417.
32. Desparmet J, Mateo J, Ecoffey C, et al. Efficacy of an epidural test dose in children anesthetized with halothane. Anesthesiology 1990;72:249–251.
33. Tobias JD. Caudal epidural block: a review of test dosing and recognition of systemic injection in children. Anesth Analg 2001;93:1156–1161.
34. Tanaka M, Kimura T, Goyagi T, et al. Evaluating hemodynamic and T wave criteria of simulated intravascular injection using bupivacaine or isoproterenol in anesthetized children. Anesth Analg 2000;91:567–572.

35. Kozek-Langenecker SA, Marhofer P, Jonas K, et al. Cardiovascular criteria for epidural test dosing in sevoflurane- and halothane-anesthetized children. Anesth Analg 2000;90:579–583.

36. Mowafi HA, Arab SA, Ismail SA, et al. Plethysmographic pulse wave amplitude is an effective indicator for intravascular injection of epinephrine-containing epidural test dose in sevoflurane-anesthetized pediatric patients. Anesth Analg 2008;107:1536–1541.

37. Doyle E, Morton NS, McNicol LR. Plasma bupivacaine levels after fascia iliaca compartment block with and without adrenaline. Paediatr Anaesth 1997;7:121–124.

38. Dadure C, Pirat P, Raux O, et al. Perioperative continuous peripheral nerve blocks with disposable infusion pumps in children: a prospective descriptive study. Anesth Analg 2003;97:687–690.

Ultrasound-Guided Brachial Plexus Blockade in Infants and Children

JOSEPH D. TOBIAS, STEFAN LUCAS, SANTHANAM SURESH, PAUL E. BIGELEISEN

Introduction: The brachial plexus is derived from the ventral (anterior) branches of spinal roots C5-C8 and T1. These spinal nerves pass through the intervertebral formina and course between the anterior and middle scalene muscles, which attach respectively to the anterior and posterior tubercles of the transverse processes of the cervical vertebrae. The brachial plexus provides sensory and motor innervation to most of the shoulder and upper extremity. A portion of the shoulder is innervated by the cervical plexus, and the medial aspect of the upper arm is innervated by the intercostobrachial nerve, a branch of the second intercostal nerve, which communicates with the medial cutaneous nerve of the arm. As the spinal roots exit the vertebral column and pass between the anterior and middle scalene muscles, they form three trunks (superior, middle, and inferior). As the trunks exit the interscalene groove, they lie in a cephaloposterior position to the subclavian artery as it courses along the upper surface of the first rib. The trunks split into anterior and posterior divisions that then unit to form cords (lateral, posterior, and medial), which are named because of their relationship to the axillary artery at the level of the coracoid process. These cords surround the axillary artery and are blocked with the infraclavicular approach to the brachial plexus. The cords further divide into the nerves of the brachial plexus (musculocutaneous, ulnar, median, and radial) as they surround the axillary artery and can be blocked with an axillary approach to the brachial plexus. The brachial plexus can be anesthetized by one of several approaches (interscalene, supraclavicular, infraclavicular, or axillary route). The site of block will be determined by the location of the surgery as well as the expertise of the anesthesia provider. With the use of ultrasound-guided techniques, it is postulated that the risks of adverse events associated with these techniques, including vascular puncture or pneumothorax, should decrease. Given that, these techniques should play an increasing role in the provision of postoperative analgesia in the pediatric-aged patient.

Younger children and infants rarely require surgery on the shoulder joint itself. When they do, an interscalene approach is appropriate. Although the axillary approach was previously the most commonly used technique, the use of ultrasound has allowed practitioners to use more proximal blocks safely. In most cases, surgery of the upper extremity distal to the shoulder can be performed with a supraclavicular or infraclavicular approach. Local anesthetic injection, using an axillary approach in small children frequently spreads cephalad. Thus, the axillary nerve is often blocked when local anesthetic is injected around the radial nerve. A selective musculocutaneous nerve block is usually required with the axillary approach. In most cases, axillary block is sufficient for anesthesia of the upper arm, forearm, and hand in small children. If the surgical site includes the medial arm, a separate subcutaneous injection along the medial arm, just below the axilla, should be made to anesthetize the intercostal brachial nerve, which is a branch of the second intercostal nerve. As with most regional anesthesia that is performed in infants and children, brachial plexus anesthesia is most frequently used as an adjunct to general anesthesia with the block placed after the induction of anesthesia either at the start or after completion of the surgical procedure.[2] In these cases, the block is used to provide postoperative analgesia. In other circumstances, axillary block can be used instead of general anesthesia to provide surgical anesthesia or even occasionally as a therapeutic modality, where the sympathetic block that accompanies the motor and sensory blockade is used to improve regional blood flow.[3–6]

Axillary Approach to the Brachial Plexus

Background and Indications: The terminal branches of the brachial plexus (musculocutaneous, median, radial, and ulnar nerves) arise from the cords relatively high in the axilla. The musculocutaneous nerve is identified as an oval hyperechoic structure cephalad to the artery, lying between the biceps and coracobrachialis muscles. The median, radial, and ulnar nerves or the cords that give rise to them may have variable positions around the artery (Figs. 28-1 and 28-2). The median nerve may lie anterior, superior, or inferior to the artery. The radial nerve often lies inferiorly to the artery, and the ulnar nerve usually lies anterior and inferior to the artery. These three nerves appear as hyperechoic clusters around the artery. The cutaneous nerves have the same appearance, although depending on the size of the patient, it may not be possible to identify these nerves. However, in many cases, the outlines of the nerves become apparent as the local anesthetic solution is injected. In children, it may be possible to anesthetize the axillary nerve as well as the radial nerve by injecting local anesthetic posterior to the axillary artery when the block is performed high in the axilla. For this reason, axillary block in children is suitable for all procedures of the upper extremity distal to the deltoid muscle. One of the major limitations of this approach is that it cannot be performed in patients who cannot abduct their arm because of pain or restricted mobility while they are awake.

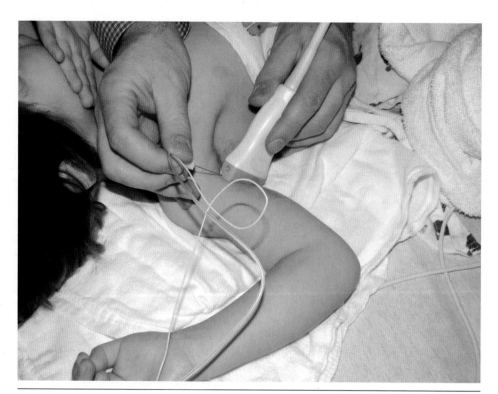

Figure 28-1. Needle and transducer position for axillary block.

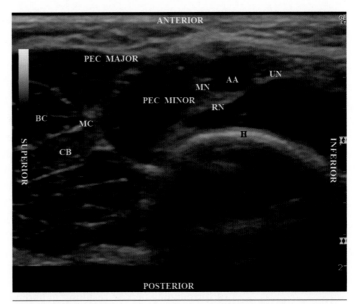

Figure 28-2. Ultrasound scan of axilla. *PMAJOR*, pectoralis major; *PMINOR*, pectoralis minor; *BC*, biceps muscle; *MC*, musculocutaneous nerve; *CB*, coracobrachialis muscle; *AA*, axillary artery; *RN*, radial nerve; *MN*, median nerve; *UN*, ulnar nerve; *H*, humerus.

 Patient Position: Supine with arm abducted 90 degrees from the body and the elbow flexed 90 degrees.

 Transducer: 25-mm linear array oscillating at 13 MHz.

 Transducer Orientation: Transverse in the axilla.

 Needle: 22- or 24-gauge, 1- or 2-inch, blunt or insulated needle.

 Local Anesthetic: For postoperative analgesia, 0.25% bupivacaine (with epinephrine 1:200,000) or 0.2% ropivacaine, 0.5% concentrations for surgical anesthesia. Volume = 0.2 to 0.4 mL/kg, total dose ≤3 mg/kg.

 Technique: For the axillary approach, the patient's arm is abducted 90 degrees from the body, and the elbow is flexed at a 90-degree angle so that the hand is over the head or behind it. For ultrasound-guided block of the axillary plexus, after the axilla is washed with a sterile prep solution, sterile ultrasound gel is placed, and the ultrasound probe is inserted into a sterile cover. A 25-mm linear transducer oscillating at 13 MHz is oriented in the transverse plane. If the procedure is performed without the use of general anesthesia, local anesthesia is provided by the subcutaneous infiltration of 0.5% lidocaine with a 27-gauge needle. The block needle is inserted in-line, cephalad to the probe and directed toward the musculocutaneous nerve. The nerve is surrounded with a small volume of the local anesthetic agent (2–3 mL). The needle is then withdrawn to a position just below the skin and directed toward the median nerve. An injection 2 to 4 mL of local anesthetic, depending on the size of the patient, is made until the nerve is surrounded. The procedure is repeated for the ulnar and radial nerves. In some patients, the artery must be pushed out of the way of the needle to reach all four nerves through the same injection site. If slightly larger volumes are injected around the radial nerve, the axillary nerve is usually blocked if the needle insertion site is in the proximal axilla.

Interscalene Approach to the Brachial Plexus

Background and Indications: Prior to the introduction of ultrasound for regional anesthesia, interscalene blocks were used less frequently in children because of the potential for adverse effects including pneumothorax and vascular puncture. As the trunks of the brachial plexus are organized in a superior to inferior direction in the interscalene groove, the lower dermatomes of the brachial plexus may be less effectively blocked than with more distal approaches.[7] In addition to the risks of pneumothorax, vertebral artery puncture with local anesthetic toxicity is a concern. In the latter cases, because there is direct flow to the central nervous system, even minute amounts of local anesthetic agents can lead to seizures should arterial injection occur. Because of the proximity of the vertebral column and spinal cord, there is also a potential for epidural or intrathecal injection. The risk of such complications should be decreased by the use of ultrasound and direct visualization of the site of local anesthetic placement. Additional issues include blockade of surrounding nerves, resulting in phrenic nerve blockade with hemidiaphragm paralysis, recurrent laryngeal nerve block with unilateral vocal cord paralysis, and sympathetic block with Horner syndrome.[8] Although phrenic/recurrent laryngeal nerve block is well tolerated in healthy, older patients, infants and patients with respiratory dysfunction may be dependent on the diaphragm for respiratory function.[9] Additionally, airway compromise can occur with unilateral vocal cord paralysis in infants and young children. In young children, our clinical experience has demonstrated that cephalad spread to the cervical plexus may also occur so that effective analgesia may be provided in these dermatomes as well.

Patient Position: Supine with the head turned away from the operator and the side of the block.

Transducer: 25-mm linear array oscillating at 13 MHz or 35-mm linear probe oscillating at 8 to 13 MHz for larger patients.

Transducer Orientation: Transverse oblique in the supraclavicular fossa and then transverse over the sternocleidomastoid muscle at the level of the thyroid cartilage.

Needle: 22- or 24-gauge, 1- or 2-inch, blunt or insulated needle.

Local Anesthetic: For postoperative analgesia, 0.25% bupivacaine (with epinephrine 1:200,000) or 0.2% ropivacaine, 0.5% concentrations for surgical anesthesia. Volume = 0.2 to 0.4 mL/kg, total dose ≤3 mg/kg.

Technique: For ultrasound-guided block, the skin is washed, and sterile ultrasound gel is placed in the supraclavicular fossa. A 25-mm linear probe oscillating at 13 MHz is placed in the supraclavicular fossa in an oblique sagittal orientation. The subclavian artery and brachial plexus are identified. The brachial plexus is traced cephalad to the level of the thyroid cartilage while the probe is rotated into an axial alignment. At this level, the roots of C5, C6, and C7 appear as hypoechoic circles sandwiched between the anterior and middle scalene muscles (Figs. 28-3 and 28-4). In small children, the carotid artery and internal jugular vein will appear medial to the brachial plexus, and the sternocleidomastoid muscle will overly the scalene muscles in some patients. Alternatively, these structures can be identified by placing the probe in a horizontal position just above the clavicle/sternum in the middle of the neck. The probe is then moved laterally to identify the carotid artery, the jugular vein, and then the

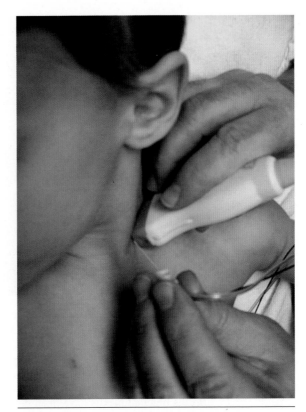

Figure 28-3. Needle and probe position for interscalene block.

anterior and middle scalene muscles. The nerve roots can also be seen adjacent to the transverse process by togging the probe, so that it has a caudal oblique angle relative the surface of the neck (Fig. 28-5). The needle can be inserted in-line with the ultrasound probe, medial to its end, and directed toward the roots. The needle can also be inserted above the probe using an out-of-plane technique. When an out-of-plane technique is used, a gentle bounce on the needle will displace the tissues and aid in identification of the needle path. Once the needle is adjacent to the roots, the local anesthetic solution is injected in aliquots of 3 mL until the plexus is surrounded. It may be necessary to insert the needle between the roots to ensure circumferential spread of local anesthetic around the plexus. Care must be exercised not to inject local anesthetic into the nerves at this level. Each nerve root is in direct communication with the cerebrospinal fluid surrounding the spinal cord.

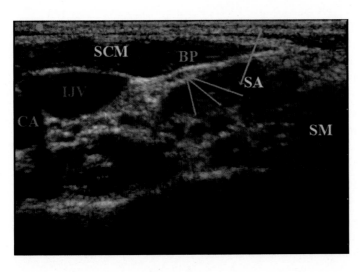

Figure 28-4. Ultrasound scan of the neck for interscalene block. *SCM*, sternocleidomastoid muscle; *IJV*, internal jugular vein; *CA* carotid artery; *BP*, nerve roots C5, C6, C7; *SA*, anterior scalene muscle; *SM*, middle scalene muscle.

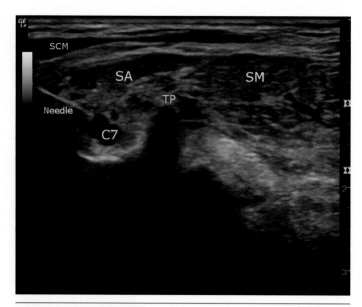

Figure 28-5. Transverse scan at nerve root C7. *TP*, transverse process; *C7*, C7 nerve root; *SA*, anterior scalene; *SM*, middle scalene.

Supraclavicular and Infraclavicular Approaches to the Brachial Plexus

Background and Indications: Both supraclavicular and infraclavicular approaches to the brachial plexus have been described and used with a high degree of success in the adult population. However, prior to the advent of ultrasound for regional anesthesia, there was a paucity of reports regarding the use of a supraclavicular approach in children.[10] In the supraclavicular fossa, block of the brachial plexus may also cause vocal cord paresis and phrenic nerve paresis. Younger patients, such as infants who are more dependent on diaphragmatic function for ventilation, or those with diminished respiratory reserve may not tolerate this insult. Vocal cord paresis has not been reported with infraclavicular block although phrenic nerve paresis does occur very infrequently when a very proximal approach is used. Both supraclavicular and infraclavicular approaches can be used to provide anesthesia for all branches of the brachial plexus. However, given the proximity of these approaches to the pleura and vascular structures, they do carry a risk of vascular puncture or pneumothorax. However, the use of these techniques will increase if ultrasound-guided block is shown to decrease the adverse effect rate in the small pediatric patient.

Patient Position: Supine with the head turned away from the practitioner.

Transducer: 25-mm linear array oscillating at 13 MHz (supraclavicular); the 35-mm linear probe may be useful in children who weigh more than 40 kg, whereas the 11-mm curved array oscillating at 10 MHz may be useful for the performance blocks where there is limited space for the placement of the probe such as the supraclavicular area.

Transducer Orientation: Transverse oblique in the supraclavicular fossa (supraclavicular block). Sagittal in the deltopectoral groove (infraclavicular block).

Local Anesthetic: For postoperative analgesia, 0.25% bupivacaine (with epinephrine 1:200,000) or 0.2% ropivacaine, 0.5% concentrations for surgical anesthesia. Volume = 0.2 to 0.4 mL/kg, total dose ≤3 mg/kg.

Technique: For the ultrasound-guided supraclavicular approach, the skin is prepped and sterile gel is placed in the supraclavicular fossa. The probe is placed in an oblique, transverse orientation in the supraclavicular fossa and the subclavian artery, and brachial plexus are identified (Figs. 28-6 and 28-7). The plexus should appear as a cluster of hypoechoic structures. The rib can be identified immediately below the plexus as a hyper-echoic streak. The pleura has a similar appearance to the rib, but the pleura lies 3 to 10 mm deep to the plexus, whereas the rib lies immediately beneath the plexus. The needle is inserted in-line at the medial end of the probe and advanced toward the subclavian artery. When the needle reaches the equator of the artery, the needle is used to push the artery away from the plexus. The needle is then advanced between the artery and plexus until the tip of the needle is immediately above the rib. Injection of a small amount of local anesthetic solution (0.05–0.1 mL/kg) should cause the entire plexus to float off the rib. The remainder of the injection is done in aliquots of 0.05 to 0.1 mL/kg as the needle is withdrawn. A total of 0.2 to 0.3 mL/kg of local anesthetic solution should be sufficient to achieve a block depending on the size of the patient and specific trajectory of the needle. Catheters are best placed through a needle that is immediately above the rib after an injection has been made to float the plexus off the rib.

For ultrasound-guided infraclavicular blockade, the skin is washed, and sterile gel is placed in the deltopectoral groove, which is also called the infraclavicular fossa. The arm may be abducted 90 degrees and flexed at the elbow as in axillary block or left at the patient's

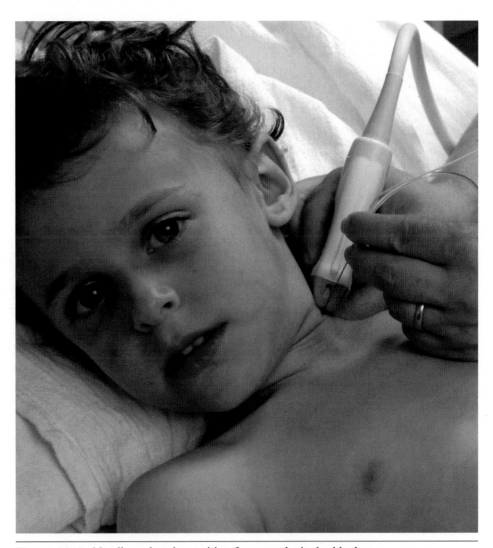

Figure 28-6. Needle and probe position for supraclavicular block.

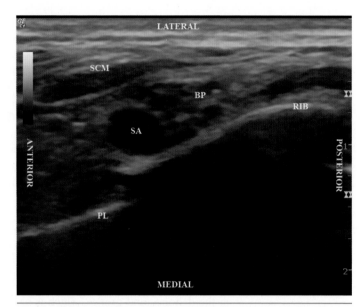

Figure 28-7. Ultrasound scan of the supraclavicular fossa. *SCM*, clavicular head of sternocleidomastoid muscle; *Pl*, pleura; *Rib*, rib; *SA*, subclavian artery; *BP*, brachial plexus.

side. A curved, 11-mm probe, oscillating at 8 to 13 MHz is placed in the fossa, and the axillary artery and vein are imaged. The pectoralis major and minor muscles are identified superficial to the artery, and the cords can be seen as hypoechoic circles superior to the artery (Figs. 28-8 and 28-9). The rib or pleura can be seen as hyperechoic lines posterior and inferior to the plexus and artery. The needle is inserted in-line with the transducer, cephalad to the probe, and directed toward the cords. Local anesthetic is injected in aliquots of 0.05 to 0.1 mL/kg superiorly, posteriorly, and inferiorly to the cords. The needle tip is very close to the pleura in this block, and it is important to keep the tip in view at all times. A total of 0.2 to 0.3 mL/kg of local anesthetic solution is required to achieve effective block depending on the size of the patient. Catheters are best placed inferior to the plexus or in the space between the lateral and posterior cords.

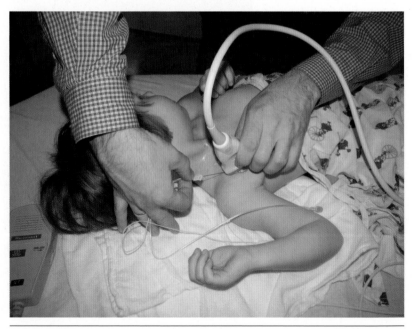

Figure 28-8. Needle and probe position for infraclavicular block.

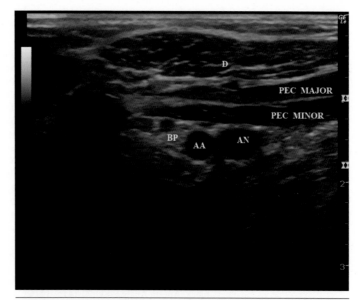

Figure 28-9. Ultrasound scan for infraclavicular block. *D,* deltoid muscle; *PMAJOR,* pectoralis major muscle; *PMINOR,* pectoralis minor muscle; *AA,* axillary artery; *AV,* axillary vein; *BP,* brachial plexus.

An additional approach to the brachial plexus, which has been recently added to the armamentarium for approaches to the brachial plexus, is the lateral infraclavicular block or the coracoid block.[12,13] This approach is a modification of the infraclavicular block where needle placement is more lateral, thereby decreasing the risk of pleural injury. The arm is adducted to the trunk and the elbow flexed at a 90-degree angle with the forearm placed on the abdomen. The coracoid process is palpated, and the site of needle insertion is 0.5 cm distal to the coracoid. The hyperechoic cords of the brachial plexus and axillary vessels are imaged as they pass 0.5 to 1 cm caudal (inferior) to the coracoid. The needle is inserted superior or inferior to the probe using an in-line approach and advanced toward each cord (Figs. 28-10 and 28-11). Local anesthetic dosing would remain the same as for any of the previously described blocks.

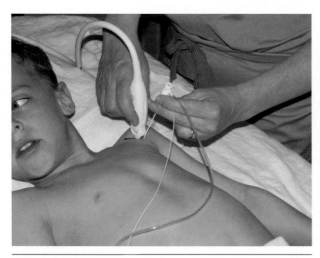

Figure 28-10. Needle and probe position for coracoid block.

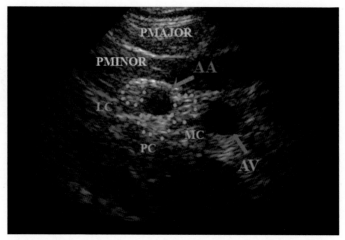

Figure 28-11. Ultrasound scan for coracoid block. *PMAJOR,* pectoralis major; *PMINOR,* pectoralis minor; *AA,* axillary artery; *AV,* axillary vein; *LC,* lateral cord; *PC,* posterior cord; *MC,* medial cord.

References

1. Tobias JD. Brachial plexus anaesthesia in children. Pediatr Anaesth 2001;11:265–275.
2. Altintas F, Bozfurt P, Ipek N, et al. The efficacy of pre- versus post-surgical axillary block on postoperative pain in paediatric patients. Paediatr Anaesth 2000;10:23–28.
3. Messeri A, Calamandrei M. Percutaneous central venous catheterization in small infants: axillary block can facilitate the insertion rate. Paediatr Anaesth 2000;10:527–530.
4. Ross DM, Williams DO. Combined axillary plexus block and basal sedation for cardiac catheterization in young children. Br Heart J 1970;32:195–197.
5. Inberg P, Kassila M, Vilkki S, et al. Anaesthesia for microvascular surgery in children: a combination of general anaesthesia and axillary plexus block. Acta Anaesthesiol Scand 1995;39:518–522.
6. Audenaert SM, Vickers H, Burgess RC. Axillary block for vascular insufficiency after repair of radial club hands in an infant. Anesthesiology 1991;74:368–370.
7. Vester-Andersen T, Christiansen C, Hansen A, et al. Interscalene brachial plexus block: area of analgesia, complications, and blood concentrations of local anesthetics. Acta Anaesthesiol Scand 1981;25:81–84.
8. Urmey WF, Talts KH, Sharrock NE. One hundred percent incidence of hemidiaphragmatic paresis associated with interscalene brachial plexus anesthesia as diagnosed by ultrasonography. Anesth Analg 1991;72:498–503.
9. Kempen PM, O'Donnell J, Lawler R, et al. Acute respiratory insufficiency during interscalene plexus block. Anesth Analg 2000;90:1415–1416.
10. Pande R, Pande M, Bhadani U, et al. Supraclavicular brachial plexus block as a sole anaesthetic technique in children: an analysis of 200 cases. Anaesthesia 2000;55:798–802.
11. Dalens B, Vanneuville G, Tanguy A. A new parascalene approach to the brachial plexus in children: Comparison with the supraclavicular approach. Anesth Analg 1987;66:1264–1271.
12. Fleishmann E, Marhofer P, Greher M, et al. Brachial plexus anaesthesia in children: lateral infraclavicular block versus axillary approach. Paediatr Anaesth 2003;13:103–108.
13. Maria B, Tielens LK. Vertical lateral infraclavicular brachial plexus block in children: a preliminary study. Pediatr Anesth 2004;14:931–935.

29

Ultrasound-Guided Regional Anesthesia of the Thorax, Trunk, and Abdomen in Infants and Children

JOSEPH D. TOBIAS, STEFAN LUCAS, SANTHANAM SURESH, JEAN-LOUIS HORN, PAUL E. BIGELEISEN

Introduction: Depending on the site of injury and the nerves that need to be anesthetized, there are several approaches for regional anesthesia of the thorax, trunk, and abdomen that are applicable to the pediatric population. Examples of these techniques are the use of thoracic paravertebral or intercostal block for analgesia following thoracotomy, ilioinguinal and iliohypogastric block following inguinal herniorrhaphy, and rectus sheath block following umbilical herniorrhaphy. Additional techniques that have been used most commonly in the adult population, but are now finding their way into the pediatric population, include lumbar paravertebral blocks for analgesia following renal surgery and the transversus abdominis block for analgesia following lower abdominal procedures. In the past, analgesia following many of these procedures was most commonly accomplished with the use of a epidural block at the caudal, lumbar, or thoracic level; however, given the data demonstrating efficacy and lower risk of adverse events with peripheral nerve block versus caudal epidural block,[1] it is likely that there will be an increasing use of peripheral nerve block of the lower extremity. Additionally, the blocks of the thorax, trunk, and abdomen, which are described in this chapter, also have the advantage of providing unilateral block, thereby eliminating the adverse effects associated with bilateral epidural block.

Transversus Abdominis Block

Background and Indications: The lateral abdominal wall contains three muscle layers, including the external oblique, internal oblique, and transversus abdominis muscles and their associated fascial sheaths. The lower thoracic and upper lumbar nerves provide sensory innervation of the skin, muscles, and parietal peritoneum of the anterior abdominal wall. These nerves course in a plane between the transversus abdominis and internal oblique muscles. Given the anatomic localization of these nerves, McDonnell et al[2-5] described a unique approach that allows for block of these nerves with the administration of local anesthetic agents in the plane between the transversus abdominis and internal oblique muscles with a single injection administered in the triangle of Petit. The triangle of Petit is bounded posteriorly by the latissimus dorsi muscle, anteriorly by the external oblique muscle, and inferiorly by the iliac crest. In clinical practice, the transversus abdominis plane (TAP) block is placed by using an ultrasound-guided technique, with the ultrasound probe placed in the axial plane just above the iliac crest. A needle is inserted in-line with the probe so that it can be demonstrated that the needle lies in the correct fascial plane prior to injection of the local anesthetic solution. The potential utility of the TAP block has been demonstrated by

McDonnell et al[3] in a cadaveric and radiological evaluation. Using a double-pop or loss-of-resistance technique with a blunt block needle in a cadaver model, the authors demonstrated that methylene blue dye could be injected between the transversus abdominis and internal oblique muscles. The correct anatomic location of the dye was demonstrated by dissection of the cadaver specimen. This was followed by the demonstration of radiopaque dye in the correct fascial plane using computed tomography and magnetic resonance imaging in three healthy, adult volunteers.

In the adult population, the TAP block has been shown to provide effective analgesia following various types of lower abdominal procedures, including retropubic prostatectomy, cesarean section, and total abdominal hysterectomy.[2,4–6] In a prospective, randomized trial of 50 adults following cesarean delivery, TAP block with 0.2 mL/kg of 0.75% ropivacaine on each side resulted in decreased postoperative-pain scores, delayed request for postoperative analgesia, and decreased morphine use during the initial 48 postoperative hours.[5] The median time to first request for postoperative analgesia was 90 minutes in the control group and 220 minutes in patients who received a TAP block. Morphine use during the initial 48-hour postoperative period was decreased by 70% in patients who received a TAP block (66 ± 26 mg in control patients versus 18 ± 14 mg in patients who received a TAP block, $p < 0.001$). The same investigators evaluated the efficacy of the TAP block following total abdominal hysterectomy in 50 women.[5] After anesthetic induction and prior to surgical incision, a bilateral TAP block was placed using 0.2 mL/kg of 0.75% ropivacaine on each side. Patients who received a TAP block had decreased postoperative-pain scores, delayed request for postoperative analgesia, and decreased morphine use during the initial 48 postoperative hours (55 ± 17 mg in control patients vs. 27 ± 20 mg in patients who received a TAP block, $p < 0.001$).

To date, there are limited data regarding the use of TAP block in infants and children.[7–9] Mukhtar and Singh reported the successful use of TAP block to provide analgesia following laparoscopic appendectomy in four patients, 14 to 17 years of age. A bilateral TAP block was placed using 20 mL of 0.25% bupivacaine per side with ultrasound guidance. No patient required supplemental analgesic agents for the initial 12 postoperative hours, with pain scores ranging from 0 to 2. Two patients required no analgesic agents during their postoperative course. Unilateral TAP block has also been shown to provide effective analgesia for inguinal hernia repair in a cohort of eight children, whereas anecdotal success demonstrated the efficacy of a TAP block in a 3.6-kg infant with vertebral, anal, cardiovascular, tracheoesophageal, esophageal, renal or radial, and limb anomalies (VACTERL) syndrome undergoing colostomy placement on day 2 of life.[8,9] In the latter case, the TAP block was chosen instead of caudal epidural blockade because of associated vertebral anomalies. We have reported successful preliminary experience with the TAP block following various surgical procedures involving the umbilicus and lower abdomen in a cohort of 10 pediatric patients, with ages ranging from 10 months to 8 years.[10] Effective postoperative analgesia was achieved in 8 of the 10 patients. The adult and pediatric data suggest that a TAP block can be used for major open abdominal surgeries involving the umbilicus and lower abdominal area. The procedure is also useful for open appendectomies, colostomy placement, transverse lower abdominal incisions (bladder and ureteral surgery), as well as for covering the access ports for various types of laparoscopic procedures.

 Patient Position: Supine.

 Transducer: 25- or 35-mm linear transducer oscillating at 8 to 13 MHz.

 Transducer Orientation: Transverse, between the ribs and iliac crest in the triangle of Petit at the midaxillary line.

Needle: 24-gauge, 2.5-cm or 22-gauge, 5-cm blunt needle; 18-gauge Tuohy needle for continuous techniques

 Local Anesthetic: 0.1 to 0.2 mL/kg of 0.2% ropivacaine or 0.25% bupivacaine. Epinephrine in a concentration of 1:200,000 is added to the solution.

 Technique: The skin between the iliac crest and the lower margin of the 12th rib over the triangle of Petit in the midaxillary line is washed, and sterile gel is applied. A 25- or 35-mm linear transducer oscillating at 10 to 13 MHz is oriented in the transverse plane. The external oblique, internal oblique, and transversus abdominis muscles are identified. The bowel can be seen immediately below the transversus abdominis muscle. For surgeries of the upper abdominal wall, the probe is moved cephalad and anteriorly until it is immediately below the costal margin. The needle is inserted posterior or anterior to the probe. For lower abdominal surgeries, the probe is placed immediately above the iliac crest. The needle is inserted in-line and anterior to the end of the ultrasound probe. The needle is directed to the fascial plane between the internal oblique and transversus abdominis muscles (Figs. 29-1 through 29-3). Once the proper plane has been entered, the local anesthetic is injected in divided doses. The procedure is repeated on the opposite side for midline or bilateral incisions. A catheter may be inserted after the plane between the muscles has been dilated.

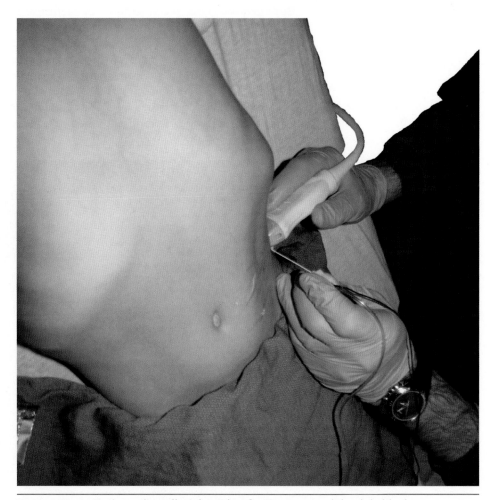

Figure 29-1. Probe and needle orientation for transversus abdominis block.

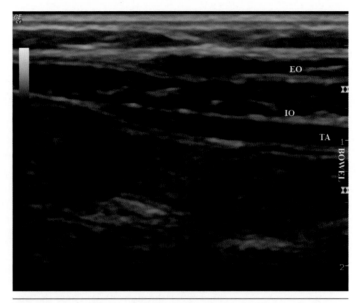

Figure 29-2. Ultrasound scan. EO, external oblique muscle; IO, internal oblique muscle; TA, transversus abdominis muscle.

Rectus Abdominis (Paraumbilical or Rectus Sheath) Block

Background and Indications: An alternative to analgesia for surgery around the umbilical area is the rectus abdominis block, otherwise known as the paraumbilical block or rectus sheath block.[11,12] The umbilical area is innervated by the right and left thoracoabdominal intercostal nerves, which are derived from the anterior rami of spinal roots T8-T12. These nerves travel in the plane between the internal oblique and transversus abdominis muscles. The transversus abdominis muscle ends in a tendon sheath that forms the posterior wall of the rectus sheath, which runs posterior to the rectus abdominis muscle. The anterior wall of the rectus sheath is formed by the merger of the tendons of the internal and

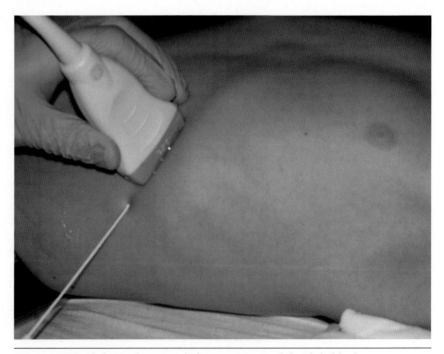

Figure 29-3. Subcostal approach for transversus abdominis block.

external oblique muscles. The anterior and posterior walls of the rectus sheath encase the rectus abdominis muscle starting at the linea alba laterally and joining in the midline of the abdomen into a single sheath. The intercostal nerves travel in the space behind the rectus abdominis muscle and posterior wall of the rectus sheath. The nerves perforate the sheath near the midline of the abdomen after traveling behind the rectus abdominis muscle. They end at the anterior cutaneous branch supplying the area around the midline of the abdomen. Alternatively, the anterior cutaneous branch arises before the rectus abdominis muscle and travels over the top of the muscle in the subcutaneous space. Given this anatomy, these nerves can be blocked by the placement of local anesthetic agent above and behind the rectus abdominis muscle.

 Patient Position: Supine.

 Transducer: 25- or 35-mm linear transducer oscillating at 8 to 13 MHz.

 Transducer Orientation: Transverse, lateral to the midline.

 Needle: 24-gauge, 2.5-cm or 22-gauge, 5-cm blunt needle; 18-gauge, Tuohy needle for continuous techniques.

 Local Anesthetic: 0.1 to 0.2 mL/kg of 0.2% ropivacaine or 0.25% bupivacaine. Epinephrine in a concentration of 1:200,000 is added to the solution.

 Technique: The skin over the umbilicus is washed, and sterile gel is placed medial and lateral to the umbilicus. The ultrasound probe, oscillating at 10 to 13 MHz, is placed in an axial orientation 2 to 5 cm lateral to the midline and slightly above the level of the umbilicus. Using ultrasound, the anterior and posterior borders of the rectus sheath are identified. Note that the peritoneum and bowel are immediately below the posterior boundary of the posterior rectus sheath. The needle is inserted in-line at the lateral end of the probe (Figs. 29-4 and 29-5). Note that the needle will pass through the rectus abdominis muscle during performance of this block. The needle is directed to the edge of

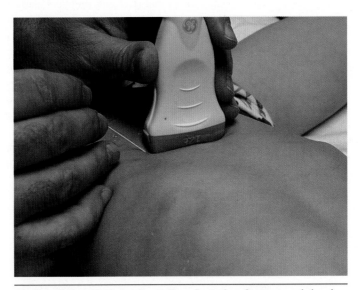

Figure 29-4. Probe and needle orientation for rectus abdominis block.

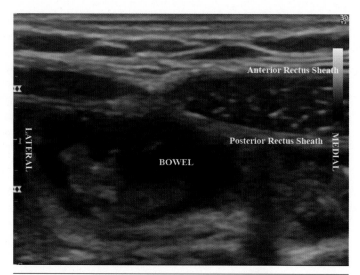

Figure 29-5. Ultrasound scan of rectus abdominis. *RA*, rectus abdominis muscle; *TS*, tendonous sheath; *B*, bowel.

the sheath, and the local anesthetic is deposited between the posterior rectus sheath and posterior border of the rectus abdominis muscle. Half of the local anesthetic is placed posterior to the muscle, whereas the other half is placed anteriorly. Alternatively, the entire volume can be placed behind the rectus abdominis muscle because it will generally spread in the space and cover the muscle anteriorly and posteriorly. The procedure is repeated on the contralateral side.

Ilioinguinal and Iliohypogastric Block

Background and Indications: Ilioinguinal and iliohypogastric (IL–IH) nerve block provides analgesia to the inguinal area for inguinal hernia repair, orchiopexy, and hydrocelectomy. This block has been shown to be equally as effective as a caudal block for these procedures.[13–15] However, the IL–IH block cannot be used as the sole anesthetic, instead of general anesthesia, for groin surgery because the stress response and visceral pain from peritoneal traction and manipulation of the spermatic cord are not covered by an IL–IH block. The ilioinguinal (L1) and iliohypogastric (T12 and L1) nerves originate from the lumbar plexus and provide innervation to the scrotum and inner thigh. The roots travel in the space between the iliacus and psoas muscle. More distally along their course, these nerves pierce the transversus abdominis muscle near the anterior superior iliac spine (ASIS) and travel in the plane between the tranversus abdominis and internal oblique muscles. Complications fro m IL–IH block are rare; however, there have been reports of colonic and small-bowel puncture when these blocks are placed blindly without ultrasound guidance. An IL–IH block may also result in motor block of the quadriceps muscle if the local anesthetic solution is placed below the inguinal ligament. Weintraud et al[16] demonstrated that when the IL–IH block is placed blindly, the local anesthetic is placed in the correct location only 14% of the time. Willschke et al[17] demonstrated that when using ultrasound guidance, the effective volume can be reduced to 0.075 mL/kg.

Patient Position: Supine.

Transducer: 25- or 35-mm linear probe oscillating at 13 MHz.

Transducer Orientation: Transverse oblique.

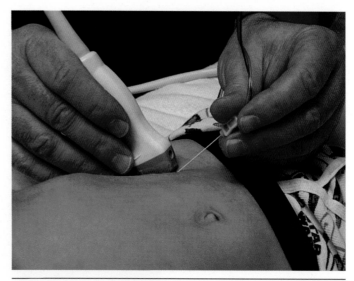

Figure 29-6. Transducer and needle position for ilioinguinal and iliohypogastric nerve block.

 Needle: 24-gauge, 2.5-cm or 22-gauge, 5-cm blunt or insulated needle.

 Local Anesthetic: 0.1 to 0.15 mL/kg of 0.2% ropivacaine or 0.25% bupivacaine with epinephrine 1:200,000.

 Technique: The skin lateral to the ASIS is washed, and sterile gel is applied. The ultrasound probe oscillating at 13 MHz is placed immediately lateral to and slightly above the ASIS. The plane between the transversus abdominis and internal oblique muscles is identified. In larger children, it may be possible to identify the nerves as deep to the internal oblique muscles. The nerves are close beside each other and often have an "owl's eyes" appearance. The needle is inserted in-line at the medial or lateral end of the probe and directed toward the nerves (Figs. 29-6 and 29-7). The local anesthetic agent is injected around the nerves. If the nerves cannot be readily identified, local anesthetic can be infiltrated between the internal oblique and transversus abdominis muscles. Because of the anatomic variation, the nerves may be found between the external and internal oblique muscles (Fig. 29-8). For this reason, some practitioners inject local anesthetic in the plane between the external and internal oblique as well as the plane between the internal oblique and transversus abdominis muscles.

Intercostal Blockade

Background and Indications: Intercostal nerve block may be useful for providing analgesia after thoracotomy, upper abdominal procedures, rib fractures, or for chest-tube pain. For these indications, intercostal block may be used either in the perioperative arena or in an emergency-room or intensive care unit (ICU) setting. Intercostal blocks are not effective for intraperitoneal procedures because they do not block the celiac plexus. The intercostal nerves arise paravertebrally from the thoracic spinal nerves (T1-T12) and may be blocked in their position between the intercostal muscles in a groove that is found underneath the corresponding rib and shared with the intercostal vessels. Gray and white rami communicantes branch off from the spinal nerves before entering the intercostal space and adjoin the sympathetic ganglia to form the thoracic sympathetic chain. A second branch, the posterior cutaneous nerve, travels posteriorly, innervating the paraspinous musculature.

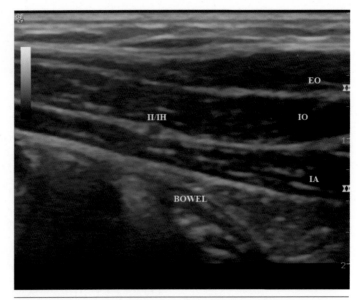

Figure 29-7. Ultrasound scan of ilioinguinal and iliohypogastric nerve between the internal oblique and transversus abdominis muscles. *IL–IH*, ilioinguinal and iliohypogastric nerves; *IO*, internal oblique muscle; *EO*, external oblique; *TA*, transversus abdominis muscle; *B*, bowel.

Although an intercostal block may be performed at any location along the lower border of the rib, an approach to the intercostal space at the posterior axillary line will provide adequate analgesia for thoracotomy, is relatively simple to perform, and is the most common approach. A more anterior approach can be used for midline procedures such as open pectus excavatum repair or sternotomy. The patient can either be in supine or sitting position. Given the cross innervation of the various interspaces, the block should be performed at the interspace of the surgical incision or injury and two interspaces above and below. Complications of intercostal

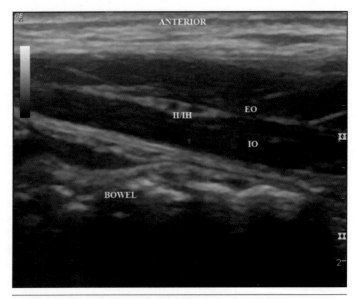

Figure 29-8. Ilioinguinal and iliohypogastric nerves between internal and external oblique muscles. *IL–IH*, ilioinguinal and iliohypogastric nerves; *EO*, external oblique; *IO*, internal oblique; *B*, bowel.

block include pneumothorax, vascular puncture, and epidural or spinal local anesthetic spread. This complication is rare and is more common in the posterior approach compared to more anterior approaches. Another complication that must be considered during intercostal nerve block is the risk of local anesthetic toxicity. Because of the proximity of vessels to the intercostal nerves, there may be increased risk of local anesthetic toxicity from systemic uptake or vascular puncture compared to other peripheral nerve blocks. In fact, the peak blood concentration of the local anesthetic agent is second only to interpleural analgesia when considering the various regional anesthetic techniques performed in anesthetic practice.

Anterior Intercostal Block

Background and Indications: The nerves to the sternum take origin from the roots of T1-T6. After exiting the lateral spinous foramina, the nerves travel in the space between the internal and innermost intercostal muscles along with the intercostal artery and vein below the inferior edge of the rib. Anterior intercostal block is most useful for analgesia after pectus excavatum repair.

Patient Position: Supine.

Transducer: 25-mm linear array oscillating at 13 MHz.

Needle: 24-gauge, 2.5-cm or 22-gauge, 5-cm blunt needle.

Local Anesthetic: Total dose of 0.2 to 0.5 mL/kg of 0.2% ropivacaine or 0.25% bupivacaine with epinephrine 1:200,000 divided in the various interspaces.

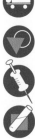

Technique: The skin is washed, and sterile gel is applied. A 25-mm linear probe oscillating at 13 MHz is initially applied in the sagittal plane several centimeters lateral to the expected site of the pectus repair. The ribs are imaged as bright hyperechoic structures. Between the ribs, the pleura appears as hyperechoic streaks approximately 2 to 10 mm deep to the anterior surface of the rib. The probe is then rotated so that it is aligned along the rib. By toggling the probe, the pleura and intercostal muscles can be seen (Figs. 29-9 through 29-11). The needle is inserted in-line at the lateral end of the probe and directed to the plane between the internal and innermost intercostal muscles at the lower border of the rib. Once the proper plane has been entered, the local anesthetic is injected. The block must be repeated at several levels and on the contralateral side.

Posterior Intercostal Block

Background and Indications: The nerves to the thorax and upper abdominal wall arise from nerve roots T1-T12. After exiting the lateral spinous foramina, the nerves travel in the space between the internal and innermost intercostal muscles along with the intercostal artery and vein. Posterior intercostal block can be used for analgesia after thoracotomy or sternotomy.

Patient Position: Prone or sitting.

Transducer: 25-mm linear array oscillating at 13 MHz.

Needle: 24-gauge, 2.5-cm or 22-gauge, 5-cm blunt needle; 18-gauge insulated Tuohy needle for catheter techniques.

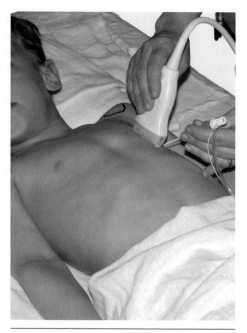

Figure 29-9. Needle and probe position for anterior intercostal block.

 Local Anesthetic: Total dose of 0.2 to 0.5 mL/kg of 0.2% ropivacaine or 0.25% bupivacaine with epinephrine 1:200,000 divided in the various interspaces.

 Technique: Depending on the size of the patient and whether they are anesthetized, the patient can be placed in supine, prone, or sitting position. The block can be placed at the posterior axillary line if the patient is in supine position or more centrally if the patient is in sitting or prone position. The skin is washed, and sterile ultrasound gel is applied. The ultrasound transducer is initially oriented in the sagittal plane, and the rib and pleura are identified. The transducer is then rotated so that it is along the long axis of the rib. In this orientation, rotating

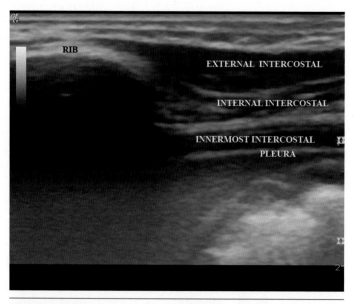

Figure 29-10. *R*, rib; *EC*, external intercostal muscle; *P*, pleura.

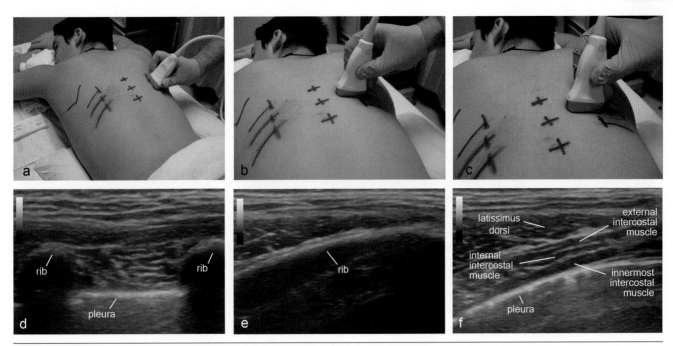

Figure 29-11. Probe position for posterior intercostal block.

the transducer back and forth allows the practitioner to identify the rib and pleura. When the patient breathes, the visceral and parietal pleura can usually be identified as they slide past each other. In thin patients, the fascia between the intercostal muscles can also be identified (Figs. 29-11 and 29-12). After sterile preparation, the needle (length dependent on the size of the child) is inserted through the skin, immediately below the lower border of the rib. The needle is introduced at the lateral border of the transducer using an in-plane approach. The

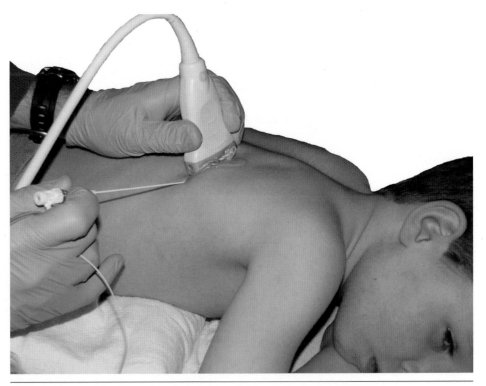

Figure 29-12. Needle and probe position for posterior intercostal block.

needle is then advanced until it lies approximately 2 mm superficial to the pleura. A small amount of local anesthetic is injected. If a tissue plane appears, this is the plane between the internal and innermost intercostal muscles. Once this plane has been identified, the total dose of local anesthetic for that interspace can be injected. At the conclusion of this injection, a catheter may be inserted 2 to 3 cm beyond the end of the needle if a continuous block is desired. If radiopaque dye is injected through the catheter, and a chest x-ray is obtained, then the dye usually spreads in a spindle-like pattern in the paravertebral space.

Paravertebral Block

Background and Indications: Thoracic paravertebral nerve block can provide perioperative analgesia for unilateral procedures, including thoracotomy, upper abdominal surgery, and renal surgery. The advantages to paravertebral block include the ability to provide unilateral analgesia without adverse effects, which may be associated with central neuraxial techniques.[18–20] Continuous paravertebral block has been shown to be superior to epidural anesthesia for unilateral renal surgery and may also be used for analgesia during inguinal surgery in children.[21,22] The paravertebral space is a wedge-shaped space along the vertebral column that is bound by parietal pleura, superior costotransverse ligament, and intercostal membrane. It contains the intercostal nerve and dorsal ramus, rami communicantes, and sympathetic chain. There is free communication between adjacent levels of the paravertebral space, making it possible to achieve multiple levels of analgesia with the use of a continuous catheter technique or a single injection. The exception to the free communication is at the level of T12 wherein the insertion of the psoas muscle may inhibit flow to the lumbar areas of the paravertebral space. This anatomical variant mandates a two-injection technique for inguinal procedures, one above and the other below the level of T12. Complications from paravertebral block in children are rare, but may include vascular puncture, pleural puncture, and pneumothorax. In older children or adults, hypotension may also occur from sympathectomy.

Patient Position: Lateral.

Transducer: 25- or 35-mm linear array oscillating at 8 to 13 MHz.

Needle: 22-gauge, 5-cm or 21-gauge, 10-cm blunt needle; 18-gauge Tuohy needle for continuous techniques.

Local Anesthetic: Total dose of 0.3 to 0.5 mL/kg of 0.2% ropivacaine or 0.25% bupivacaine with epinephrine 1:200,000.

Technique: The skin is washed, and sterile ultrasound gel is applied. The transducer is initially placed in the midline, along the back and the spinous processes identified. It is then moved slightly laterally to identify the transverse processes. Slight angulation (toggling) of the tip of the probe back to the midline allows the identification of the superior costotransverse ligament, and thereby, will guide the depth of needle insertion (Figs. 29-13 and 29-14).

The spinous process of the desired primary dermatome to be blocked is identified. The point of needle insertion is lateral to the midline across this spinous process, at a distance that is approximately equal to the distance from spinous process to spinous process. Alternatively, the approximate lateral distance in millimeters from the spinous process to the point of needle insertion is $(0.12 \times \text{body weight in kilogram}) + 10.2$.[23] After sterile preparation and draping, the needle is inserted and advanced using a loss-of-resistance technique to saline. With the needle perpendicular to the skin, the transverse process of the lamina is contacted, and the needle is then walked over the cephalad margin of this process. The approximate depth

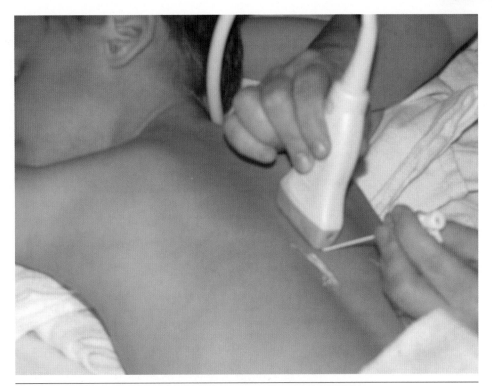

Figure 29-13. Needle and probe position for paravertebral block.

from the skin to the paravertebral space in millimeters is (0.48 × body weight in kilogram) + 18.7. As the transverse process is passed, there should be a light loss of resistance felt as entry into the paravertebral space is gained. Local anesthetic may be injected after negative aspiration for blood or cerebrospinal fluid, and a catheter is threaded if desired. In infants and children, only 2 to 4 cm of the catheter should be threaded into the paravertebral space to avoid placing the tip laterally into an intercostal space, which would result in analgesia of a single dermatome. If radiopaque dye is injected through the catheter and a chest x-ray is obtained, the catheter can be seen in the paravertebral space.

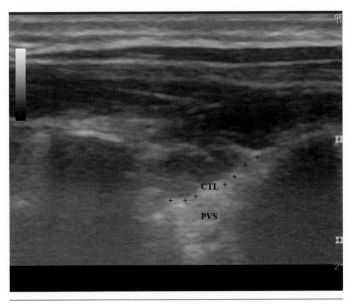

Figure 29-14. *TP*, transverse process; *CT*, costotransverse ligament.

References

1. Giaufre E, Dalens B, Gombert A. Epidemiology and morbidity of regional anesthesia in children: a one-year prospective survey of the French-language society of pediatric anesthesiologists. Anesth Analg 1996;83:904–912.
2. O'Donnell BD, McDonnell JG, McShane AJ. The transversus abdominis plane (TAP) block in open retropubic prostatectomy. Reg Anesth Pain Med 2006;31:91.
3. McDonnell JG, O'Donnell BD, Farrell T, et al. Transversus abdominis plane block: a cadaveric and radiological evaluation. Reg Anesth Pain Med 2007;32:399–404.
4. McDonnell JG, O'Donnell BD, Curley G, et al. Analgesic efficacy of transversus abdominis plane block after abdominal surgery: a prospective, randomized controlled trial. Anesth Analg 2007;104;193–197.
5. McDonnell JG, Curley G, Carney J, et al. The analgesic efficacy of transversus abdominis plane block after cesarean delivery: a randomized controlled trial. Anesth Analg 2008;106:186–191.
6. Carney J, McDonnell JG, Ochana A, et al. The transversus abdominis plane block provides effective postoperative analgesia in patients undergoing total abdominal hysterectomy. Anesth Analg 2008;107:2056–2060.
7. Mukhtar K, Singh S. Transversus abdominis plane block for laparoscopic surgery. Br J Anaesth 2008;102:143–144.
8. Frederickson M, Seal P, Houghton J. Early experience with the transversus abdominis plane block in children. Pediatr Anesth 2008;18:891–892.
9. Hardy CA. Transverse abdominis plane block in neonates: is it a good alternative to caudal anesthesia for postoperative analgesia following abdominal surgery? Pediatr Anaesth 2009;19:56.
10. Tobias JD. Preliminary experience with transversus abdominis plane block for postoperative pain relief in infants and children. Saudi J Anesth 2009;3:2–6.
11. Ferguson S, Thomas V, Lewis I. The rectus sheath block in paediatric anaesthesia: new indications for an old technique. Paediatr Anaesth 1996;463–466.
12. Courreges P, Poddevin F, Lecoutre D. Para-umbilical block: a new concept for regional anaesthesia in children. Paediatr Anaesth 1997;7:211–214.
13. Hannallah RS, Broadman LM, Belman AB, et al. Comparison of caudal and ilioinguinal/iliohypgastric nerve blocks for control of post-orchiopexy pain in pediatric ambulatory surgery. Anesthesiology 1987;66:832–834.
14. Casey WF, Rice LJ, Hannallah RS, et al. A comparison between bupivacaine instillation versus ilio-inguinal/iliohypogastric nerve block for postoperative analgesia following inguinal herniorrhaphy in children. Anesthesiology 1990;72:637–639.
15. Fisher QA, McComiskey CM, Hill JL, et al. Postoperative voiding interval and duration of analgesia following peripheral or caudal nerve blocks in children. Anesth Analg 1993;76:173–177.
16. Weintraud M, Marhofer P, Boenberg A, et al. Ilioinguinal/iliohypogastric blocks in children: where do we administer the local anesthetic without direct visualization? Anesth Analg 2008;106:89–93.
17. Willschke H, Bosenberg A, Marhofer P, et al. Ultrasonographic-guided ilioinguinal/iliohypogastric nerve block in pediatric anesthesia: what is the optimal volume? Anesth Analg 2006;102:1680–1684.
18. Lönnqvist PA. Continuous paravertebral block in children: initial experience. Anaesthesia 1992;47:607–611.
19. Lönnqvist PA, MacKenzie J, Soni AK, et al. Paravertebral blockade. Failure rate and complications. Anaesthesia 1995;50:813–815.
20. Lönnqvist PA, Olsson GL. Paravertebral vs epidural block in children. Effects on postoperative morphine requirements after renal surgery. Acta Anesthesiol Scand 1994;38:346–349.
21. Naja ZM, Raf M, El Rajab-M, et al. Nerve stimulator-guided paravertebral blockade combined with sevoflurane sedation versus general anesthesia with systemic analgesia for post-herniorrhaphy pain relief in children. Anesthesiology 2005;103:600–605.
22. Naja ZM, Raf M, El-Rajab M, et al. A comparison of nerve stimulator guided paravertebral block and ilio-inguinal nerve block for analgesia after inguinal herniorrphaphy in children. Anaesthesia 2006;61:1064–1068.
23. Lönnqvist PA, Hesser U. Location of the paravertebral space in children and adolescents in relation to surface anatomy assessed by computed tomography. Paediatr Anaesth 1992;2:285–289.

30

Ultrasound-Guided Lower Extremity Block in Children

JOSEPH D. TOBIAS, STEFAN LUCAS, GIOVANNI CUCCHIARO, PAUL E. BIGELEISEN

Introduction: Depending on the site of injury and the nerves that need to be anesthetized, there are several approaches for regional anesthesia of the lower extremity that are applicable to the pediatric population. These techniques may be used for procedures on the foot and ankle, such as club foot repair or tendon lengthening of the lower aspect of the lower extremity, or for major procedures on the femur and hip, such as the treatment of traumatic femoral fractures or open reduction and internal fixation of the hip because of traumatic or congenital conditions.[1-4] In addition to their use for postoperative analgesia, isolated block of the lower extremity may be used, instead of anesthesia, in patients with comorbid diseases, which may increase the risk of general anesthesia, such as patients with undiagnosed myopathy.[5-8] In these patients, muscle biopsy can generally be accomplished with a 3-in-1 block or a fascia iliaca block. Alternatively, there are also isolated case reports of the use of regional anesthesia to induce sympathectomy in the lower extremity for the treatment of vascular compromise of various etiologies.[9] In the past, analgesia following lower extremity procedures was most commonly accomplished with the use of a caudal epidural block; however, given data demonstrating efficacy and lower risk of adverse events with peripheral nerve blockade versus caudal epidural block,[10] it is likely that there will be an increasing use of peripheral nerve blockade of the lower extremity. This process will be facilitated by the use of ultrasound guidance in such techniques. As with upper extremity techniques, these regional blocks may be performed as a single-shot approach, or alternatively, a catheter may be placed to allow for repeated dosing or continuous infusion.

Lumbar Plexus Block

Background and Indications: The sensory and motor innervation of the lower extremity is derived from the lumbar and sacral plexuses. The lumbar plexus is formed by the union of the anterior rami of the first 4 lumbar nerves (L1-L4) with variable input from the 12th thoracic nerve (T12) and L5. The lumbar plexus lies in the "psoas compartment" in the paravertebral space. The anterior border of this compartment is formed by the psoas major muscle and the posterior border is formed by the quadratus lumborum/erector spinae muscles (Fig. 30-1). In many cases, the lumbar plexus lies within the psoas muscle. As the lumbar plexus emerges from psoas compartment, it divides into the three nerves that innervate the anterior portion of the upper aspect of the lower extremity: (a) the femoral, (b) the lateral femoral cutaneous, and (c) the obturator nerve. The femoral nerve provides sensory innervation to the anterior and medial aspects of the thigh and motor innervation to the quadriceps muscles (Fig. 30-2). The lateral femoral cutaneous nerve is purely sensory, providing sensory innervation to the lateral aspect of the thigh. It braches from the lumbar plexus and enters the thigh deep to the inguinal ligament, medial to the anterior superior iliac spine. The obturator nerve provides motor innervation to the adductors of the leg as well as sensory innervation to part of the medial aspect of the lower portion of the

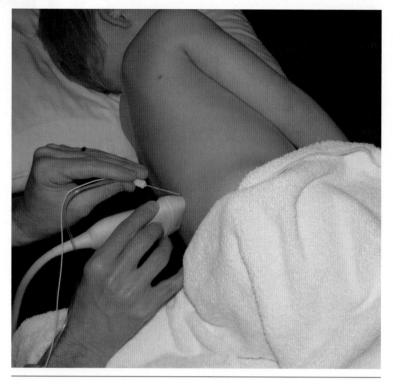

Figure 30-1a. Needle and probe position for transverse lumbar plexus block.

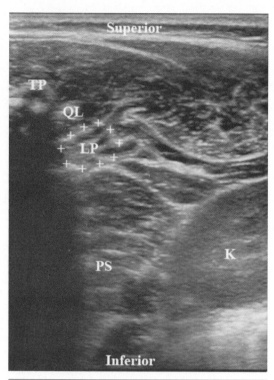

Figure 30-1b. Transverse ultrasound scan. *QL,* quadratus lumborum muscle; *PS,* psoas muscle; *NP,* nerve plexus; *K,* kidney.

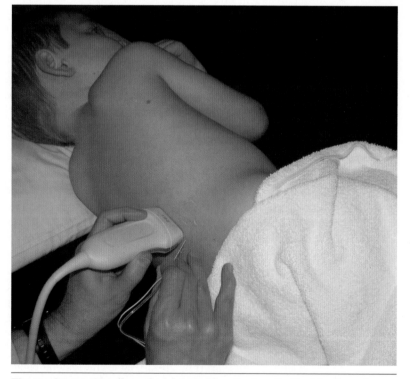

Figure 30-1c. Needle and probe position for longitudinal lumbar plexus block.

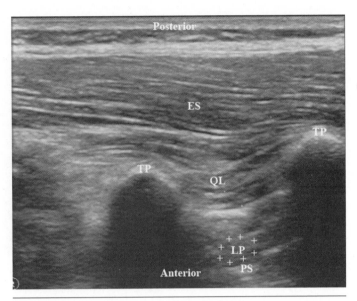

Figure 30-1d. Longitudinal ultrasound; *TP*, transverse process; *QM*, quatrautus lumborum muscle; *PM*, psoas muscle; *NP*, nerve plexus.

thigh. The obturator nerve also innervates the knee joint, making it necessary to anesthetize it to achieve analgesia following procedures involving the knee.

The most central approach to the lumbar plexus is direct block at the lumbar plexus. The technique provides anesthesia of the three nerves of the lumbar plexus (femoral, lateral femoral cutaneous, and obturator) with a single injection (also known as the "psoas

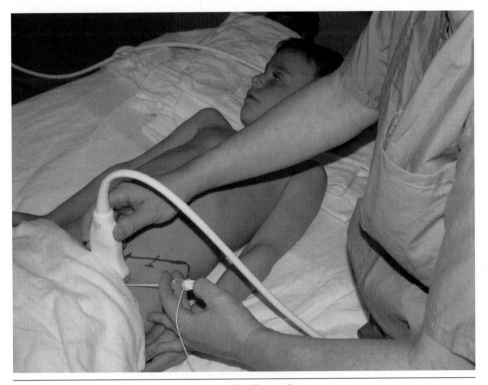

Figure 30-2a. Needle and probe position for femoral nerve.

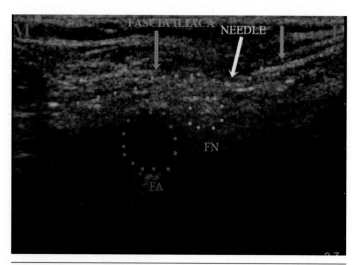

Figure 30-2b. *M*, medial; *L*, lateral; *FV*, femoral vein; *FA*, femoral artery; *FN*, femoral nerve.

compartment block.") As the lumbar and sacral plexuses lie in the same anatomic planes, variable analgesia of the sacral plexus occurs, making it suitable for femoral osteotomies as well as surgical procedures of the hip. Sacral plexus anesthesia is not achieved with other approaches to the lumbar plexus such as the 3-in-1 or fascia iliaca block of the femoral nerve. Dalens et al compared two techniques of lumbar plexus block in a prospective study in a cohort of 50 children.[11] The technique included either a modification of that described by Chayen (group 1) or Winnie (group 2).[12,13] The local anesthetic included a combination of equal volumes of 0.5% bupivacaine and etidocaine 1% with epinephrine 1:200,000. Dosing was based on weight: 0.75 mL/kg up to 20 kg, 20 mL for 20 to 30 kg, and 25 mL for 30 to 55 kg. In group 1, the needle was inserted at a 90-degree angle to the skin at the midpoint of a line connecting the spinous process of the 5th lumbar vertebra and the posterior superior iliac spine (PSIS). In group 2, the site of needle insertion was at the intersection of the intercristal line with a line drawn through the PSIS and parallel to the spinous processes. In group 1, difficulties inserting the needle were noted in 7 of 25 cases so that the needle had to be inserted more medially in 2 cases and more laterally in 5. In group 2, no difficulties were encountered with needle insertion. Success rates were comparable between the two groups (96% in group 1 and 100% with group 2); however, the authors noted a significant difference in the sensory distribution with the techniques. Additionally, the depth of needle insertion was greater (by 6–10 mm) in group 2 versus group 1. In group 1, the sensory involvement included only the lumbar plexus in 2 patients whereas 23 patients had bilateral blockade indicative of epidural spread of the local anesthetic. This was confirmed by dye study demonstrating spread into the epidural space. Conversely, in group 2, the sensory distribution included the lumbar and sacral plexus in 23 and the lumbar plexus in 2. The authors concluded that both techniques provided effective postoperative analgesia with the caveat that the technique described by Chayen et al was more of an epidural technique. Although there are limited data in the pediatric population, the lumbar plexus analgesia can be used following major orthopedic surgical procedures of the hip or upper femur. In our experience, we have advocated a slightly more medial approach to needle insertion than that described in the adult population (Fig. 30-2). As with the techniques of Winnie and Chayen, a line is drawn through the PSIS, parallel to the spine. A second line is drawn connecting the two iliac crests (the intercristal line). The point of intersection of these two lines is identified and the needle is moved slightly (1–2 cm) medially along the intercristal line. The needle is inserted at a 90-degree angle to the skin and advanced using a nerve stimulator. As the psoas compartment is entered, a loss of resistance is felt, and a muscle response in the quadriceps muscle will be obtained. During needle insertion, if the transverse process is contacted, the needle is walked off the transverse process in either a caudad or cephalad direction.

Patient Position: Lateral decubitus with knees and hip flexed as feasible.

Transducer: 35-mm linear array oscillating at 13 MHz (small patients), curved 11-mm probe oscillating at 5 to 10 MHz (larger patients).

Transducer Orientation: Transverse, just below the site of needle insertion.

Needle: 21-gauge, 10-cm blunt needle; 18-gauge insulated Tuohy needle for continuous infusion.

Local Anesthetic Agent: 0.25% bupivacaine or 0.2% ropivacaine (analgesia), 0.5% concentration for profound motor block. Volume is 0.2 to 0.4 mL/kg, total dose ≤3 mg/kg. Epinephrine (1:200,000) is added to bupivacaine.

Technique: For use of ultrasound to guide the lumbar plexus block, sterile preparation of the skin is performed and sterile ultrasound gel is placed over the skin below the inguinal ligament. The ultrasound probe is placed in a transverse position and the needle is inserted superior to the probe using an in-line approach. The bony elements of the vertebral body and the muscles that border the psoas compartment (the quadratus lumborum/erector spinae and the psoas major muscles) are identified (Fig. 30-1). The kidney can usually be identified superior (cephalad) to the psoas muscle. In many cases, the lumbar plexus can be visualized within the psoas major muscle or between the psoas and quadratus lumborum muscles. The needle is inserted and advanced until it pierces the quadratus lumborum/erector spinae muscles and enters the psoas compartment. Once the psoas compartment is entered, the ultrasound transducer can turned into a longitudinal plane to verify the location of the tip of the needle at the lumbar plexus if desired. Electrostimulation may also be used to confirm needle placement. Once the correct placement of the needle is confirmed, local anesthetic is injected until the plexus is surrounded.

Some practitioners prefer a longitudinal approach (Fig. 30-1). In this case, a parasagittal scan is obtained that identifies the transverse processes and quadratus lumborum and psoas muscles. In slim patients, the nerve plexus may also be identified. The needle is inserted in-line with the probe until the lumbar plexus compartment is entered. Needle position may be confirmed with electrostimulation. Once proper needle placement is confirmed, local anesthetic is injected until the nerve plexus is surrounded.

Femoral Nerve Block

Background and Indications: The femoral nerve is the largest branch of the lumbar plexus. It arises from the dorsal division of the anterior rami of L2-4 and descends into the pelvis lateral to the psoas major muscle where it passes deep to the inguinal ligament. In the anterior compartment of the thigh, the femoral nerve divides into multiple branches supplying the muscle, joints, and skin of the anterior thigh. The inguinal crease is generally several centimeters caudad to the inguinal ligament. Below the inguinal crease is the level at which the block is performed. At this level, the nerve lies deep to the fascia lata and the fascia iliaca and is separated from the femoral artery and vein by the iliopectineal ligament (Cooper's ligament). The anterior branch of the femoral nerve innervates the pectineus muscle and is responsible for thigh adduction on stimulation. The posterior branch innervates the quadriceps femoris muscles and provides leg extension and patellar elevation on stimulation. The superficial branch lies deep to the fascia lata and superior to the fascia iliaca. It provides contraction of the sartorius muscle on contraction. Because this branch lies above the fascia iliaca, it is not a suitable stimulation endpoint for femoral nerve block. The saphenous nerve is a cutaneous branch of the femoral nerve that supplies innervation to the skin over the medial aspect of the leg and foot. Block of the femoral nerve can be used to provide analgesia following surgical procedures on the anterior or lateral aspect of the thigh as well as traumatic femur fracture or following femoral osteotomies.[16]

There are two basic approaches described for femoral nerve blockade. The first involves direct blockade of the nerve just below the inguinal crease and lateral to the femoral artery. This technique can also be modified to provide what has been termed a 3-in-1 block or the inguinal perivascular approach whereby blockade of the femoral, lateral femoral cutaneous, and obturator nerve may be feasible (Fig. 30-2). As originally described, the theory behind the block is that the fascial sheath that surrounds the femoral nerve can be used as a conduit to carry local anesthetic centrally to the lumbar plexus. This is accomplished by the use of larger volume of local anesthetic than is used for isolated femoral nerve blockade as well as holding pressure distal to the site of injection. Aside from these two modifications, the technique for femoral nerve blockade is the same regardless of whether an isolated femoral nerve block or a 3-in-1 block is desired. An insulated needle with a nerve stimulator with detection of contraction of the quadriceps muscle or a blunt-tip needle with ultrasound guidance can be used. The needle is inserted lateral to the pulsation of the femoral artery, 1 to 2 cm below the inguinal ligament and advanced at a 45-degree angle with the skin, aiming in the cephalad direction. A double "pop" or loss of resistance can be felt as the fascia lata and fascia iliaca are penetrated.

The second approach to the femoral nerve is the fascia iliaca block. As the fascia iliaca extends lateral, it is possible to inject the local anesthetic solution more laterally and get spread medially to the femoral nerve and superiorly (centrally) to the obturator and lateral femoral cutaneous nerves. As this technique is performed away from the femoral nerve, a nerve stimulator is not used. The technique is the same as with femoral nerve block except that the point of needle entry is at the junction of the outer and middle third of the line connecting the symphysis pubis and the anterior superior iliac crest (Fig. 30-2). Dalens et al compared the fascia iliaca block with the 3-in-1 approach to the femoral nerve in 120 pediatric patients with age ranging from 0.7 to 17 years who were undergoing surgical procedures of the lower extremity.[14] A nerve stimulator was used to locate the femoral nerve during the 3-in-1 block. The local anesthetic agent included a mixture of 1% lidocaine and 0.5% bupivacaine with the dose based on body weight. Analgesia was effective in 90% of patients receiving a fascia iliaca block compared with only 20% of patients receiving a 3-in-1 block. Although the ability to achieve femoral nerve blockade was 60/60 with either technique, lateral femoral cutaneous and obturator sensory blockade were achieved in 9/60 and 8/60 patients with the 3-in-1 technique versus 55/60 and 53/60 patients with the fascia iliaca block. The difference in the success of these two techniques is that the ability of the local anesthetic solution to actually spread up the femoral nerve sheath to the lumbar plexus, and block the obturator nerve has been questioned by subsequent studies that evaluated cephalad spread with the 3-in-1 block using radiographic dye.

Femoral block at the inguinal crease:

 Patient Position: Supine.

 Transducer: 25-mm linear array oscillating at 13 MHz or 35-mm linear probe, oscillating at 8 to 13 MHz for larger patients.

 Transducer Orientation: Transverse, below the inguinal ligament.

Needle: 22- or 24-gauge, 2.5- or 5-cm, blunt needle for single-shot technique; 18-gauge insulated Tuohy needle for continuous block.

 Local Anesthetic: Analgesia, 0.25% bupivacaine or 0.2% ropivacaine, motor block 0.5% concentrations. Volume is 0.2 to 0.4 mL/kg, total dose ≤3 mg/kg. Epinephrine (1:200,000) is added to bupivacaine.

 Technique: For use of ultrasound to guide femoral nerve block, sterile preparation of the skin is performed, and sterile ultrasound gel is placed over the skin below the inguinal ligament. A high-frequency 10- to 13-MHz linear probe is placed transversely in the inguinal crease. The femoral artery is identified and the nerve is imaged lateral to the artery and deep to the fascia iliaca (Fig. 30-2). The nerve is of variable size and may be triangular in shape. The needle is inserted at the lateral end of the probe using an in-line technique. Once the fascia iliaca has been pierced, the local anesthetic is injected and observed to surround the nerve. If a fascia iliaca block is used, the point of needle insertion is more lateral (Fig. 30-3). A line is drawn connecting the anterior pubic tubercle and the anterior superior iliaca spine. The point of needle insertion is where the lateral one third of this line meets the medial two thirds. From this point, a line is drawn at a 90-degree angle to below the inguinal ligament. As the needle is inserted, a double loss of resistance may be felt as the fascia lata and fascia iliaca are penetrated. The use of ultrasound during needle placement allows visualization of the local anesthetic solution because it is injected deep to the fascia iliaca ligament and surrounds the femoral nerve.

Distal Block of the Femoral Nerve

The femoral nerve can also be blocked more distal at a point where it transitions into the saphenous nerve. This technique can be combined with a sciatic block at the knee (popliteal fossa block) to provide analgesia of the entire leg below the knee. At the level of the distal or mid-thigh, the saphenous nerve is located between the sartorius and gracilis muscles adjacent to the femoral or geniculate artery. A high-frequency probe is placed over the medial aspect

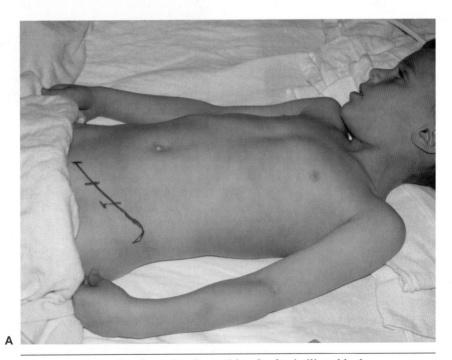

Figure 30-3a,b. Needle and probe position for fascia iliaca block.

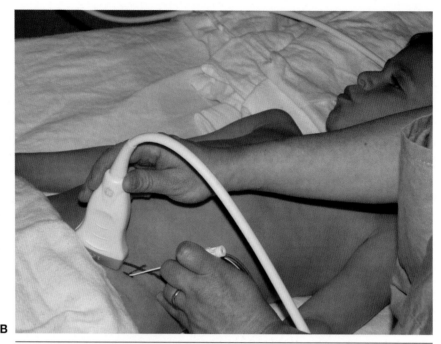

B

Figure 30-3b. *(continued).*

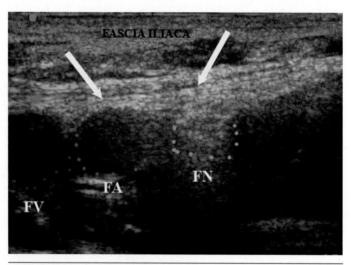

Figure 30-3c. *M*, medial; *L*, lateral; *FV*, femoral vein; *FA*, femoral artery; *FN*, femoral nerve.

of the thigh in a transverse orientation. Once the nerve has been located, the needle is inserted at the lateral aspect of the probe using an in-line approach (Fig. 30-4). A 2 to 3 mL of local anesthetic solution is injected until the nerve is surrounded. In smaller patients, given the size of the nerve, ultrasound visualization may be difficult. In that setting, infiltrating around the artery is the appropriate technique. At more distal sites, the nerve may be found between the sartorius muscle and gracilis muscle adjacent to the geniculate artery (Fig. 30-5).

Sciatic Nerve Block

Background and Indications: The sacral plexus is formed by the anterior rami of lumbar nerves 4 and 5 and sacral nerves 1-3 with variable input from the 4th sacral nerve. The sacral plexus lies on the surface of the sacrum anterior to the piriformis muscle. The sacral plexus gives rise to the posterior cutaneous nerve of the thigh (small sciatic nerve) and the

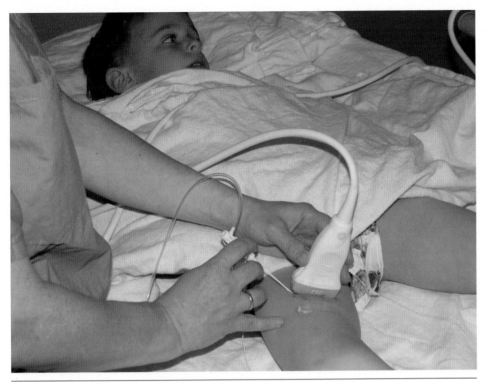

Figure 30-4a. Gross anatomy of the saphenous nerve. Needle and probe position for saphenous block.

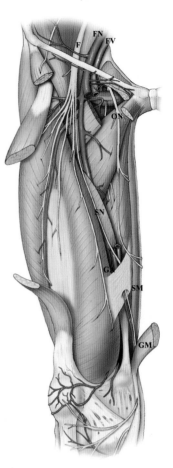

Figure 30-4b. Gross anatomy of the saphenous nerve. *FA*, femoral artery; *FV*, femoral vein; *GA*, geniculate artery; *SN*, saphenous nerve; *SA*, sartorius muscle; *GM*, gracilis muscle; *ON*, obturator nerve.

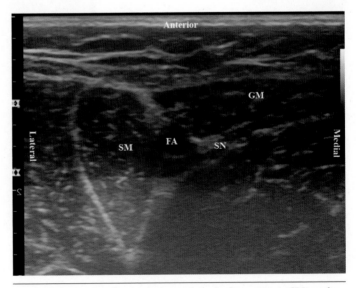

Figure 30-5. *FA*, femoral artery / geniculate artery; *SN*, saphenous nerve; *SA*, sartorius muscle; *GM*, gracilis muscle.

sciatic nerve, two other nerves that innervate the lower extremity. The sciatic nerve provides sensory and motor innervation to the posterior aspect of the thigh and the majority of the leg below the knee. The only other nerve that provides sensory innervation below the knee is the saphenous nerve, a branch of the femoral nerve. The saphenous nerve provides sensory innervation to the medial aspect of the leg below the knee and the medial aspect of the foot. The remainder of the leg below the knee is innervated by the sciatic nerve as it divides at a variable distance from the popliteal fossa into the common peroneal and the posterior tibial nerve.

The sciatic nerve is part of the sacral plexus (L_4, L_5, S_{1-3}) and is the largest nerve in the body. The sacral plexus forms on the anterior surface of the lateral sacrum and gives rise to the sciatic nerve on the ventral surface of the piriformis muscle. The sciatic nerve exits the pelvis through the grater sciatic foramen. Below the piriformis muscle, the nerve descends medial to the midpoint of a line drawn between the greater trochanter of the femur and the ischial tuberosity. Inferior to the border of the gluteus maximus muscle, the nerve is relatively superficial and is generally easily blocked with a posterior approach (Figs. 30-6 and 30-7). At the level of the lesser trochanter, the sciatic nerve lies posterior to the femur (Fig. 30-8). Near the apex of or within the popliteal fossa, the sciatic nerve divides into the tibial nerve that passes medially down the back of the leg and the common peroneal nerve, which travels laterally and eventually wraps around the head of the fibula. The sciatic nerve can be blocked at various levels along its course depending on the patient and the site of the surgical procedure.

Commonly used approaches include the subgluteal (posterior) approach, the anterior approach, a midfemoral approach, and blockade in the popliteal fossa. A sciatic nerve block is used most commonly to provide analgesia following contracture release of the thigh, leg, ankle, or surgical repair of fractures of the leg and ankle. The posterior approach (subgluteal and posterior popliteal) remain the most popular, perhaps, because these were the most common approaches before the advent of ultrasound guidance. The lateral approach at the mid-thigh and anterior approach have gained popularity because of their relative ease with ultrasound guidance and because the patient's lower extremity does not have to be elevated to perform the block.

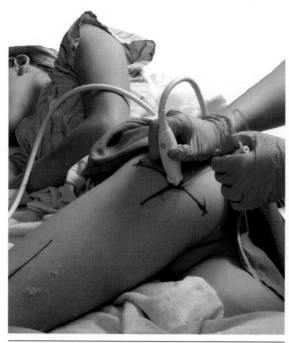

Figure 30-6a. Needle and probe position for subgluteal block.

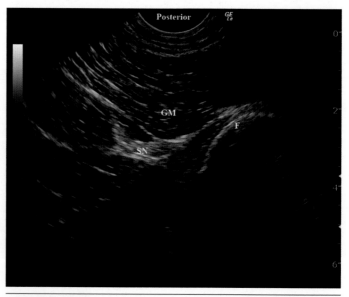

Figure 30-6b. *F*, femur; *SN*, sciatic nerve; *GMM*, gluteus maximus muscle.

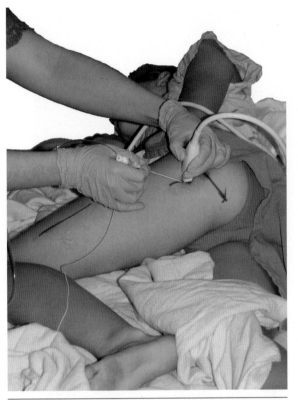

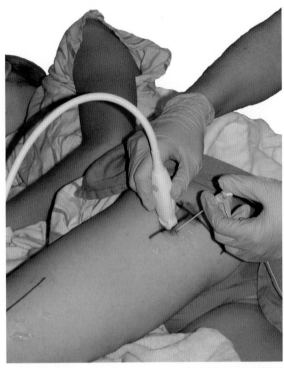

Figure 30-7a. Needle and probe position for out of plane block (lateral).

Figure 30-7b. Needle and probe position or in line block (lateral).

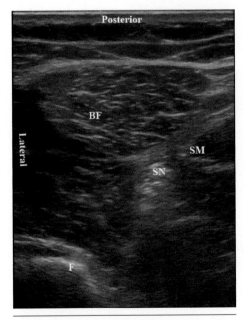

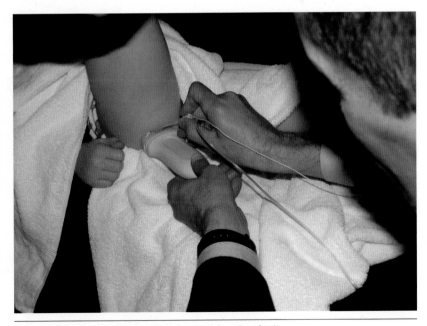

Figure 30-7c. Ultrasound for subgluteal block (lateral). *BF,* biceps femoris; *SN,* sciatic nerve; *F,* femur.

Figure 30-7d. Needle and probe position (supine).

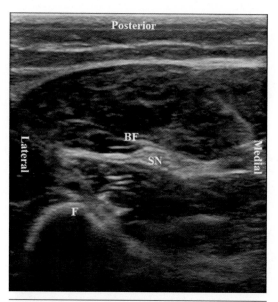

Figure 30-7e. Subgluteal ultrasound (supine). *BF*, biceps femoris; *F*, femur; *SN*, sciatic nerve.

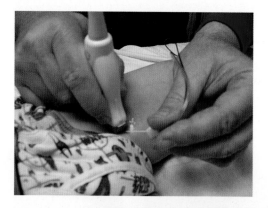

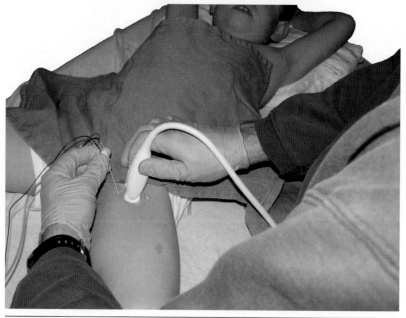

Figure 30-8a,b. Needle and probe position for anterior sciatic block.

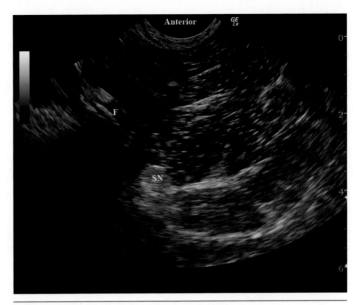

Figure 30-8c. *F*, femur; *SN*, sciatic nerve.

Subgluteal Sciatic Block

 Patient Position: Supine, lateral, or prone.

 Transducer: Children ≤30 kg, 25- or 38-mm linear probe oscillating at 10 to 14 MHz. Children ≥30 kg, 11-mm curved probe (5–10 MHz).

 Transducer Orientation: Transverse in the gluteal crease.

 Needle: 24-gauge, 2.5-cm blunt needle, 22-gauge, 5-cm blunt needle, or 21-gauge, 10-cm blunt needle, depending on patient size; 18-gauge insulated Tuohy needle for continuous techniques.

 Local Anesthetic: 0.1 to 0.2 mL/kg of 0.2% ropivacaine or 0.25% bupivacaine. Epinephrine in a concentration of 1:200,000 is added to the solution.

 Technique: The subgluteal approach is the most proximal approach. The nerve is located between the quadratus femorus (lateral) and the biceps femoris (medial) muscles. The patient may be positioned supine, lateral, or prone. In small patients, the patient is usually positioned supine, and the thigh and leg are elevated by an assistant. In larger patients, the lateral position is preferred. The skin is washed, and the probe is positioned in a transverse orientation at the gluteal crease. The nerve is imaged with the appropriate transducer, and the needle is inserted caudal (distal) to the probe using an out of plane approach or using an inline approach (Fig. 30-7). The needle tip is positioned adjacent to the nerve, and the local anesthetic is injected until the nerve is surrounded. Some physicians prefer a modification of the block when the patient is in the lateral position. In that setting, the ischium and greater trochanter are palpated. The probe is sited at the midpoint drawn along the line between the ischium and trochanter. The sciatic nerve is imaged and traced distally until it appears between the ham string muscles (Figs. 30-6 and 30-7). The needle may be inserted in line or out of plane and advanced until it is adjacent to the nerve. Local anesthetic is injected until the nerve is surrounded.

Anterior Sciatic Block

Patient Position: Supine with the operative extremity in the frog-leg position.

Transducer: 25-mm probe oscillating at 8 to 13 MHz for smaller patients or 11-mm, 6 to 10 Hz probe for larger patients.

Transducer Orientation: Transverse, 3 to 5 cm below the inguinal ligament.

Needle: 24-gauge, 1 2.5-cm needle ; 22-gauge, 2 5-cm needle, or 21-gauge, 10-cm needle, depending on patient size; 18-gauge insulated Tuohy needle for continuous techniques.

Local Anesthetic: 0.1 to 0.2 mL/kg of 0.2% ropivacaine or 0.25% bupivacaine. Epinephrine in a concentration of 1:200,000 is added to the solution.

Technique: The anterior sciatic block is one of the most difficult blocks in adults because of the distance from the skin to the target nerve. However, in children, the sciatic nerve is usually only 3 to 5 cm deep to the skin. This makes ultrasound-guided block very practical in the pediatric population. The operative lower extremity is placed in the frog-leg position (Fig. 30-8). This maneuver rotates the sciatic nerve from a position posterior to the femur into a position where the nerve is now medial and deep to the femur. For smaller patients, a high-frequency (10–13 MHz) linear probe will suffice, but for most patients, an 11-mm curved probe oscillating at 6 to 10 MHz provides the best working image. The probe is placed 3 to 5 cm below the inguinal crease in a transverse orientation. The hypoechoic shadow of the lesser trochanter is imaged. Medial and anterior to the trochanter, the femoral artery is imaged. The sciatic nerve usually lies on a line drawn perpendicularly through the artery at a depth that is 2 to 3 cm deep to the posterior border of the femur in Figure 30-8. In some patients, the hyperechoic nerve lies in a position that is deep to the femur at a point that is midway between the femur and the femoral artery. The appropriate length needle is inserted, in-line at the medial end of the probe. The needle is directed laterally until its tip is adjacent to the nerve. The local anesthetic agent is injected until the nerve is surrounded.

Midfemoral Sciatic Nerve Block

Patient Position: Supine with the thigh and leg internally rotated.

Transducer: 11-mm curved array oscillating at 6 to 10 MHz.

Transducer Orientation: Transverse, between the vastus lateralis and biceps femoris muscles.

Needle: 22-gauge, 5-cm blunt needle or 21-gauge, 10-cm blunt needle, depending on patient size; 18-gauge insulated Tuohy needle for continuous techniques.

Local Anesthetic: 0.1 to 0.2 mL/kg of 0.2% ropivacaine or 0.25% bupivacaine. Epinephrine in a concentration of 1:200,000 is added to the solution.

Technique: The skin is washed, and a small curved probe (6–10 MHz) is positioned in a transverse orientation between the vastus lateralis and biceps femoris muscles. The nerve is a round hyperechoic structure imaged posterior to the femur (Fig. 30-9). The needle is inserted

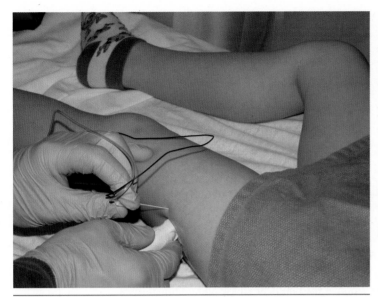

Figure 30-9a. Needle and probe position for lateral sciatic block.

Figure 30-9b. Ultrasound scan of lateral sciatic block. *F*, femur; *SN*, sciatic nerve.

superior to the probe using an in-line approach and advanced at a 45-degree angle to the skin until it is adjacent to the nerve. Local anesthetic is inserted until the nerve is surrounded.

Popliteal Block (Sciatic at the knee)

 Patient Position: Supine, lateral, or prone.

 Transducer: 25- or 35-mm linear array oscillating 8 to 13 MHz or 11-mm curved array oscillating at 6 to 10 MHz.

 Transducer Orientation: Transverse.

 Needle: 22-gauge, 5-cm blunt needle or 21-gauge, 10-cm blunt needle, depending on patient size; 18-gauge insulated Tuohy needle for continuous techniques.

 Local Anesthetic: 0.1 to 0.2 mL/kg of 0.2% ropivacaine or 0.25% bupivacaine. Epinephrine (1:200,000) is added to the bupivacaine.

 Technique: The patient can be positioned supine, lateral, or prone. If the patient is positioned supine, the leg is elevated and bent 90 degree at the hip and at the knee. A modest amount of further extension at the knee can be used to better delineate the tendons and the boundaries of the popliteal fossa. The skin is washed, and the transducer is positioned in a transverse orientation at the level of the popliteal crease. The popliteal artery and vein and bones are imaged. The tibial nerve is an oval hyperechoic structure, lying superficial to the vein (Fig. 30-10). The probe is advanced cephalad until the tibial nerve is joined by the common peroneal nerve. This is generally several centimeters above the popliteal crease. Once the junction of the two nerves has been identified, the needle is inserted at the lateral end of the probe using an in-line approach. When the tip of the needle is adjacent to the round hyperechoic sciatic nerve, local anesthetic is injected until the nerve is surrounded.

Caudal Block

 Patient Position: Prone or lateral decubitus.

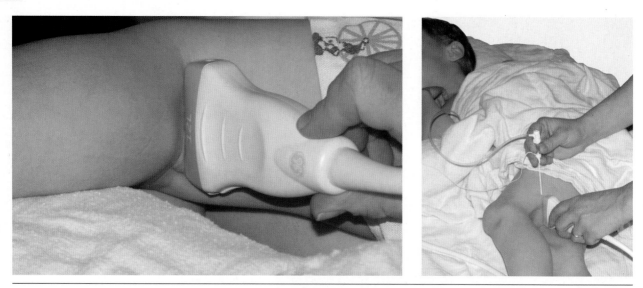

Figure 30-10a,b. Ultrasound probe and needle position at the popliteal crease and popliteal fossa.

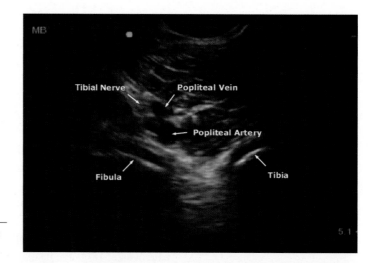

Figure 30-10c. Ultrasound image at the popliteal crease.

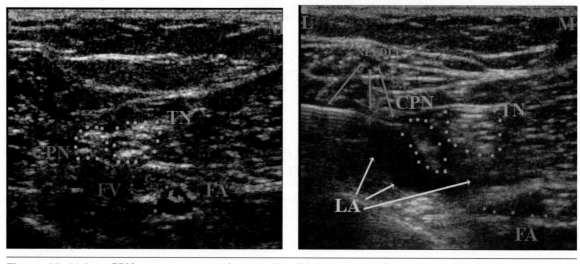

Figure 30-10d,e. *CPN*, common peroneal nerve; *TN*, tibial nerve; *FV*, femoral vein; *FA*, femoral artery; *LA*, local anesthetic; *L*, lateral; *M*, medial.

Transducer: 25-mm linear transducer oscillating at 13 MHz.

 Transducer Orientation: Transverse over the sacral hiatus.

 Needle: 22-gauge, 5-cm blunt needle or 18-gauge, 5-cm blunt needle.

 Local Anesthetic: 3 to 10 mL of 0.2% ropivacaine or 0.25% bupivacaine with epinephrine.

 Technique: Caudal block is the most distal of the approaches to the epidural space. Before the advent of ultrasound-guided blocks, this block was used extensively for anesthesia of the lower extremities as well as pelvic, abdominal, and thoracic surgery. For lower extremity surgery, caudal block has largely been replaced by peripheral nerve blocks. For surgery of the abdomen or thorax, the caudal approach has been largely replaced by blocks of the abdominal wall or paravertebral space. Nonetheless, the caudal canal is easily imaged on ultrasound, and all practitioners should master this approach. A high-frequency (10–13 MHz) linear transducer is placed in a transverse orientation over the sacral cornu (Fig. 30-11). The cornu is hyperechoic structures that lie 1 to 2 cm lateral to the midline. In the midline, the sacral hiatus and its hyperechoic membrane are imaged as well as the posterior wall of the caudal canal (Fig. 30-11). A 22-gauge, 5-cm needle is inserted through the skin at the midpoint of the transducer using an out-of-plane approach. Once the sacral membrane has been pierced, the needle hub is lowered, and the needle is advanced an additional 1 cm into the caudal canal. A 5 to 10 mL of local anesthetic is then injected in ali-

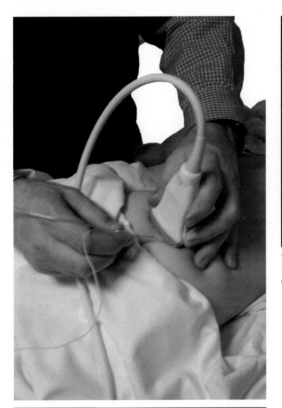

Figure 30-11a. Needle and probe position for caudal block.

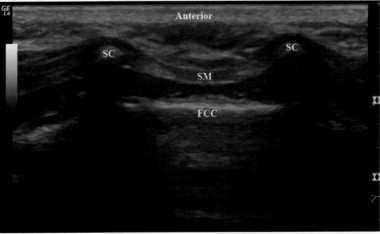

Figure 30-11b. *SC*, sacral cornu; *SM*, sacral membrane; *FCC*, floor of caudal canal.

quots of 2 to 3 mL. The practitioner should aspirate between injections. For continuous infusions, an 18-gauge, 5-cm Tuohy needle can be used with a 20-gauge epidural catheter.

Some practitioners prefer to rotate the probe to sagittal position once the caudal canal has been identified. In this approach, the needle is inserted in line at the caudal end of the transducer. This approach allows the practitioner to visualize the catheter entering the canal as well as the injection of local anesthetic. In principle, this may minimize the risk of intravascular injection.

References

1. Tobias JD, Mencio GA. Regional anesthesia for club foot surgery in children. Amer J Ther 1998;5:273–277.
2. Manion SC, Tobias JD. Lumbar plexus blockade in children. Am J Pain Manage 2005;15:120–126.
3. Johnson CM. Continuous femoral nerve blockade for analgesia in children with femoral fractures. Anaesth Intensive Care 1994;22:281–283.
4. Tobias JD. Continuous femoral nerve block to provide analgesia following femur fractures in a Paediatric ICU population. Anaesth Intensive Care 1994;22:616–618.
5. Gielen M, Viering W. 3-in-1 lumbar plexus block for muscle biopsy in malignant hyperthermia patients. Amide anaesthetics may be used safety. Acta Anaesthesiol Scand 1986;30:581–583.
6. Maccani RM, Wedel DJ, Melton A, et al. Femoral and lateral femoral cutaneous nerve block for muscle biopsies in children. Paeditr Anaesth 1995;5:223–227.
7. Ion T, Cook-Sather SD, Finkel RS, et al. Fascia iliaca block for an infant with arthrogryposis muliplex congenital undergoing muscle biopsy. Anesth Analg 2005;100:82–84.
8. Vincent CR, Turchiano J, Tobias JD. Fascia iliaca block for a muscle biopsy in an infant with undiagnosed hypotonia. Saudi J Anesth 2008;2:22–24.
9. Sanchez V, Segedin ER, Moser M, et al. Role of lumbar sympathectomy in the Pediatric Intensive Care Unit. Anesth Analg 1988;67:794–797.
10. Giaufré E, Dalens B, Gombert A. Epidemiology and morbidity of regional anesthesia in children: a one-year prospective survey of the French-Language Society of Pediatric Anesthesiologists. Anesth Analg 1996;83:904–912.
11. Dalens B, Tanguy A, Vanneuville G. Lumbar plexus block in children: A comparison of two procedures. Anesth Analg 1988;67:750–758.
12. Chayen D, Nathan H, Chayen M. The psoas compartment block. Anesthesiology 1976;45:95–99.
13. Winnie AP, Ramamurthy S, Durrani X, et al. Plexus blocks for lower extremity surgery. Anesthesiol Rev 1974;1:11–16.
14. Dalens B, Vanneuville G, Tanguy A. Comparison of the fascia iliaca compartment block with the 3-in-1 block in children. Anesth Analg 1989;69:705–713.

Section *VI*

Pain Blocks

31 Ultrasound-Guided Maxillary Nerve Block

32 Ultrasound-Guided Mandibular Nerve Block

33 Stellate Ganglion Block

34 Ultrasound-Guided Cervical Sympathetic Block

35 Endoscopic Celiac Ganglion Block

36 Ultrasound-Guided Superior Hypogastric Plexus Block

37 Ultrasound-Guided Lumbar (L1–L4) Zygapophysial Medial Branch and L5 Dorsal Ramus Block

38 Use of Ultrasonography in Rheumatology

Ultrasound-Guided Maxillary Nerve Block

PAUL E. BIGELEISEN

 Background and Indications: Maxillary nerve block is used primarily for diagnosis of trigeminal neuralgia and for postoperative pain relief in children having cleft palate repairs. The block can also be used as the sole block for facial surgery in patients who are poor candidates for general surgery.

 Anatomy: The maxillary nerve is the second division (V2) of cranial nerve V (trigeminal nerve). The nerve exits the base of the skull through the foramen rotundum and travels into the pterygopalatine fossa (Fig. 31-1). The nerve is found anterior and deep to the lateral pterygoid plate. The nerve supplies sensory innervation to the skin of the face including the cheeks, upper lip, and nasolabial folds as well as sensory innervation to the maxillary sinuses, upper teeth, and the hard and soft palate.

 Patient Position: Supine with the head turned away from the operator.

 Transducer: 25- or 38-mm linear probe oscillating at 10 to 13 MHz.

 Transducer Orientation: Transverse oblique below the zygoma.

 Needle: 22-gauge, 5-cm blunt-tip needle.

 Local Anesthetic: Ropivacaine 0.2%, bupivacaine (Marcaine) 0.25%.

 Technique: The patient is positioned supine with the head turned away from the practitioner. The patient is sedated and the skin is washed. The transducer is sited below the zygoma and the lateral pterygoid plate is imaged (Fig. 31-2). Anterior and deep to the pterygoid plate, the nerve is seen as a round or triangular hyperechoic structure. The needle is placed at the posterior end of the probe and advanced through the skin toward the nerve. Once the needle is adjacent to the nerve, 2 to 5 mL is injected until the nerve is surrounded with local anesthetic. The patient should be monitored closely for 30 minutes after the injection because spread of local anesthetic to the brain stem or other cranial nerves is a possibility. For small children, the dose should be reduced and the nerve must be blocked bilaterally for palate repair.

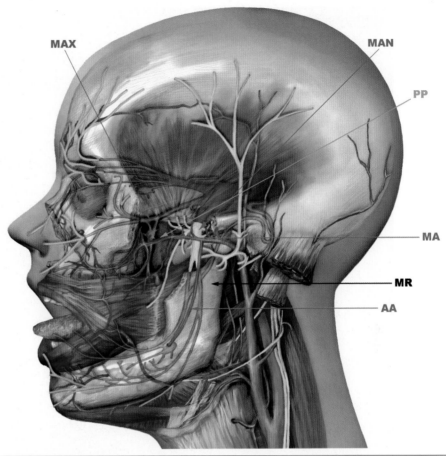

Figure 31-1. Anatomy of the maxillary nerve. *Max*, maxillary nerve; *MA*, maxillary artery; *PP*, pterygoid plate; *Man*, mandibular nerve; *AA*, alveolar artery.

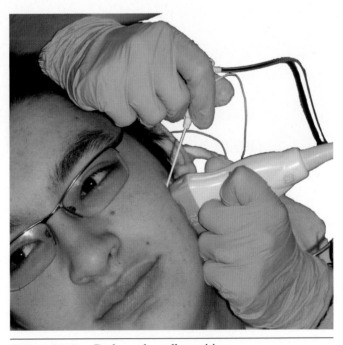

Figure 31-2a. Probe and needle position.

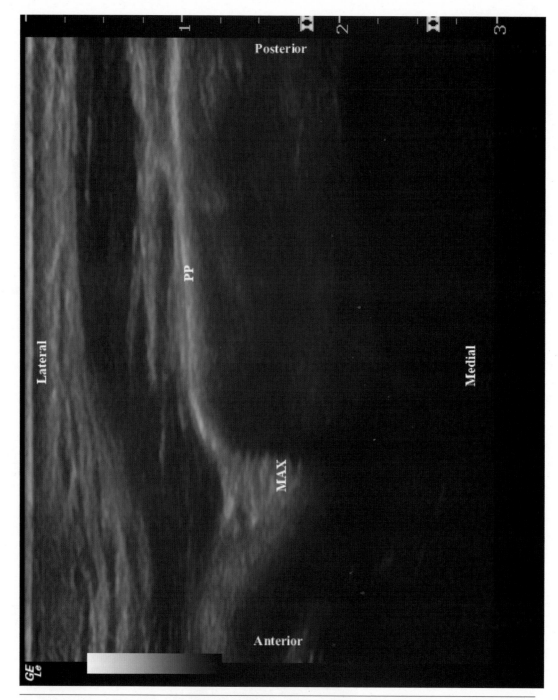

Figure 31-2b. Ultrasound scan of the maxillary nerve. *PP*, pterygoid plate; *Max*, maxillary nerve.

32

Ultrasound-Guided Mandibular Nerve Block

PAUL E. BIGELEISEN, MILENA MORENO

 Background and Indications: Mandibular nerve block was traditionally done using a blind approach wherein a needle was inserted inferior to the zygoma until the pterygoid plate was contacted. The needle was then withdrawn and advanced posterior and 1 cm deep to the pterygoid plate. Some practitioners sought a paresthesia in the lower jaw as they inserted the needle. Once the needle was assumed to be in the correct position, 5 mL of local anesthetic was injected. Another technique was to insert the needle inferior to the zygoma until the pterygoid plate was contacted. Once bony contact was made, 10 mL of local anesthetic was injected. This approach had a high success rate. In many cases, the local anesthetic spread beyond the intended distribution to anesthetize the maxillary nerve as well as other cranial nerves including cranial nerves VI and VII. The use of ultrasound to facilitate mandibular nerve block has not been studied, but it has the potential to increase success rate and decrease the incidence of intravascular injection.

The block is usually employed as a diagnostic or therapeutic procedure for trigeminal neuralgia. The block may also be used for dental procedures or repair of mandibular fractures.

 Anatomy: The mandibular nerve is the third division (V_3) of cranial nerve V (trigeminal nerve) (Fig. 32-1). It exits from the base of the skull through the foramen ovale and runs parallel to the posterior margin of the lateral ptygeroid plate where it divides into two branches. The anterior divison is primarily motor and supplies the muscles of mastication. The posterior division is sensory and supplies the skin over the lower jaw, cheek, anterior ear, and the skin above the ear. It also innervates mucous membranes overlying the lower jaw, the cheek, the mandible, and the teeth. The lingual branch of the posterior division joins the chorda tympani and supplies taste to the anterior two thirds of the tongue.

 Patient Position: Supine with the head turned away from the operator.

 Transducer: 25-mm linear probe oscillating at 13 MHz, 11-mm curved probe oscillating at 10 MHz.

 Transducer Position: Transverse inferior to the zygoma and anterior to the ramus of the mandible.

 Needle: 22-gauge, 5-cm needle with a blunt tip.

 Local Anesthetic: Ropivacaine 0.2%, bupivacaine 0.25%.

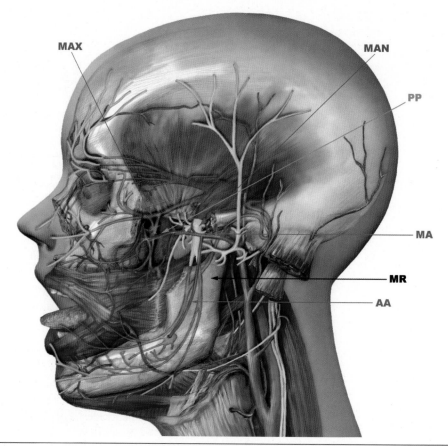

Figure 32-1. Anatomy of the mandibular nerve. *AA*, alveolar artery; *MC*, mandibular condyle; *MA*, maxillary artery; *PP*, pterygoid plate; *MAN*, mandibular nerve; *MAX*, maxillary nerve.

Technique: The skin is washed. If a linear probe is chosen, the probe is sited superior to the mandible in a transverse orientation (Fig. 32-2A). The condyle of the mandible is imaged. Anterior to the condyle, the alveolar artery and vein may be seen next to the nerve (Fig. 32-2B). The needle is inserted superior to the probe using an out-of-plane technique. The needle is advanced toward the nerve that is ovoid and hyperechoic. Three milliliters of local anesthetic are injected until the nerve is surrounded. If a curved probe is chosen, the probe is placed in an oblique transverse position below the zygoma and anterior to the mandibular condyle (Fig. 32-3). The lateral pterygoid plate is imaged. Posterior to the pterygoid plate, the maxillary artery or its branch, the alveolar artery is imaged. Deep to the artery, and posterior to the pterygoid plate, the nerve is seen as a hyperechoic round or oval structure. The needle is inserted posterior to the probe using an in-line technique. The needle is advance until it is adjacent to the nerve. Three milliliters of local anesthetic are injected until the nerve is surrounded.

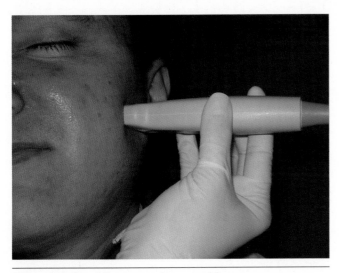

Figure 32-2a. Linear transducer position.

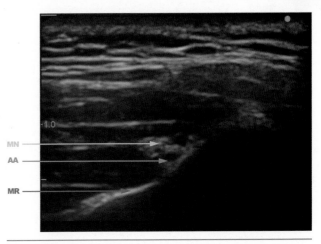

Figure 32-2b. Mandibular nerve and alveolar vessels.

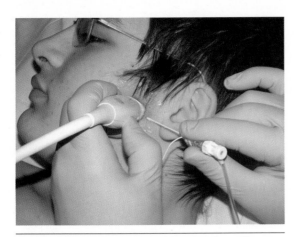

Figure 32-3a. Curved transducer and needle position.

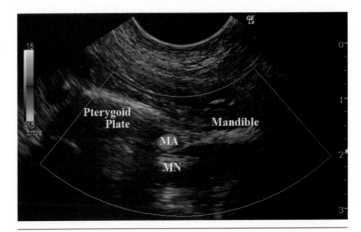

Figure 32-3b. *MA*, maxillary artery; *MN*, mandibular nerve.

33

Stellate Ganglion Block

YASUYUKI SHIBATA, TORU KOMATSU, NIZAR MOAYERI, GERBRAND J. GROEN

Background and Indications: Ultrasound-guided stellate ganglion block was first introduced in 1995 with promising results.[1] The main advantages of ultrasound over the traditional technique are direct visualization of the stellate ganglion and adjacent structures and visualization of the spread of the local anesthetic. Although more clinical reports are needed, the use of ultrasound in stellate ganglion block is reported to reduce the risk of vascular puncture, reduction of the amount of the injected anesthetic solution, and a faster onset time.[1] An important prerequisite is good clinical experience of the anesthesiologist in the practice of ultrasound.

Stellate ganglion block is usually used for the diagnosis and treatment of complex regional pain syndrome of the upper extremity.[2,3] Other uses include treatment of acute or postherpetic neuralgia of the face and[4-6] neck and poor perfusion of the upper extremity as seen in Raynaud and other vascular diseases.[7,8]

Anatomy: The cervical sympathetic ganglia consist of the superior, middle, and inferior ganglia. The inferior cervical ganglion is located at the level of C7 and C8. It joins with the first thoracic ganglion to form the stellate ganglion. The cervical ganglia lie deep to the prevertebral fascia. The prevertebral fascia overlies the vertebral body, the longus colli muscle, and the anterior scalene muscle (Figs. 33-1 and 33-2). The three cervical ganglia give off grey rami communicantes that travel through and around the longus colli to join with spinal nerves C1-C8 and T1. The carotid artery lies anterior and lateral to the cervical ganglia. The recurrent laryngeal nerve is sandwiched between the thyroid and trachea. At the level of C6, the transverse process has a bony process (Chassaignac tubercle), which may be palpated with deep pressure by retracting the carotid artery laterally. This has traditionally been the landmark used to perform stellate block before ultrasound was available.

No major changes have been suggested on the initial reported procedure for ultrasound-guided stellate ganglion block. The use of curved instead of linear transducers is advocated because linear transducers are generally too large for this procedure. In addition, similar high success rates are reported after injecting the local anesthetic around the fascia[1] compared to injecting the local anesthetic under the fascia of the longus colli muscle.[9]

Patient Position: Supine, with a towel between the shoulders.

Transducer: Small curved array (11 mm) oscillating at 5 to 10 MHz.

Transducer Position: Transverse position between the carotid artery and trachea at the level of the 6th cervical vertebra.

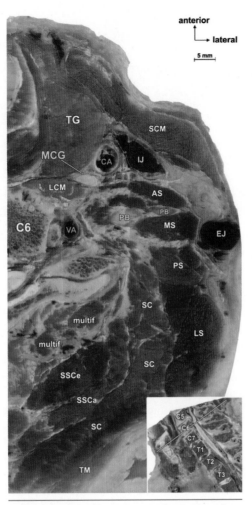

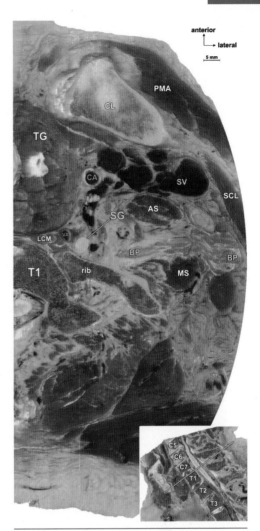

Figure 33-1a. Reconstructed cross-section of the neck at the level of the vertebral corpus C6. *C6*, vertebral corpus of C6; *TG*, thyroid gland; *CA*, common carotid artery; *IJ*, internal jugular vein; *EJ*, external jugular vein; *VA*, vertebral artery; *PB*, brachial plexus; *SCM*, sternocleidomastoid muscle; *LCM*, longus colli muscle; *AS*, anterior scalene muscle; *MS*, middle scalene muscle; *PS*, posterior scalene muscle; *MCG*, middle cervical ggl; *LS*, levator scapulae muscle; *SC*, splenius capitis muscle; *TM*, trapezius muscle; *SSCa*, semispinalis capitis muscle; *SSCe*, semispinalis cervicis muscle; multifidus muscle.

Figure 33-1b. Reconstructed cross-section of the neck at the level of the vertebral corpus C7. *C7*, vertebral corpus of C7; *T*, trachea; *TG*, thyroid gland; *C*, common carotid artery; *IJ*, internal jugular vein; *EJ*, external jugular vein; *VA*, vertebral artery; *VV*, vertebral vein; *PB*, brachial plexus; *SCM*, sternocleidomastoid muscle; *LCM*, long colli muscle; *AS*, anterior scalene muscle; *MS*, middle scalene muscle; *ICG*, inferior cervical ganglion/stellate ganglion.

Needle: 5-cm, 22-gauge blunt needle.

Local Anesthetic: 0.2 % ropivacaine or 0.25 % bupivacaine (3–10 mL).

Procedure: The patient is placed supine with a towel or small pillow placed behind the shoulders. This allows the practitioner to extend the neck and jaw. The patient is asked to open her mouth slightly, which makes it easier for the patient to relax her neck muscles

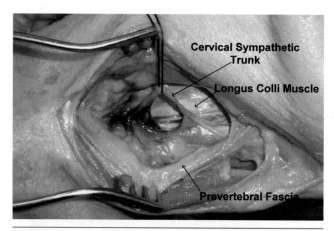

Figure 33-2. Anatomy of the sympathetic nerve trunk in the right cervical region.

during the procedure. After aseptic preparation of the skin, an 11-mm curved transducer oscillating at 8 to 10 MHz is placed adjacent to the trachea to identify the carotid artery and transverse process of C6 (Figs. 31-3 through 31-5). In most patients, the practitioner will need to apply some pressure with the transducer between the carotid artery and trachea to retract the carotid artery laterally. Once the transverse process is identified, the longus colli muscle covered with the prevertebral fascia can usually be seen immediately anterior to the transverse process. A 5-cm, 22-gauge (short- or long-bevel) needle is placed between the trachea and transducer and advanced in line until the tip of the needle is anterior to the longus colli muscle. After aspiration, 5 to 10 mL of local anesthetic is injected until the longus colli muscle is surrounded with local anesthetic (Fig. 31-5). In obese patients, it may be difficult to identify the longus colli muscle. In this case, the practitioner should advance the needle until it contacts the transverse process. The needle should then be withdrawn 1 to 2 mm, and the injection should proceed under ultrasound

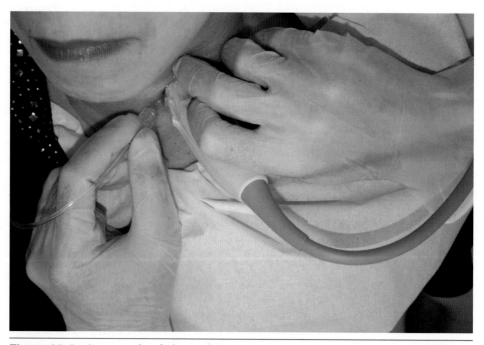

Figure 33-3. An example of ultrasound-guided needle-advancement technique in the right cervical region.

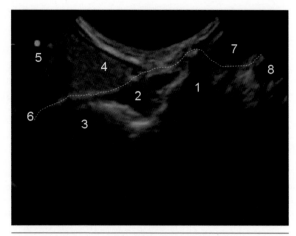

Figure 33-4. Ultrasound image of the right neck at the level of C6 before stellate ganglion block. *1*, anterior tubercle of transverse process; *2*, longus colli muscle; *3*, vertebral body of C6; *4*, thyroid gland; *5*, trachea; *6*, prevertebral fascia; *7*, common carotid artery; *8*, root of C6.

guidance. The triad of anhydrosis, miosis of the pupil, and ptosis of the upper lid, usually within 5 minutes, are evidences of successful block.

 Tips

1. Because the spinal nerve travels in the gutter of the transverse process, paresthesia may occur when the needle is advanced toward the transverse process of C6. When this occurs, the needle should be withdrawn 3 to 4 mm and then the injection may proceed.
2. The brachial plexus lies close by. Some of the local anesthetic may spill over onto the nerve roots or trunks causing a partial plexus block.

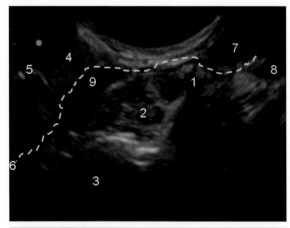

Figure 33-5. Ultrasound image during C6-stellate ganglion block injection posterior to the prevertebral fascia in the longus colli muscle; *1*, anterior tubercle of transverse process; *2*, longus colli muscle; *3*, vertebral body of C6; *4*, thyroid gland; *5*, trachea; *6*, prevertebral fascia; *7*, common carotid artery; *8*, root of C6; *9*, local anesthetic.

3. The recurrent nerve also lies nearby, and ipsilateral vocal cord paralysis may also occur. This is thought to occur when local anesthetic is injected or spreads superficial to the prevertebral fascia and reaches the space between the trachea and esophagus where the recurrent laryngeal nerve resides.

4. In rare instances, epidural block has been reported as well as spread beneath the prevertebral fascia producing bilateral stellate block.

References

1. Kapral S, Krafft P, Gosch M, et al. Ultrasound imaging for stellate ganglion block: direct visualization of puncture site and local anesthetic spread. A pilot study. Reg Anesth 1995;20:323–328.

2. Ackerman WE, Zhang JM. Efficacy of stellate ganglion blockade for the management of type 1 complex regional pain syndrome. South Med J 2006; 99:1084–1088.

3. Chaturvedi A, Dash HH. Sympathetic blockade for the relief of chronic pain. J Indian Med Assoc 2001; 99:698–703.

4. Colding A. The effect of regional sympathetic blocks in the treatment of herpes zoster. Acta Anesth Scand 1969;13:133–141.

5. Olson ER, Ivy HB. Stellate block for trigeminal zoster. J Clin Neuroophthalmol 1981;1:53–55.

6. Winnie AP, Hartwell PW. Relationship between time of treatment of acute herpes zoster with sympathetic blockade and prevention of post-herpetic neuralgia: clinical support for a new theory of the mechanism by which sympathetic blockade provides therapeutic benefit. Reg Anesth 1993;18:277–282.

7. Yildirim V, Akay HT, Bingol H, et al. Pre-emptive stellate ganglion block increases the patency of radial artery grafts in coronary artery bypass surgery. Acta Anaesthesiol Scand 2007;51:434–440.

8. Gupta MM, Bithal PK, Dash HH, et al. Effects of stellate ganglion block on cerebral haemodynamics as assessed by transcranial Doppler ultrasonography. Br J Anaesth 2005;95:669–673.

9. Shibata Y, Fujiwara Y, Komatsu T. A new approach of ultrasound-guided stellate ganglion block. Anesth Analg 2007;105:550–551.

Ultrasound-Guided Cervical Sympathetic Block

MICHAEL GOFELD

Background and Indications: Stellate ganglion block technique was first described in the 1930s. First implemented by Leriche, and further refined by Findley and Patzer, the method has been practiced without major modifications since that time.[1] It is a common intervention in the diagnosis and management of sympathetically maintained pain and vascular insufficiency of upper extremities. In addition, the block has been advocated in various medical conditions, such as phantom pain, postherpetic neuralgia, cancer pain, cardiac arrhythmias, orofacial pain, and vascular headache.[2]

The anatomy and position of the stellate ganglion has been confirmed by dissection, magnetic resonance, and computed tomography.[3–8] The stellate ganglion, or cervicothoracic ganglion, is described as a structure of 1 to 2.5 cm in length, approximately 1 cm in width, and 0.5 cm thick. It is present in about 80% of the population as a fusion of the inferior cervical ganglion and the first thoracic ganglion. The shape of the ganglion may be fusiform, triangular, or globular.[6] The ganglion sits just anterior to the transverse process of C7 and superior or anterior to the neck of the first rib.

An inferior C7 approach for stellate ganglion block has been described.[9] The more common approach is administered according to anatomical landmarks: the prominent anterior tubercle of the C6 vertebra (Chassaignac tubercle), the cricoid cartilage, and the carotid artery.[4] At the level of C6, only the traversing sympathetic fibers or middle cervical ganglion can be found.[10] Thus, the procedure at this level should be named as *cervical sympathetic block*. In 1995, ultrasound-guided stellate ganglion block was described[12] but has recently gained popularity. A new lateral approach to the cervical sympathetic trunk has been recently described and validated against fluoroscopy.[11,13]

Anatomy: The cervical sympathetic trunk is situated on the lateral surface of the longus colli muscle beneath the deep cervical fascia. The cervical sympathetic trunk lies medial to the anterior scalene muscle, lateral to the longus colli muscle, esophagus, trachea, recurrent laryngeal nerve, and anterior to the transverse process of C6. A classic anterior neck sonogram at the level of the cricoid cartilage reveals the trachea medially, the carotid artery laterally, and thyroid gland between those two structures. Immediately medial to the carotid artery, the inferior thyroid artery or the recurrent laryngeal nerve can be located (Fig. 34-1). The longus colli muscle is usually seen posterior to the thyroid gland on the anterolateral surface of the C6 vertebral body. On the left side of the neck, the esophagus is positioned just anterior to the longus colli muscle. Thus, insertion of a block needle in the usual trajectory would result in traversing the thyroid gland and esophagus. Although displacement of the carotid artery and thyroid by a pediatric-type curved transducer creates a passage for needle placement (Fig. 34-2), this approach requires application of pressure that may be very unpleasant and does not eliminate the chance for vascular and visceral damage.

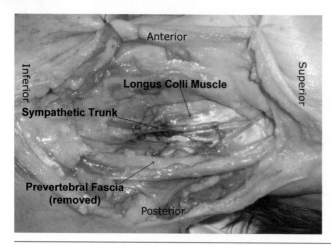

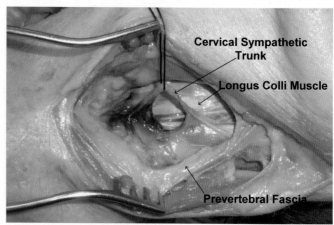

Figure 34-1a,b. Dissection of the neck showing sympathetic trunk and prevertebral fascia.

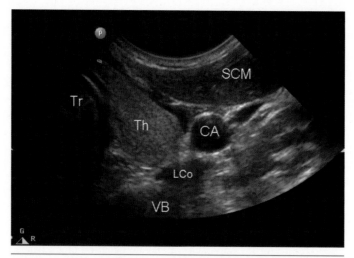

Figure 34-1c. Axial view of neck structures at C6 level. *Tr*, trachea; *Th*, thyroid gland; *SCM*, sternocleidomastoid muscle; *CA*, carotid artery; *Lco*, longus colli muscle; *VB*, C6 vertebral body.

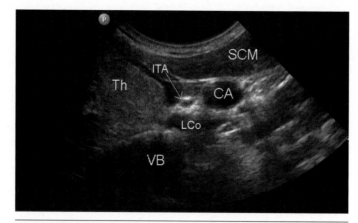

Figure 34-2. Axial view of neck structures at C6 level with application of pressure. Separation of the thyroid gland (*Th*) and the carotid artery (*CA*) is appreciated. The inferior thyroid artery (*ITA*) is clearly seen.

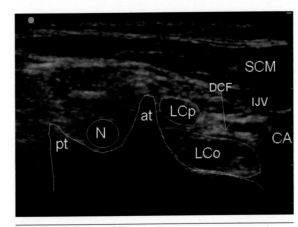

Figure 34-3. Axial view of the neck at the level of C6 vertebra. *N*, C6 nerve root; *pt*, C6 posterior transverse process; *at*, C6 anterior transverse process; *Lco*, longus colli muscle; *LCp*, longus capitis muscle; *DCF*, deep cervical fascia; *IJV*, internal jugular vein; *SCM*, sternocleido mastoid muscle; *CA*, carotid artery.

The lateral approach has the advantage of in-plane needle placement and sparring of visceral and vascular structures from damage. A lateral axial scan usually reveals the C6 transverse process with the prominent anterior and shorter posterior tubercles as well as the exiting C6 nerve root (Fig. 34-3). At the level of C6, the longus colli muscle is seen as an oval-shaped structure adjacent to the base of the transverse process and vertebral body. Sometimes, a caudal part of the longus capitis muscle can be seen as well. In 30% of patients, the middle cervical ganglion can be visualized as a spindle-shaped structure, situated on the postero-lateral surface of the longus colli muscle.[10] Otherwise, a widening of the tissue plane below the deep cervical fascia is appreciated (Fig. 34-4). Scanning caudally and slightly dorsally brings the C7 transverse process into the view. The C7 transverse process has only one tubercle, and its nerve root is situated anterior to the transverse process (Fig. 34-4).

Patient Position: Anterior approach: Supine with a towel beneath the shoulders, neck extended, mouth open.

Lateral approach: Lateral decubitus postion with the operative side up.

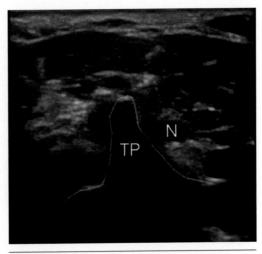

Figure 34-4. Axial view of the neck at the level of C7 vertebra. *N*, C7 nerve root; *TP*, transverse process.

Transducer: Anterior approach: Small curved transducer (C11) oscillating at 5 to 10 MHz.

Lateral approach: Small curved transducer (C11) or linear transducer (L25) oscillating at 10 to 13 MHz.

 Transducer Orientation: Anterior approach: The transducer is placed at the level of the cricoid cartilage medially to the carotid artery in the axial plane (Fig. 34-5).

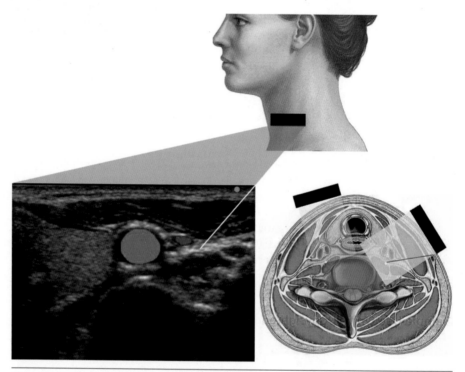

Figure 34-5a. Axial section of the neck showing lateral and anterior paths to the cervical sympathetic chain.

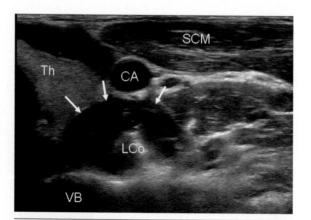

Figure 34-5b. Local anesthetic (arrows) injected anteriorly to the longus colli muscle utilizing the anterior out-of-plane approach. *Lco*, longus colli muscle; *VB*, C6 vertebral body; *SCM*, sternocleidomastoid muscle; *CA*, carotid artery; *Th*, thyroid gland.

Lateral approach: The probe is positioned at the level of the cricoid cartilage above the sternocleidomastoid muscle in the axial plane (Fig. 34-5). Usually, the transducer is moved slightly laterally or medially, cephalad, or caudad to provide the optimal image of the C6 transverse process and the longus colli muscle.

Needle: 22-gauge 5 to 10 cm blunt needle.

Local Anesthetic: 0.2% ropivacaine or 0.25% bupivacaine (3–10 mL), normal saline for test injection.

Other Equipment: 3 mL, 5 mL, and 10 mL Luer lock syringes, three-way stopcock, extension tubing, 25-gauge hypodermic needle.

Technique: Cardiovascular monitors are placed, and an intravenous catheter is inserted on the contralateral side of the block. A temperature monitor can be attached to the palm on the block side. Sedation is usually not required. An antiseptic is utilized to prepare the skin of the block area. The ultrasound transducer is covered by a sterile transparent adhesive or sleeve and positioned at the level of the cricoid cartilage. The block needle is attached to the connecting tubing and to two syringes connected via a three-way stopcock. A 5-mL syringe is filled with NaCl (0.9%), and a 10-mL syringe is filled with local anesthetic. The tubing and needle are flushed with NaCl (0.9%).

When the anterior approach is chosen, the patient is positioned supine with the neck slightly extended. The pediatric curved transducer is placed medial to the carotid artery, and gentle pressure is applied to separate the carotid artery and the thyroid gland. This technique also decreases the distance from the skin to the target. The longus colli muscle is seen as a flattened muscular structure anterior to the C6 vertebral bone shadow. The color Doppler mode should be applied at this time to identify the inferior thyroid and vertebral arteries. Skin anesthesia is performed at the point inferior (caudad) to the transducer, and the block needle is advanced using an out-of-plane technique aiming at the fascial plane of the longus colli muscle. When the needle tip is seen immediately beneath the deep cervical fascia, 0.5 to 1 mL of NaCl (0.9%) is injected. The spread of hypoechoic solution in this fascial plane typically creates a double hyperechoic line, with the deep cervical fascia superior and the colli muscle fascia inferior (Fig. 34-5). If no spread is observed, the needle tip is positioned outside of the ultrasound beam or within a vessel, and the needle should be repostioned. Needle repositioning is also required if an intramuscular injection is seen. In this case, only one hyperechoic line is visualized. Moreover, intramuscular injection is usually associated with discomfort and a retropharyngeal sensation of pressure. Once the spread is seen within the fascial plane, the analgesic solution is administered. Usually, an injection of 5 mL will result in spread from C4 to T1, reliably blocking the midneck sympathetic trunk and the stellate ganglion.[13]

If the lateral approach is performed, the patient is placed in the lateral decubitus position with the block side up. A high-frequency linear transducer is positioned in the axial orientation. The C6 anterior tubercle is brought into view. If the nerve root is also seen, it may be damaged by an in-plane approach (Fig. 34-6). Skin anesthesia is performed posterior to the probe, and the block needle is advanced under continuous in-plane viewing. The needle traverses the sternocleidomastoid and occasionally the anterior scalene and the longus capitis muscles. The needle is advanced beneath the deep cervical fascia and lateral to the longus colli muscle. Verification of the correct spread of NaCl solution is performed prior to injection of local anesthetic solution (Fig. 34-7).

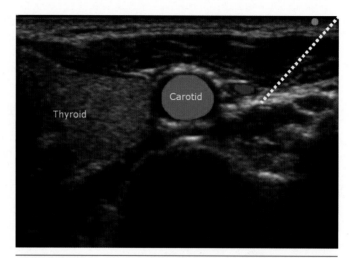

Figure 34-6. Lateral "safe-track" (dotted line) of the projected needle path. Note: the path is traversing muscles only and neither nerve roots nor blood vessels lie within the needle course.

After the block, the patient should remain in the head up supine position. Usually the first sign of a successful sympathetic blockade is the Horner syndrome, which can be seen several minutes following the injection. The patient should be closely monitored for adverse effects.

Summary of Evidence: Traditionally, the block was done as a blind injection and was associated with complications, such as intravascular injection, hematoma formation, temporary paralysis of the recurrent laryngeal nerve, and esophageal injury.[2,13-14] Ultrasound guidance can effectively reduce the volume of local anesthetic to achieve reliable block and may also prevent puncture of blood vessels and esophagus.[13,16] Ultrasound guidance has advantages compared with flouroscopic guidance. Fluoroscopic guidance relies on identification of a bony landmark (transverse process) and a contrast dye injection. A successful fluoroscopic block also relies on the assumed thickness and anatomical location of the longus colli muscle. There is some controversy about the location of the sympathetic

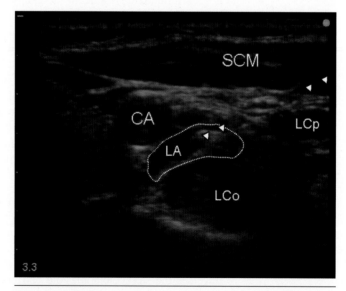

Figure 34-7. Block needle (arrowheads) placed under the deep cervical fascia and local anesthetic (dotted loop) is injected. *SCM*, sternocleido mastoid muscle; *LCp*, longus capitis muscle; *Lco*, longus colli muscle; *CA*, carotid artery.

trunk location with respect to the deep cervical fascia. The majority of anatomy atlases and regional anesthesia texts cite its position as superficial to the deep cervical fascia.[3] The subfascial position of the cervical sympathetic trunk has been confirmed by both anatomical dissection[10,13] and ultrasound imaging.[13] In addition, these texts imply that the longus colli muscle is very thin and advocate withdrawing the needle 2 to 5 mm once the transverse process has been identified and contacted by the needle using fluoroscopy. However, the longus colli muscle is actually about 10 mm in thickness.[13] Thus, a standard fluoroscopic approach would likely result in an intramuscular injection. Block of the cervical sympathetic trunk would then only be accomplished by overflow or diffusion of the injectate. Because the cervical sympathetic trunk is adjacent to soft tissues (longus colli muscle, thyroid, esophagus) ultrasound guidance should logically be a better technique.

References

1. Bonica JJ. The Management of Pain. Philadelphia: Lea & Febiger, 1953:410–432.
2. Elias M. Cervical sympathetic and stellate ganglion blocks. Pain Physician 2000;3:294–304.
3. Moore K, Dalley A. Clincally Oriented Anatomy. 5th ed. Philadelphia: Lippincott Williams & Wilkins, 2006: 1051–1082.
4. Raj PP. Stellate ganglion block. In: Waldman, Wenner, eds. Interventional Pain Management. Philadelphia: Saunders, 1996.
5. Ellis H, Feldman S. Anatomy for Anesthetists. 3rd ed. Oxford: Blackwell Scientific Publications, 1979: 256–262.
6. Hogan QH, Erickson SJ. MR imaging of the stellate ganglion: normal appearance. AJR Am J Roentgenol 1992;158:655–659.
7. Perlow S, Vehe KL. Variations in the gross anatomy of the stellate and lumbar sympathetic ganglia. Am J Surg 1935;30:454–458.
8. Erickson SJ, Hogan QH. CT-guided injection of the stellate ganglion: description of technique and efficacy of sympathetic blockade. Radiology 1993;188:707–709.
9. Abdi S, Zhou Y, Patel N, et al. A new and easy technique to block the stellate ganglion. Pain Physician 2004;7:327–331.
10. Kiray A, Arman C, Naderi S, et al. Surgical anatomy of the cervical sympathetic trunk. Clin Anat 2005; 18(3):179–185.
11. Gofeld M. Ultrasonography in pain medicine: a critical review. Pain Pract 2008;8:226–240.
12. Kapral S, Krafft P, Gosch M, et al. Ultrasound imaging for stellate ganglion block: direct visualization of puncture site and local anesthetic spread. A pilot study. Reg Anesth 1995;20:323–328.
13. Gofeld M, Bhatia A, Abbas S. Three-dimensional ultrasonography of the cervical sympathetic trunk and validation of a new ultrasound-guided technique. Reg Anesth Pain Med 2008;32:2.
14. Higa K, Hirata K, Hirota K, et al. Retropharyngeal hematoma after stellate ganglion block: analysis of 27 patients reported in the literature. Anesthesiology 2006;105(6):1238–1245.
15. Mahli A, Coskun D, Akcali DT. Aetiology of convulsions due to stellate ganglion block: a review and report of two cases. Eur J Anaesthesiol 2002;19(5):376–380.
16. Narouze S, Vydyanathan A, Patel N. Ultrasound-guided stellate ganglion block successfully prevented esophageal puncture. Pain Physician 2007;10:747–752.

35

Endoscopic Celiac Ganglion Block

PAUL E. BIGELEISEN

 Background and Indications: Celiac ganglion block is usually used for the diagnosis of visceral pain syndromes or the treatment of pain from visceral malignancies.

The traditional approach to celiac ganglion block uses a bilateral posterior approach in which the needle was placed anterior to the aorta using a transcrural approach. This was done either blind or with fluoroscopy. Subsequently, practitioners used a transaortic approach, again with a blind, fluoroscopic, or computed tomography (CT) guided technique. Other practitioners have used a transabdominal approach using fluoroscopy, CT, or ultrasound guidance.

The advent of endoscopic ultrasound has made celiac block and neurolysis simple and very safe. An endoscopic ultrasound probe consists of two imaging modalities placed into one probe. The first part of the probe is a flexible endoscope, which is identical to any flexible endoscope used for upper gastroenterological procedures. The second part of the probe is an ultrasound imaging device, which functions in the same way as a transesophageal echocardiogram (Fig. 35-1). Thus, the practitioner must be familiar with the basics of gastrointestinal endoscopy as well as transesophageal echocardiography to employ the technique. Many university gastroenterology departments have endoscopic ultrasound machines, but the technology has not diffused into the private community at this time.

 Anatomy: The celiac ganglion is predominantly a sympathetic plexus with afferent pain fibers from the foregut. Foregut organs from the distal esophagus to the splenic flexure are innervated by afferents traveling through the celiac ganglion (Fig. 35-1). Efferent fibers from the vagus also traverse the ganglion. The ganglion surrounds the celiac artery and spreads over the anterior surface of the aorta at the level of the 12th thoracic vertebra and first lumbar vertebra.

 Transducer: Endoscopic approach: 120-cm endoscopic ultrasound probe oscillating at 2 to 5 MHz. Transabdominal approach: 40- to 60-mm curved array oscillating at 2 to 5 MHz.

 Transducer Orientation: Endoscopic: The probe is passed through the mouth and placed along side the lesser curvature of the stomach. Transabdominal: Transverse, 2 cm above the umbilicus.

 Needle: Endoscopic: 22-gauge flexible needle (150 cm). Transabdominal: 20-gauge, 10- to 15-cm blunt needle.

 Local Anesthetic: 0.2% or 0.5% ropivacaine (10–20 mL).

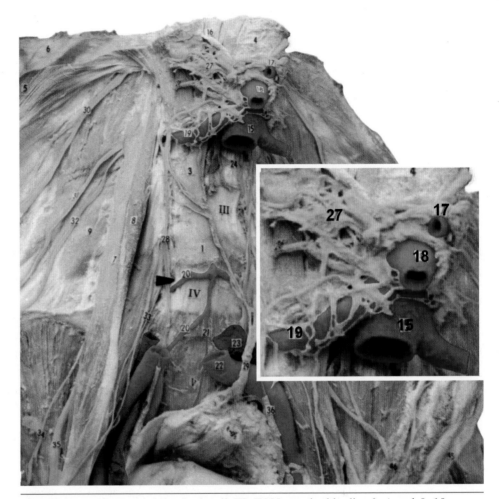

Figure 35-1. Posterior abdominal wall. III, IV, V, vertebral bodies *3*, *4*, and *5*; *15*, abdominal aorta; *17*, celiac artery; *18*, superior mesenteric artery; *19*, right renal artery; *22*, common iliac artery; *23*, common iliac vein; *24*, cisterna chili; *27*, celiac plexus; *28*, lumbar sympathetic trunk; *29*, hypogastric plexus.

Technique

Endoscopic Approach

After appropriate sedation and topicalization of the hypopharynx, the endoscopic ultrasound probe is passed orally into the stomach of the patient and then placed alongside the lesser curvature of the stomach under endoscopic guidance (Fig. 35-2). The ultrasound part of the probe is then used to visualize the aorta and celiac artery (Fig. 35-3). Once the celiac artery is identified, a flexible 22-gauge needle is passed through the wall of the stomach, and the tip of the needle is placed adjacent to the celiac artery. Ten mL of local anesthetic is then injected through the needle around the celiac artery under direct ultrasound visualization.

Transabdominal

For practitioners who do not have access to an endoscopic ultrasound device, celiac plexus block can be performed from the anterior approach using a traditional ultrasound platform. Because the needle traverses the peritoneum and small bowel, the patient should receive broad spectrum antibiotic prophylaxis prior to the block. The author's preference is 2 gm of cofoxitin. The abdomen is washed with sterile cleanser, and a 60-cm curved array oscillating at 2 to 5 MHz is placed 2 cm cephalad to the umbilicus (Fig. 35-4). The pulsatile aorta is identified and then the practitioner must scan cephalad until the celiac artery is identified (Fig. 35-5). Once the celiac artery is identified, the skin and abdominal wall is anesthetized

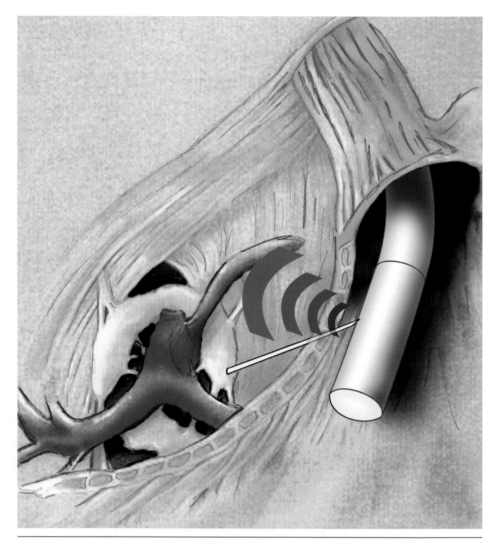

Figure 35-2. Sonoendoscopy probe emerging from esophagus into stomach.

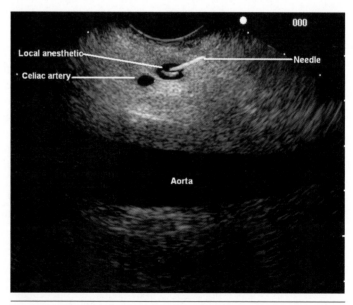

Figure 35-3. Sonogram of aorta and celiac artery using sonoendoscopy.

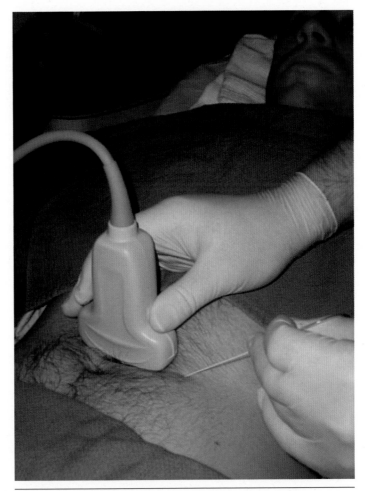

Figure 35-4. Position of abdominal probe and needle.

with local anesthetic. A 10-cm 20-gauge needle is advanced through the abdominal wall in line with the probe. When the needle tip is adjacent to the celiac artery, 10 mL of local anesthetic is injected under ultrasound vision. If the celiac artery can not be identified, the practitioner may inject the local anesthetic immediately anterior to the aorta. In this case, a volume of 30 mL of local anesthetic is required.

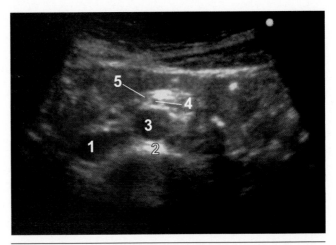

Figure 35-5. Transabdominal sonogram. *1*, vena cava; *2*, vertebral body; *3*, aorta; *4*, celiac artery; *5*, celiac plexus.

Suggested Reading

Caratozzolo M, Lirici MM, Consalvo M, et al. Ultrasound-guided alcoholization of the celiac plexus for pain control in oncology. Surg Endosc 1997;11(3):239–244.

Hoffman BJ. EUS-guided celiac plexus block/neurolysis. Gastrointest Endosc 2002;56(4):S26–S28.

Wiersema MJ, Wiersema LM. Endosonography-guided celiac plexus neurolysis. Gastrointest Endosc 1996;44(6):656–662.

Ultrasound-Guided Superior Hypogastric Plexus Block

PAUL E. BIGELEISEN

 Background and Indications: Traditionally, hypogastric plexus block was performed by anesthesiologists from a posterior approach using fluoroscopy or computed tomography (CT) guidance. This procedure was technically difficult because it required the practitioner to advance the needle between the wing of the posterior iliac crest and vertebral body into a position anterior to the vertebra at the L5, S1 junction. Radiologists often used an anterior approach with fluoroscopy or CT guidance in which the needle was advanced through the abdominal wall until it was immediately anterior to the anterior longitudinal ligament of the vertebrae. This same approach is easy to perform with ultrasound and has the advantage over fluoroscopy that the aorta and iliac arteries are readily imaged. Because this approach requires the needle to traverse the small bowel and peritoneum, the patient should be treated with broad spectrum antibiotic prophylaxis prior to the procedure. The author's preference is 2 gm of cefoxitin.

Block of the superior hypogastric plexus is used as a diagnostic procedure or therapeutic treatment of pain syndromes related to the testes, ovaries, uterus, cervix, vagina, bladder, sigmoid colon, and rectum. Ultrasound guidance can be used for the anterior approach to the superior hypogastric plexus. When neurolytic blocks are intended, the practitioner must be aware that bowel and bladder incontinence or dysfunction may ensue. For this reason, neurolytic blocks are usually reserved for patients with terminal cancer of the organs mentioned above.

 Anatomy: The superior hypogastric plexus contains contributions from the intermesenteric plexus that descends over the aortic bifurcation. It also receives branches from the two lower lumbar splanchnic nerves. The plexus caries visceral efferents to and somatic afferents from the testes, ovaries, uterus, cervix, vagina, bladder, sigmoid colon, and rectum. The plexus lies anterior to the fourth and fifth lumbar and the sacrum (Fig. 36-1). Below the junction of the lumbar vertebrae and sacrum, the plexus bifurcates into the right and left hypogastric nerves.

 Transducer: 40 to 60 mm curved array oscillating at 2 to 5 MHz.

 Transducer Orientation: Transverse below the umbilicus.

 Needle: 20-gauge needle. In slim patients, a 10-cm needle will suffice. In larger patients, a needle 15 to 20 cm in length will be required.

 Local Anesthetic: 10 to 20 mL of 0.2% or 0.5% ropivacaine.

237

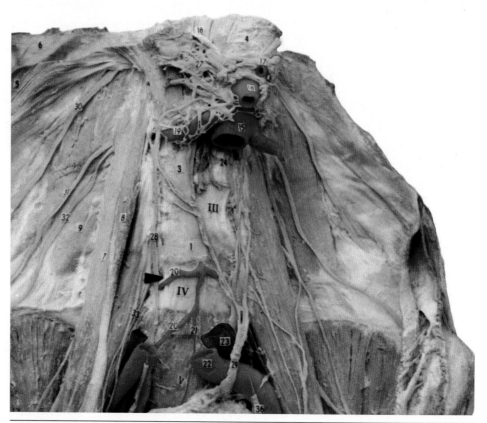

Figure 36-1. Celiac and superior hypogastric plexuses. *III, IV, V,* vertebral bodies 3, 4, and 5; *15,* abdominal aorta; *17,* celiac artery; *18,* superior mesenteric artery; *19,* right renal artery; *22,* common iliac artery; *23,* common iliac vein; *24,* cysterna chili; *27,* celiac plexus; *28,* lumbar sympathetic trunk; *29,* hypogastric plexus.

Technique: The patient's abdomen is washed with sterile solution. The probe is placed about 2 cm cephalad to the umbilicus in a transverse orientation (Fig. 36-2A). The spine is seen as a white, hyperechoic curved line (Fig. 36-2B). The pulsatile aorta is identified anterior to the spine. In many cases, the celiac artery can also bee seen immediately anterior to the aorta. The inferior vena cava is seen to the right of the aorta. The probe is moved caudad until the practitioner views the aorta bifurcating into the right and left common iliac arteries (Fig. 36-3A,B). The spine may now be seen lying between the iliac arteries.

The needle is introduced through the skin, inline with the probe. Under direct visualization, the needle is advanced until its tip contacts the anterior surface of the L4 vertebra (Fig. 36-3B). For unilateral blocks, the practitioner will need to place the needle tip to the right or left of the midline of the vertebra. Once the vertebra has been contacted, the needle is withdrawn 2 to 3 mm, and local anesthesia is injected under direct vision. A hypoechoic puddle of local anesthetic should appear anterior to the spine (Fig. 36-3C). When unilateral block is desired, the dose should be limited to 3 to 5 mL of local anesthetic.

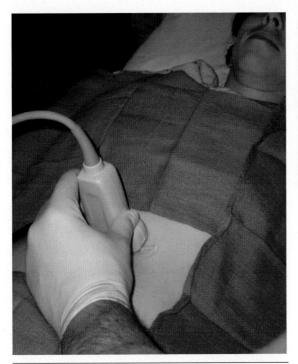

Figure 36-2a. Probe orientation above the umbilicus.

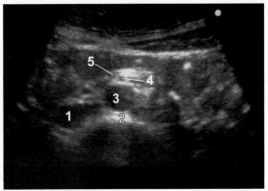

Figure 36-2b. Ultrasound scan above the umbilicus. *1*, vena cava; *2*, L; vertebral body; *3*, aorta; *4*, celiac artery; *5*, celiac plexus.

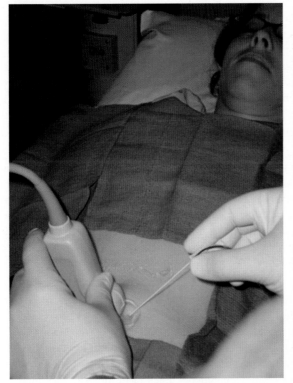

Figure 36-3a. Probe orientation below umbilicus.

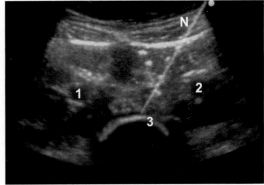

Figure 36-3b. *N*, needle; *1*, right iliac artery; *2*, left iliac artery; *3*, L4 vertebral body.

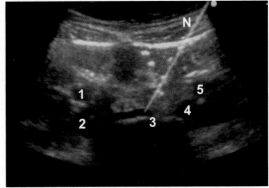

Figure 36-3c. *N*, needle with local anesthetic injection; *1*, right iliac artery; *2*, right iliac vein; *3*, L4 vertebral body; *4*, left iliac vein; *5*, left iliac artery.

37

Ultrasound-Guided Lumbar (L1–L4) Zygapophysial Medial Branch and L5 Dorsal Ramus Block

YOSHIRO FUJIWARA, TORU KOMATSU, MICHAEL GOFELD

Background and Indications: In the past decade, ultrasound has been applied to regional anesthesia, helping to visualize neuroaxial structures. For example, the distance from the skin to epidural space can be measured to estimate the needle depth for obstetric anesthesia.[1,2] In thin patients and children, the ligamentum flavum epidural space, dura mater, and nerve roots have been imaged. However, the application of ultrasound to chronic spinal pain is still an emerging tool. Diagnostic and therapeutic lumbar zygapophysial (facet) joint interventions are among the most commonly performed injections in pain management. At present fluoroscopic guidance is the standard of care, but several studies have validated ultrasound as an imaging tool for facet injection.[3–6] Imaging is necessary to ensure precise needle position and to exclude vascular injection. When fluoroscopy is employed, it may be difficult to image the site on the sacrum for injection as a result of shadowing caused by the iliac bone. Although ultrasound-guided block of the L5 ramus has not been studied, its technique has been described and it may turn out to be an easier technique than fluoroscopic guidance. Moreover, facet block is considered a low-risk intervention. Thus, the use of the ultrasound is an attractive alternative to fluoroscopy because the patient and practitioner are no longer exposed to radiation.

Zygapophysial injection is used for the diagnosis and treatment of spinal pain caused by inflammation or degeneration of the facet joint. The technique may be used to treat pain in the sacral, lumbar, thoracic, or cervical regions. Today, ultrasound is only used for the sacral and lumbar regions. Facet joint injections and facet nerve blocks have been shown to be of equal value in the management of facet syndrome. In 10% to 20% of patients, visualization of the joint is not possible because of hypertrophy and ossification of the joint. Thus, facet nerve block is considered to be the block of choice.

Anatomy: The lumbar facet joints consist of the superior and inferior articular surfaces of the vertebral bodies at the lateral recess of the spinal nerve root (Fig. 37-1). The superior facet surface has a concave shape that articulates with the convex surface of the inferior facet (Fig. 37-1A). These articulations allow flexion but limit rotation. The median branch of the dorsal primary ramus of the spinal nerve innervates the facet joint as well as the supraspinous and interspinous ligaments. Each facet joint receives innervation from its own spinal nerve (median branch) as well as the median branch from the spinal nerve above it (Fig. 37-1B). The median branch courses along the lateral surface of the superior process and the cephalad surface of the transverse process. The median nerve wraps around to innervate the joint and ligaments. The median branch is usually blocked here. If the pathology

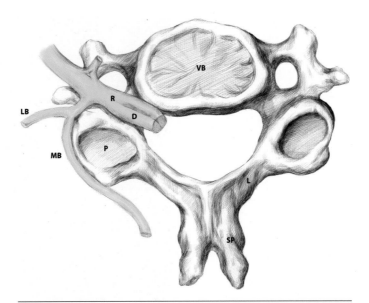

Figure 37-1a. *VB*, vertebral body; *D*, dorsal root; *R*, spinal nerve root; *MB*, medial branch nerve; *L*, lamina; *SP*, spinous process.

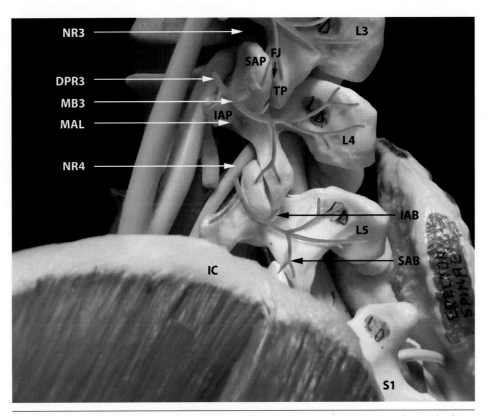

Figure 37-1b. *IAP*, inferior articular process; *FJ*, facet joint; *SAP*, superior articular process; *TP*, transverse process; *MB3*, medial branch from nerve root 3; *IAB*, inferior articular branch; *SAB*, superior articular branch; *DPRS1*, dorsal primary ramus of S1; *DPRL5*, dorsal primary ramus of L%; *IC*, iliac crest; *NR4*, nerve root 4; *NR3*, nerve root 3.

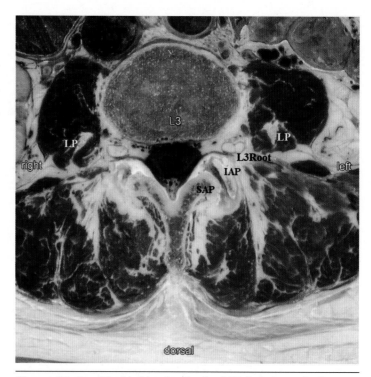

Figure 37-1c. *L3*, third lumbar body; *IAP*, inferior articular process; *SAP*, superior articular process; *LP*, lumbar plexus.

exists at a single lumbar level, the median branch at that level as well as at the level above it must be blocked to provide pain relief because of the dual innervation of the joint.

 Patient Position: Prone with pillows under the hips.

 Transducer: 40- to 60-mm curved array oscillating at 3 to 5 MHz. A transducer guide has a limited value, because it is necessary to rotate the transducer to verify needle position before the injection is performed.

 Transducer Orientation: Longitudinal and transverse over the lumbar vertebrae and sacrum.

 Needle: 22-gauge, 10-cm blunt needle.

 Local Anesthetic: 0.5% bupivacaine (0.5–1 mL per nerve), methylprednisolone (4 mg) for the intra-articular block.

Other Equipment: Two 3-mL Luer-lock syringes, 25-g hypodermic needle. Lidocaine 2%, for skin anesthesia.

 Technique: Ultrasound image acquisition of the lumbar spine requires imaging either soft tissue (i.e., paraspinal muscles, ligaments, dura) and/or bony contours. Typically, both longitudinal and axial scanning are required to identify structures and to position the needle next to the nerve. A 3- to 8-MHz curved transducer is routinely used. A linear high-frequency probe may be used on a lean person to avoid the creation of "air pockets" between skin and a large curved transducer.

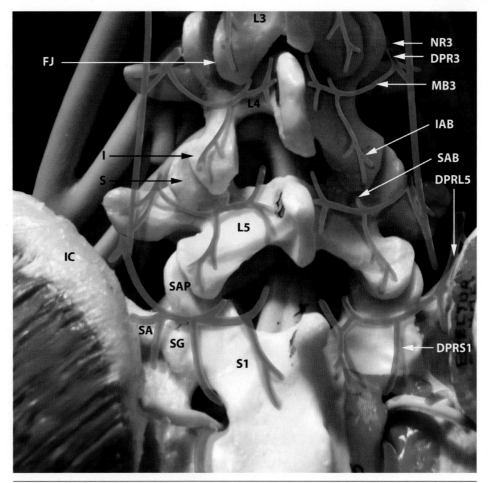

Figure 37-2a. Anatomy of the L5 dorsal ramus. *SAP*, superior articular process; *IC*, iliac crest; *SA*, sacral ala; *SG*, sacral groove; *FJ*, facet joint; *I*, inferior articular process; *S*, superior articular process; *NR3*, nerve root 3; *DPR3*, dorsal primary ramus of nerve root 3; *MB3*, medial branch of nerve root 3; *IAB*, inferior articular branch; *SAB*, superior articular branch; *DPRL5*, dorsal primary ramus of L5; *DPRS1*, dorsal primary ramus of S1.

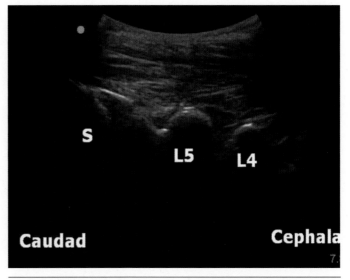

Figure 37-2b. *S*, sacrum; *L5*, transverse process of L5; *L4*, transverse process of L4.

The probe is positioned just lateral to the midline longitudinally to identify the different spinal levels. The cephalad part of the sacrum is identified via a paravertebral sonogram. Then, the target lumbar transverse process is confirmed by counting upward from the sacrum (Fig. 37-2). After the transverse process of the target lumbar vertebra is confirmed, the probe is rotated 90 degrees and a transverse sonogram is obtained. The target point for the needle is the bottom of the fossa between the lateral surface of the superior articular process and the cephalad margin of the transverse process (Figs. 37-1, 37-3, and 37-4). By adjusting and toggling the probe, the facet joint can be visualized as a hypoechoic slit just medial to the superior articular process (Fig. 37-5). The needle is inserted in-line until

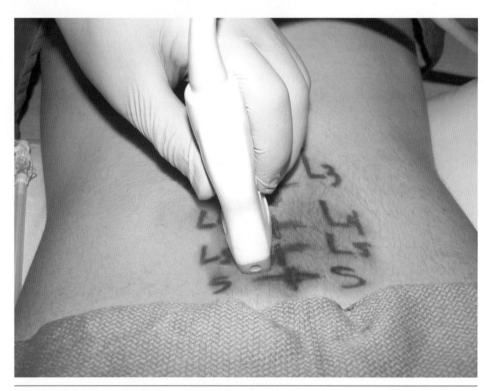

Figure 37-3a. Longitudinal probe position.

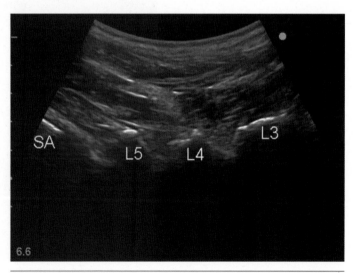

Figure 37-3b. *S*, sacrum; *L5*, transverse process of L5; *L4*, transverse process of L4; *L3*, transverse process of L3.

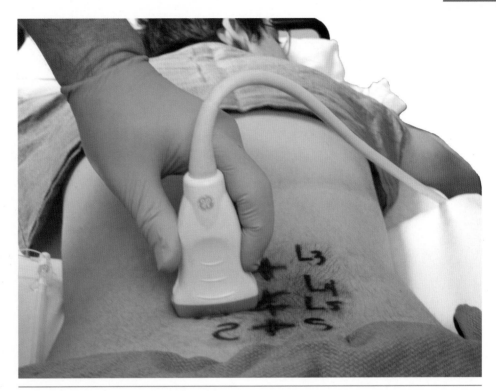

Figure 37-3c. Transverse probe position.

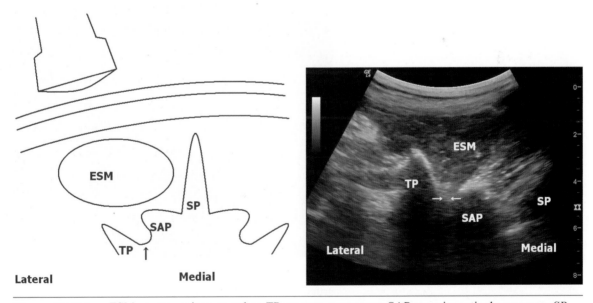

Figure 37-3d,e. *ESM*, erector spinae muscles; *TP*, transverse process; *SAP*, superior articular process; *SP*, spinous process; *arrows*, needle tip target.

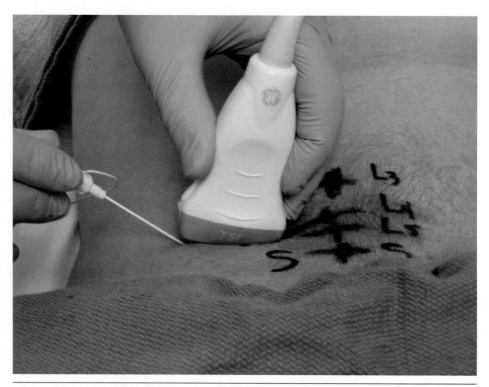

Figure 37-4a. In-line needle placement.

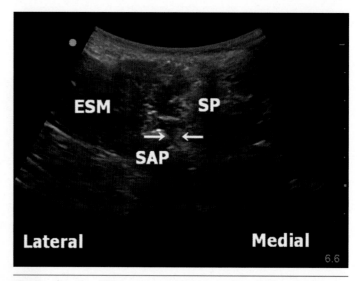

Figure 37-4b. *ESM,* erector spinae muscles; *SAP,* superior articular process; *SP,* spinous process; *arrows,* needle tip target.

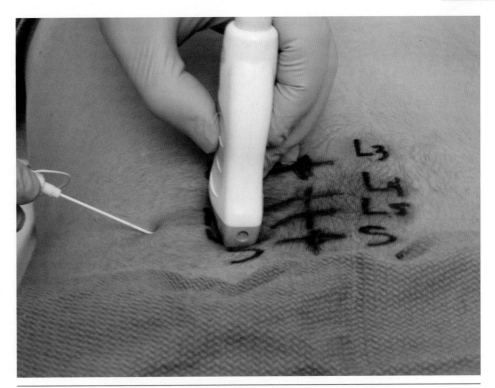

Figure 37-5a. Out-of-plane needle placement.

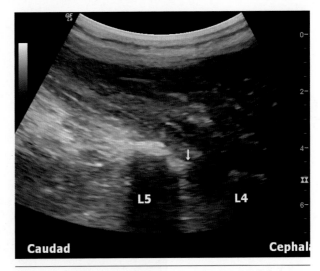

Figure 37-5b. *L4*, L4 transverse process; *L5*, L5 transverse process; *arrow*, target for needle tip.

boney contact is made. Once the bone has been contacted, the probe may be rotated back to the long axis and the shadows of the transverse processes are imaged (Fig. 37-6). The tip of the needle should be evident by moving the needle and the tip should be seen at the upper part of the transverse process. Failure to image the tip may result in transforaminal injection or nerve root injury. Once the proper location of the needle tip is confirmed, local anesthetic is injected.

L5 Nerve Root Block: L5 dorsal ramus blockade can be technically challenging because of a high iliac crest. The sacrum and transverse processes are imaged in the longitudinal plane (Fig. 37-7). If the iliac crest is obscuring the view, the injection should be

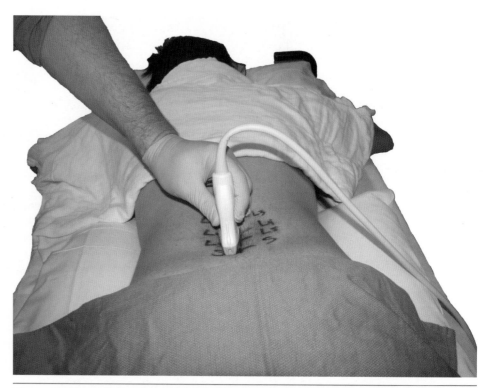

Figure 37-6a. L5 dorsal ramus block, probe position.

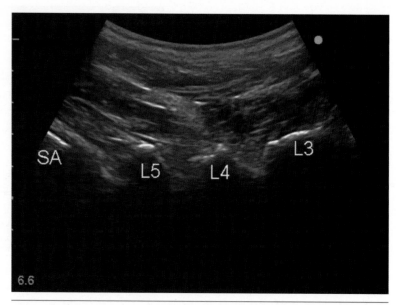

Figure 37-6b. *S*, sacrum; *L5*, transverse process of L5; *L4*, transverse process of L4; *L3*, transverse process of L3.

done as the out-of-plane approach. The transducer is rotated to transverse position at the level L5/S1 (Fig. 37-8). The base of the S1 superior articular process (the angle between S1 superior articular process and the sacral ala) is kept in the middle of image. The block needle is inserted in caudocephalad direction until the tip contacts the target—S1/sacral ala junction (Fig. 37-8). If necessary, the probe can be rotated back to a longitudinal view to verify that the tip is not positioned beyond the sacral ala into the L5/S1 intervertebral foramen. If the needle is within the L5/S1 foramen, it should be withdrawn 2 to 3 mm

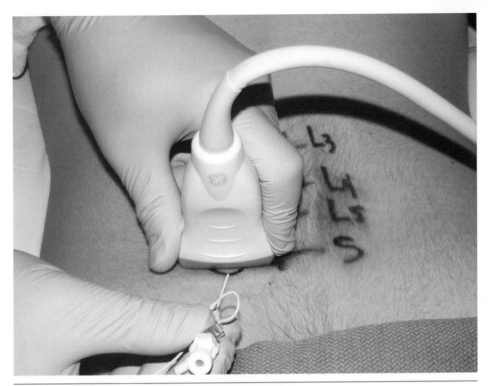

Figure 37-7a. L5 dorsal ramus block, probe position.

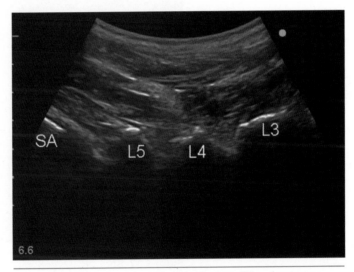

Figure 37-7b. *IC*, iliac crest; *SA*, sacrum; *SP*, spinous process.

to prevent transforaminal injection. Once the proper needle position is confirmed, local anesthetic is injected.

Facet Joint Injection: A needle is inserted via an in-line technique at an angle of 45 degrees to the skin. The needle is advanced toward the target joint, and the tip of the needle is placed in the joint space (Fig. 37-5). Once the needle has entered the joint space, local anesthetic is injected. In cases in which injection is impossible resulting from high resistance, local anesthetic is administered around the joint space.

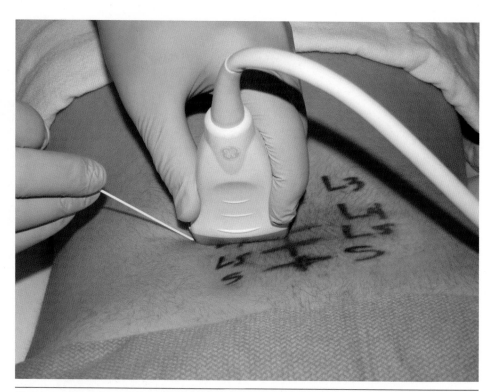

Figure 37-8a. Facet joint injection.

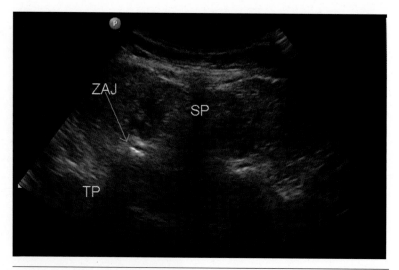

Figure 37-8b. *ZAG*, zygopophysial joint (facet joint);
SP, spinous process; *TP*, transverse process.

Summary of Evidence: Lumbar zygapophysial joint pain is routinely diagnosed by comparative block of the sensory nerves. This is one of the most common diagnostic procedure in the management of spinal pain.[3] Ultrasound guidance of such injections has been studied with healthy volunteers[4] and validated against computed tomography (CT).[5] In a recently published clinical study with fluoroscopic control,[6] all 101 needles were placed in the correct lumbar segment, and 96 (95%) of the needles were in the correct position. Two of the needles were associated with intravascular spread of the contrast dye. The mean pain score on a visual analog scale was reduced from 52 before to 16 after block.[6] The study had several limitations, in particular the relatively low body mass index of the study patients, which facilitated visualization of the spine and a high success rate. However, in the earlier study by Greher et al,[4] ultrasound imaging was of adequate quality in a patient with a 36 kg/m², so body mass index is not necessarily a limiting factor. It is also worth mentioning that patients with pain related to the lumbosacral zygapophysial joint were excluded from the study,[6] and L5 dorsal ramus block has therefore not been evaluated.

Periarticular injection of lumbar zygapophysial joints was probably the first application of ultrasound guidance to be describe,[7] and the method was recently validated against CT-guided injection in a randomized controlled study.[8]

Although fluoroscopy and CT should remain the standard image guidance tools for patients whose anatomic features pose particular challenges (e.g., obesity, severe degenerative changes, malformation), ultrasound can be implemented in the office-based practice for diagnostic and therapeutic injections.

References

1. Grau T, Leipold RW, Horter J, et al. The lumbar epidural space in pregnancy: visualization by ultrasonography. Br J Anaesth 2001;86:798–804.
2. Arzola C, Davies S, Rofaeel A, et al. Ultrasound using the transverse approach to the lumbar spine provides reliable landmarks for labor epidurals. Anesth Analg 2007;104:1188–1192.
3. Boswell MV, Shah RV, Everett CR, et al. Interventional techniques in the management of chronic spinal pain: evidence-based practice guidelines. Pain Physician 2005;8:1–47.
4. Greher M, Scharbert G, Kamolz LP, et al. Ultrasound-guided lumbar facet nerve block: a sonoanatomic study of a new methodologic approach. Anesthesiology 2004;100:1242–1248.
5. Greher M, Kirchmair L, Enna B, et al. Ultrasound-guided lumbar facet nerve block: accuracy of a new technique confirmed by computed tomography. Anesthesiology 2004;101:1195–1200.
6. Shim JK, Moon JC, Yoon KB, et al. Ultrasound-guided lumbar medial-branch block: a clinical study with fluoroscopy control. Reg Anesth Pain Med. 2006;31:451–454.
7. Küllmer K, Rompe JD, Löwe A, et al. [Ultrasound image of the lumbar spine and the lumbosacral transition. Ultrasound anatomy and possibilities for ultrasonically-controlled facet joint infiltration] [Article in German] Z Orthop Ihre Grenzgeb 1997;135(4):310–314.
8. Galiano K, Obwegeser AA, Walch C, et al. Ultrasound-guided versus computed tomography-controlled facet joint injections in the lumbar spine: a prospective randomized clinical trial. Reg Anesth Pain Med 2007;32:317–322.

38

Use of Ultrasonography in Rheumatology

RALF THIELE

Musculoskeletal ultrasonography is increasingly recognized as a useful tool in rheumatology practice. Proficiency in this imaging modality has been a requirement for board eligibility in some European countries for more than 15 years. Since then, the number of scientific publications on musculoskeletal ultrasound has been rising steadily (Fig. 38-1). Ultrasonography provides the highest image resolution of all available imaging modalities, is safe, inexpensive, and can be repeated at every office visit. As with conventional radiography, magnetic resonance imaging (MRI), and computerized tomography (CT), performance and interpretation of ultrasound imaging requires training and standardized protocols. Guidelines for musculoskeletal ultrasound in rheumatology and criteria for pathological findings have been suggested.[1,2] When trained rheumatologists perform reliability exercises using such guidelines, they regularly achieve good to excellent interobserver agreement.[3–5]

In musculoskeletal imaging, conventional radiography provides an overview over bony structures but gives little information about soft tissues. There is limited information about blood flow and inflammation. In contrast, ultrasonography visualizes only a small sector at one time but gives detailed tissue resolution and provides information about inflammation when Doppler imaging is used. MRI would be placed between these other imaging modalities on a continuum from overview to detail (Fig. 38-2).

In rheumatology, B-mode (or *brightness modulated*) and Doppler ultrasound are used. In B-mode or grayscale ultrasound, tissues are distinguished by their brightness or echogenicity, with bony structures, tendons and crystals being bright or hyperechoic, synovial tissue gray or hypochechoic, and synovial fluid black or anechoic. Doppler ultrasound detects shifts in the frequency of sound waves reflected from moving objects, which in the human body are largely erythrocytes. Doppler ultrasound is therefore an ideal tool to assess increased blood flow in inflamed synovial tissue.[6]

What are important indications for ultrasound in rheumatology?

- Early detection of erosive disease
- Assessment of effusions
- Assessment of synovial tissue
- Assessment of treatment response
- Detection of enthesitis in seronegative spondyloarthropathy
- Diagnosis of large vessel vasculitis
- Assessment of salivary glands
- Assessment of crystal arthropathy
- Needle guidance in aspiration and injection

Figure 1

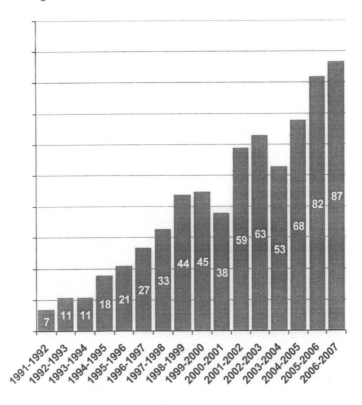

Number of publications on musculoskeletal ultrasound, two year periods. Database: OVID

Figure 38-1. Publications in ultrasonography and rheumatology.

1. Early detection of erosive disease: Conventional radiography has traditionally been used to detect bony erosions. Radiographs project three-dimensional structures on a two-dimensional plane. This summation effect makes conventional radiography less sensitive in the detection of bony erosions when compared with cross-sectional imaging such as MRI and ultrasound (Figs. 38-3 and 38-4). Ultrasonography detects early erosions with higher sensitivity than radiography, and detects more erosion in later disease stages.[7] This imaging modality is therefore useful in early detection of erosive arthritis and may facilitate early institution of disease modifying treatment (Fig. 38-4). MRI is also used in assessing erosions but has the disadvantage of considerable higher cost. In addition, MRI may overestimate or underestimate the size of the actual erosion. Infiltration of the erosion with fatty tissue may mimic normal trabecular bone, whereas bone sclerosis, resulting from a lack of signal on MRI, may mimic erosion.[8]

2. Assessment of effusions: Ultrasonography is superior to clinical examination in the detection and localization of knee joint effusions in rheumatoid arthritis (Fig. 38-5).[9,10] When compared with MRI, sonography detects more joint and tendon sheath effusions.[11] Detection of small joint effusions is more effective with US compared with MRI.[12]

3. Assessment of synovial tissue: Ultrasonography was found to be a valid and reproducible technique for detecting synovitis.[10] Synovial hypervascularity can be assessed with power Doppler or color Doppler.[13] Power Doppler provides information about the strength of blood flow and is sensitive in low-flow states such as vascularized synovial tissue (Fig. 38-6). Color Doppler encodes direction and velocity of blood flow, which are of lesser interest in rheumatology. In newer machines, sensitivities are often equal for power and color Doppler, so that either modality is used.[6]

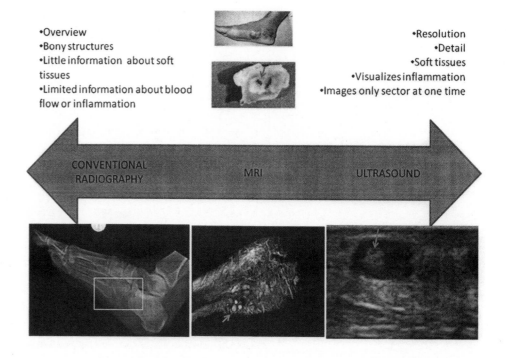

- Overview
- Bony structures
- Little information about soft tissues
- Limited information about blood flow or inflammation

- Resolution
- Detail
- Soft tissues
- Visualizes inflammation
- Images only sector at one time

CONVENTIONAL RADIOGRAPHY   MRI   ULTRASOUND

30 year old male with granulomatous condition of the midfoot contracted in Africa over 5 years ago (top). Resection yielded a mycetoma. Hyphae are seen on biopsy specimen (arrow, below) and ultrasound image (arrow, bottom right). Less detail is seen on MRI (bottom, middle), and conventional radiograph (bottom, left).

Figure 38-2. Comparison of x-ray, MRI, and ultrasound.

4. Assessment of treatment response: Ultrasound is inexpensive and user friendly (Fig. 38-7). Examination of pathological findings in a given patient can therefore be repeated at every office visit. This makes US an ideal tool to assess treatment response. Erosion size can be measured, and an increase in number and size may serve as an indicator that remission has not been achieved. Conversely, stability of erosions or healing of erosions can indicate efficacy of treatment. Thickness of hypertrophic synovial tissue can be measured from the hyperechoic capsular tissue to the anechoic synovial fluid, with synovium having a hypoechoic echogenicity. A decrease of this thickness corresponds to treatment response. An increase or decrease of hyperemia seen on Doppler studies corresponds to disease activity.[6]

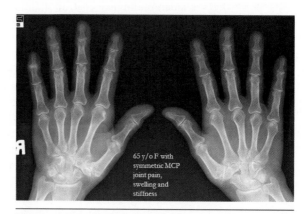

65 y/o F with symmetric MCP joint pain, swelling and stiffness

Figure 38-3. Conventional radiograph appears normal.

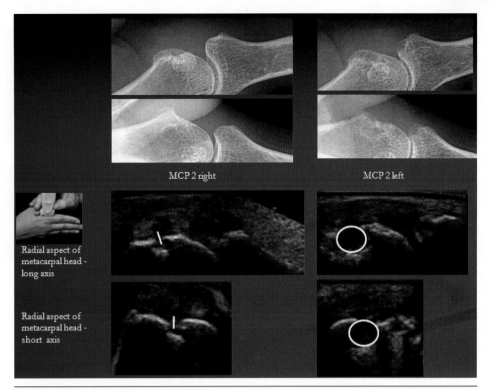

MCP 2 right   MCP 2 left

Radial aspect of
metacarpal head -
long axis

Radial aspect of
metacarpal head -
short axis

Figure 38-4. Ultrasound shows erosive disease.

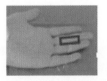

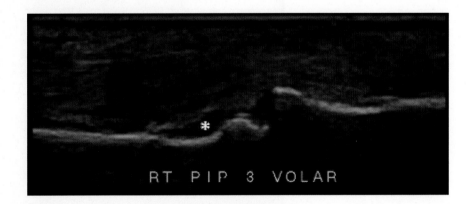

RT PIP 3 VOLAR

Inflammatory arthritis: Minute effusion in PIP joint

Figure 38-5. Joint effusion.

- Tenosynovitis: Hypoechoic tissue surrounding the hyperechoic tendons on the dorsal, volar, ulnar or radial aspect, seen in long and short axis.

- Synovitis: Hypoechoic, poorly compressible tissue distending the more hyperechoic joint capsules of radiocarpal and midcarpal joints, with or without the presence of displaceable anechoic synovial fluid.

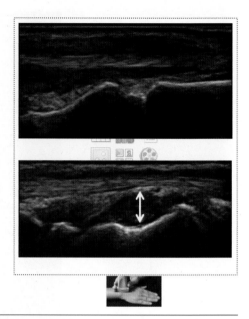

Figure 38-6. Diagnosis of synovitis and tenosynovitis.

5. Detection of enthesitis in seronegative spondyloarthropathy: Enthesitis is one of the hallmark findings in spondyloarthropathies, in particular psoriatic arthritis, ankylosing spondylitis and reactive arthritis (Fig. 38-8). Entheseal pain and swelling can be appreciated on clinical exam, but visualization of characteristic findings will increase specificity. Characteristic sonographic findings in enthesitis include edema of the tendon insertion with increased thickness when compared with normal values, synovial inflammation of adjacent bursae, erosive changes at or near the enthesis, and blood flow at

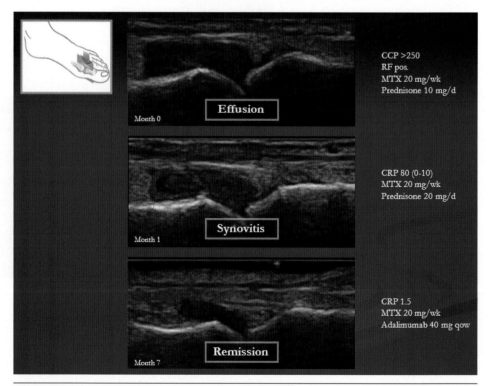

Figure 38-7. Stages of recovery documented on ultrasound.

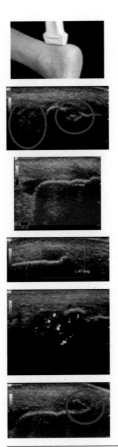

Detection of enthesitis in seronegative spondyloarthropathy

Criteria for enthesitis:

1. Erosion at calcaneus

2. Retrocalcaneal bursitis

3. Thickening of Achilles tendon
   (normal: f <4.1 mm, m<4.6 mm)
   Schmidt, WA 2006

4. Power Doppler signal at insertion or within bursa

5. New bone formation

   OMERACT 2005

Figure 38-8. Detection of enthesitis.

the interface of tendon and bone (a normally avascular area).[14] It is currently not known if MRI or ultrasonography provides a higher sensitivity, but characteristic changes can be seen on ultrasound even in the absence of enthesitis or bone marrow edema on MRI. Ultrasonography can assist with early diagnosis and assessment of treatment response. It may help decide which patients are adequately treated with disease modifying medication such as methotrexate alone, and which patients require biologic treatment.

6. Assessment of large vessel vasculitis: Grayscale and Doppler sonography can assess superficial large arteries. Aortic branches can be evaluated in Takayasu arteritis and temporal arteries can be evaluated in temporal arteritis. Intima, media, and adventitia layers can be distinguished, and concentric thickening of media structures can be appreciated sonographically. The "halo-sign" of concentric thickening around the vascular lumen distinguishes arteritis from atherosclerotic disease.[15–17] Sensitivity of 87% and specificity of 96% were found in a metaanalysis of 23 studies.[18]

7. In Sjögren syndrome, assessment of salivary glands may be of interest (Fig. 38-9). Measurement of volume and detection of parenchymal inhomogeneity of the major salivary glands resulted in high specificity for the diagnosis of primary and secondary Sjögren's syndrome.[19]

8. Assessment of crystal arthropathy: Gout is one of the most common forms of inflammatory arthritis with a rapidly growing incidence and prevalence worldwide. Diagnosis rests on needle aspiration and polarizing microscopy. However, this is often not done because it results in a dry aspiration. Urate crystals in and around joints are very echogenic and can readily be appreciated sonographically. In contrast, urate crystals are radiolucent and can therefore not be seen on conventional radiographs. MRI can see larger tophaceous deposits (but not small deposits), yet findings are often nonspecific. Using MRI, tophi adjacent to tendons cannot readily be distinguished from giant cell tumors, so that surgical biopsies are often requested if an MRI is ordered in this setting.

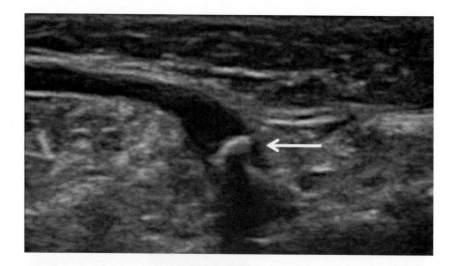

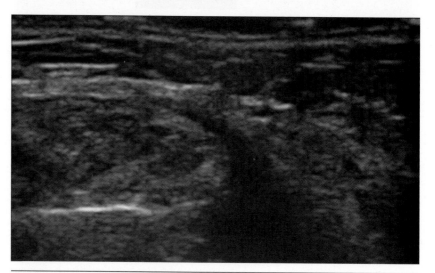

Figure 38-9. Detection of a stone in a dilated salivary duct.

Early use of ultrasonography in suspected gout can therefore facilitate effective treatment with urate-lowering drugs. Urate crystals can be distinguished sonographically from calcium pyrophosphate crystals by their characteristic pattern of distribution.[20]

9. Needle guidance in aspiration and injection: Most rheumatologists will feel very comfortable injecting large and small joints without imaging guidance. However, accurate intra-articular or intrabursal placement of the needle is not always certain with blind injections. Correct intra-articular needle placement was achieved in 32% and 59%, respectively, when clinical examination alone was used. Ultrasound-guided injections achieved 96% to 97% accuracy, when Roentgen arthrography was used as the gold standard.[21,22] But does it change the clinical outcome whether a steroid is placed in or around a joint or bursa? In one study comparing blind shoulder injections with ultrasound-guided injections, visual analog pain scores and functional assessment scores improved more in the group that received the ultrasound-guided injections.[23]

Conclusion

• Office-based musculoskeletal ultrasound has a wide spectrum of useful indications.
• There is a good potential for research.
• Patient care is improved through precise, early diagnosis.

- Treatment response can be quickly assessed.
- Standardization of the exam is essential to minimize operator variability.
- Musculoskeletal ultrasound is a promising diagnostic tool that belongs in the hands of the practitioner.

References

1. Backhaus M, Burmester GR, Gerber T, et al. Guidelines for musculoskeletal ultrasound in rheumatology. Ann Rheum Dis 2001;60(7):641–649.
2. Wakefield RJ, Balint PV, Szkudlarek M, et al. Musculoskeletal ultrasound including definitions for ultrasonographic pathology. J Rheumatol 2005;32(12):2485–2487.
3. Scheel AK, Schmidt WA, Hermann KG, et al. Interobserver reliability of rheumatologists performing musculoskeletal ultrasonography: results from a EULAR "Train the trainers" course. Ann Rheum Dis 2005;64(7):1043–1049.
4. Naredo E, Moller I, Moragues C, et al. Interobserver reliability in musculoskeletal ultrasonography: results from a "Teach the Teachers" rheumatologist course. Ann Rheum Dis 2006;65(1):14–19.
5. Koski JM, Saarakkala S, Helle M, et al. Assessing the intra- and inter-reader reliability of dynamic ultrasound images in power Doppler ultrasonography. Ann Rheum Dis 2006;65(12):1658–1660.
6. Thiele R. Doppler ultrasonography in rheumatology: adding color to the picture. J Rheumatol 2008;35(1): 8–10.
7. Wakefield RJ, Gibbon WW, Conaghan PG, et al. The value of sonography in the detection of bone erosions in patients with rheumatoid arthritis: a comparison with conventional radiography. Arthritis Rheum 2000;43(12):2762–2770.
8. Dohn UM, Ejbjerg BJ, Hasselquist M, et al. Rheumatoid arthritis bone erosion volumes on CT and MRI: reliability and correlations with erosion scores on CT, MRI and radiography. Ann Rheum Dis 2007;66(10):1388–1392.
9. Kane D, Balint PV, Sturrock RD. Ultrasonography is superior to clinical examination in the detection and localization of knee joint effusion in rheumatoid arthritis. J Rheumatol 2003;30(5):966–971.
10. Karim Z, Wakefield RJ, Quinn M, et al. Validation and reproducibility of ultrasonography in the detection of synovitis in the knee: a comparison with arthroscopy and clinical examination. Arthritis Rheum 2004;50(2):387–394.
11. Hoving JL, Buchbinder R, Hall S, et al. A comparison of magnetic resonance imaging, sonography, and radiography of the hand in patients with early rheumatoid arthritis. J Rheumatol 2004;31(4): 663–675.
12. Szkudlarek M, Narvestad E, Klarlund M, et al. Ultrasonography of the metatarsophalangeal joints in rheumatoid arthritis: comparison with magnetic resonance imaging, conventional radiography, and clinical examination. Arthritis Rheum 2004;50(7):2103–2112.
13. Strunk J, Heinemann E, Neeck G, Schmidt KL, Lange U. A new approach to studying angiogenesis in rheumatoid arthritis by means of power Doppler ultrasonography and measurement of serum vascular endothelial growth factor. Rheumatology (Oxford) 2004;43(12):1480–1403.
14. D'Agostino MA, Said-Nahal R, Hacquard-Bouder C, et al. Assessment of peripheral enthesitis in the spondylarthropathies by ultrasonography combined with power Doppler: a cross-sectional study. Arthritis Rheum 2003;48(2):523–533.
15. Schmidt WA, Kraft HE, Volker L, Vorpahl K, Gromnica-Ihle EJ. Colour Doppler sonography to diagnose temporal arteritis. Lancet 1995;345(8953):866.
16. Schmidt WA, Kraft HE, Vorpahl K, Volker L, Gromnica-Ihle EJ. Color duplex ultrasonography in the diagnosis of temporal arteritis. N Engl J Med 1997;337(19):1336–1342.
17. Schmidt WA. Takayasu and temporal arteritis. Front Neurol Neurosci 2006;21:96–104.
18. Karassa FB, Matsagas MI, Schmidt WA, et al. Meta-analysis: test performance of ultrasonography for giant-cell arteritis. Ann Intern Med 2005;142(5):359–369.
19. Wernicke D, Hess H, Gromnica-Ihle E, et al. Ultrasonography of salivary glands—a highly specific imaging procedure for diagnosis of Sjogren's syndrome. J Rheumatol 2008;35(2):285–293.
20. Thiele RG, Schlesinger N. Diagnosis of gout by ultrasound. Rheumatology (Oxford) 2007;46(7): 1116–1121.
21. Balint PV, Kane D, Hunter J, et al. Ultrasound guided versus conventional joint and soft tissue fluid aspiration in rheumatology practice: a pilot study. J Rheumatol 2002;29(10):2209–2213.
22. Raza K, Lee CY, Pilling D, et al. Ultrasound guidance allows accurate needle placement and aspiration from small joints in patients with early inflammatory arthritis. Rheumatology (Oxford) 2003; 42(8):976–979.
23. Naredo E, Cabero F, Beneyto P, et al. A randomized comparative study of short term response to blind injection versus sonographic-guided injection of local corticosteroids in patients with painful shoulder. J Rheumatol 2004;31(2):308–314.

Section *VII*

The Future of Ultrasound

39 The Future of Sonography

40 Identification of Nerves on Ultrasound Scans Using Artificial Intelligence and Machine Vision

41 Acoustic Radiation Force Imaging In Regional Anesthesia

42 Impedance Neurography

43 Evaluation of Thoracic Paravertebral And Lumbar Plexus Anatomy Using a 3D Ultrasound Probe

44 Optimum Design of Echogenic Needles for Ultrasound-Guided Nerve Block

45 Medical Image Segmentation Using Modified Mumford Segmentation Methods

The Future of Sonography

PAUL E. BIGELEISEN

Getting Started: In 1992, anesthesiologists in the United States began to use primitive ultrasound machines to assist with axillary blocks. These machines were designed to guide vascular cannulation. Some anesthesiologists used these machines to image the axillary artery. That allowed the user to direct the injection of local anesthetic around the artery. This technique showed modest improvements over transarterial, stimulation guided, and paresthesia techniques. I did not have access to one of these devices, but I thought with a better machine I might be able to see some or all of the nerves. I enlisted the help of two vascular sonographers who had access to an ATL platform. We used a linear probe oscillating at 6 MHz and imaged the infraclavicular fossa in 20 healthy, fit volunteers all of whom had body mass indices of less than 21. The vascular anatomy was clear, but I could not identify any nerves. Part of the problem was that I did not have a proper idea of where the cords or branches should lie or what they should look like on ultrasound. I abandoned the concept.

By 2002, the world had changed. Portable ultrasound platforms, costing about $25,000 were available and several authors had reported excellent results performing infraclavicular blocks with this technology in the United States. My colleague, Rajbala Thakur encouraged me to give this new technology a try. I was skeptical based on my experience a decade earlier. But Thakur invited N.P. Sandhu to give us a demonstration in Rochester. Lacking patients that day, Sandhu gave me an infraclavicular block with ultrasound guidance. He was able to anesthetize my arm and forearm with 3 mL of 2% lidocaine. He convinced me that ultrasound was the wave of the future.

Now with my own machine, I had to teach myself how to perform these blocks. There were no courses to take, no books to study, and there was little consensus in the literature regarding what the images really depicted. I went back to the cadaver lab and made sagittal and axial cross sections of the brachial, lumbar, and sciatic plexuses. These dissections would enable me to interpret the images I saw on ultrasound. I also paid my children to lie still for hours and scanned them from head to toe so that I could make some real time correlations with the cadaver dissections I had created. After 2 years of trial and error, I felt that I could reliably image and perform interscalene, supraclavicular, infraclavicular, axillary, femoral, and popliteal blocks.

Still, the portable ultrasound platforms we used were adequate at best and I had difficulty teaching this new technology to my peers and residents. Seasoned faculty were especially skeptical. I decided to work on enhancing the images. I recruited two engineers at Rochester Institute of Technology (Maria Helgera, Steven Gold) in imaging science and two applied mathematicians at the National Science Foundation (Steven Damelin, Yungha An). Together we developed a technique using a Mumford Shaw algorithm that enabled us to improve the resolution of still images. This was an imaging triumph, but had little practical application because the image analysis could not be done in real time. In fact, it took about 25 minutes to process each image. Nonetheless, the improved images did give me some unusual insights that other practitioners did not have. When I performed ultrasound-guided blocks, it seemed to me that the needle was often intraneural and that the nerve would swell when I injected local anesthetic. I took some of these images of probable intraneural injection, enhanced them with the Mumford Shaw technique, and I became convinced that I was frequently injecting nerves. Armed with this additional information, I brought the enhanced and unenhanced images to a radiologist who specialized in ultrasound imaging. She assured me that the injections were intraneural.

After several hundred intraneural injections, I became convinced that intraneural injections in peripheral nerves were unlikely to cause nerve damage. In fact, they provided excellent surgical anesthesia with very low doses of local anesthetic. In 2005, I decided to study this phenomenon in a prospective study of axillary blocks. I presented some early results to my colleagues at Rochester. I showed them videos of intraneural injections that did not reliably produce paresthesiae or dysaesthesiae and in which there were no permanent complications. I published the material in late 2006, and a firestorm erupted. All prejudice aside, I think that ultrasound will continue to provide information about the risks and benefits of intraneural injections,

In 2006, I took leave of Rochester and went to Pittsburgh at the invitation of Jacques Chelly. The University of Pittsburgh has the largest regional anesthesia department in the world, performing over 20,000 peripheral nerve blocks a year. The university, along with Carnegie Mellon University also has the greatest expertise using artificial intelligence to perform image enhancement and pattern recognition of images. I enlisted CC Li and James Chien from the department of electrical engineering to help me. Dr. Williams funded the study, and in about a year we had trained a computer to recognize static images of nerves on an ultrasound scan using artificial intelligence. At the same time, Nizar Moayeri came to work with me on a Fulbright fellowship and used his background in computer science and medicine to make better correlations between gross anatomy and ultrasound scans.

The Future: A few years ago, Phil Cory asked me to look at a new technique he had developed using radiofrequency energy to image nerves. The concept is similar to an electrocardiogram (EKG). Nerves, even at rest, give off electrical signals. With a proper surface antenna and processing, one can image the nerves. I allowed Cory to test the device on me and became convinced that it had merit. Work continues to develop this very useful and potentially inexpensive technology. At the same time, I recognized that we needed better needles to enhance ultrasound-guided block. I made a few protoypes myself and enlisted Assad Oberai and Yun Jing at Rensselaer Polytechnic Institute to study the problem using a formal physics foundation. This enabled us to quickly zero in on the most likely designs. Prototypes have been tested, and likely candidates have been identified for commercial production. At Duke University, Stuart Grant enlisted several engineers to study the use of radiation force ultrasonography. This technique, which measures the elasticity of tissue, shows great potential in allowing us to image needles and nerves for much deeper blocks. Sugantha Ganapathy had begun some interesting studies using 3D ultrasound and graciously shared her ideas with me. All of these advances are discussed in the next chapters. The future of regional anesthesia with ultrasound guidance is robust. The addition of new needles, artificial intelligence, radiation force sonography, three-dimensional ultrasound, and impedance neurography will certainly allow users to quickly identify nerves and anesthetize them.

40

Identification of Nerves on Ultrasound Scans Using Artificial Intelligence and Machine Vision

PAUL E. BIGELEISEN, JONG-CHIH CHIEN

Background: One of the skills necessary to conduct ultrasound-guided nerve blocks is the ability to recognize nerves, vessels, muscles, bones, and viscera in sagittal and axial cross sections. In fit, healthy patients, these structures are relatively easy to recognize. In obese patients, this can be a challenge because adipose tissue rapidly attenuates the ultrasound signal. Moreover, adipose tissue, both within and outside the nerve plexus, causes speculation that degrades the resolution of the image.

In each region of the body, nerves have a different set of textures and appearances on ultrasound scans. Near the spinal cord (above the clavicle), the nerves are usually hypoechoic. Further from the spinal cord (below the clavicle), the nerves are usually hyperechoic.[1] Fortunately, the nerves lie near to arteries, veins, bones, muscles, and viscera that can serve as easily recognizable landmarks. When populations of patients are studied, a map of the distribution of nerves relative to these landmarks can be made.[2–4] Once this map has been made, it can be used as the domain in which nerves can be identified using standard texture analysis. This process is also called artificial intelligence or machine vision. An example of machine vision familiar to most physicians is the identification and counting of red and white blood cells in a Coulter counter.[5] This device uses electrical impedance to measure the size of cells in a blood sample. Using the statistical variation in the size of blood cells, the machine is able to count the number and type of each cell (red cells and white cells) as well as anomalies in a blood sample. We have used standard techniques in image processing and artificial intelligence to develop a process that will identify nerves on ultrasound scans in fit patients.[6–9]

Materials and Methods: For brevity, we will focus on the supraclavicular and midinfraclavicular regions of the brachial plexus. The nerves in these areas represent hypoechoic and hyperechoic regions of interest. The nerves are superficial and adjacent to easily recognized landmarks. For the supraclavicular region, these landmarks are the subclavian artery and first rib. For the infraclavicular region, these landmarks are the axillary artery and vein, the pectoral muscles and the second rib.

Five ultrasound images of the supraclavicular and midinfraclavicular region from our ultrasound archive were taken from five patients whose ages ranged from 18 to 78 years and whose body mass indices ranged from 18 to 26. For the supraclavicular and infraclavicular approaches, three physicians were asked to identify the landmarks and nerves in each scan. From this data set, the position of the brachial plexus relative to the artery, vein, rib/pleura, and muscles were determined. The boundary of this area for all patients was then determined to be the search domain (region of interest) for the identification of the nerve plexus. This region of interest was defined as the positive data set.

Within each region of interest, textures that were similar to the positive data set but that were deemed to be nonneural tissue by the experts were also identified. These textures were defined as the negative data set. Using both positive and negative data sets, a Bayesian analysis was implemented in the machine vision algorithm to exclude nonneural tissue from the machine identification of nerves.[10,11]

Each image was processed using Law's texture analysis.[6] In this process, texture energy measures are evaluated from microtextures. The microtextures are computed from a set of 25 texture kernels of size 5 × 5 pixels applied to a small 5 × 5 region centered around each pixel. Each of these 2-dimensional kernels is constructed from the convolution of 1-dimensional kernels. That is a 5 × 1 pixel, vertical 1-demensional kernel is convoluted with a 1 × 5 pixel, horizontal 1-dimensional kernel. Five types of 1-dimensional kernels representing level, edge, spot wave, and ripple characteristics were used. This gave 25 different combinations for 2-dimensional kernels yielding the microtexture information (level, edge, spot, wave, and ripple). Once the microtexture kernels were built, a large macro window of size 15 × 15 pixels was placed around each pixel to generate a texture energy measure for each pixel. From the texture energy map and the search domain, the contour of the brachial plexus in each scan was determined. All programming was done in MATLAB.

Results: Figure 40-1 shows the region of interest for the infraclavicular region. Figure 40-2 shows a scan of the infraclavicular fossa. Figure 40-3 shows the negative (blue) data set. Figure 40-4 shows the areas identified as neural tissue. Figure 40-5 shows another scan of the infraclavicular fossa. Figure 40-6 shows the texture energy map of this scan that is used to identify the neural and nonneural tissue. Red and yellow are highly predictive of neural tissue. Figure 40-7 shows the neural tissue identified by machine vision.

Figure 40-8 shows the supraclaviular region of interest. Figure 40-9 shows a scan superimposed on the region of interest. The rib is identified by machine vision and used to narrow the region of interest. Figure 40-10 shows the texture analysis used to search for neural tissue in this scan. Figure 40-11 shows the neural tissue identified by human and machine vision.

Discussion: The boundaries of nerves (regions of interest) determined in our data set match those described in the anesthesia and radiology literature. The latter have been determined by CT and magnetic resonance imaging (MRI) scanning as well as cadaver dissection. The boundaries of the neural tissue identified by machine vision closely match those that were determined by human vision (skilled sonographers). In Figures 40-4, 40-6, and 40-11, a small amount of nonneural tissue appears to be identified as neural tissue by machine vision. This represents a failure of the Baysian filter. Further work in this field will be required to improve the Baysian filter and to extend this approach to obese patients and to other regions of the body.

Search Range: Infraclavicular

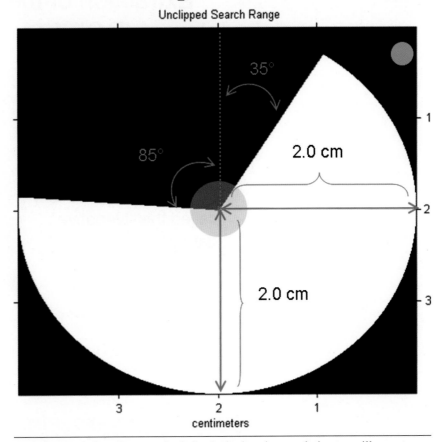

Figure 40-1. Search range for infraclavicular plexus relative to axillary artery.

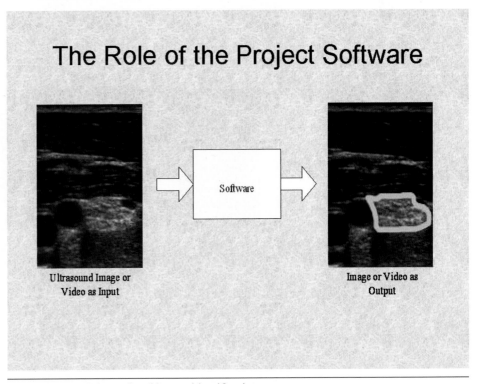

Figure 40-2. Schematic of image identification process.

Extraction of the Regions-of-Interest (ROI) from Samples, cont.

- The ensemble of the regions that do not contain nerve or nerves but resemble the regions that do is called the "Negative" data set.

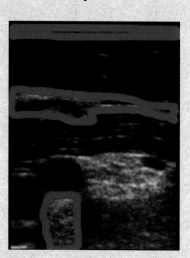

Figure 40-3. Identification of the negative set for infraclavicular block.

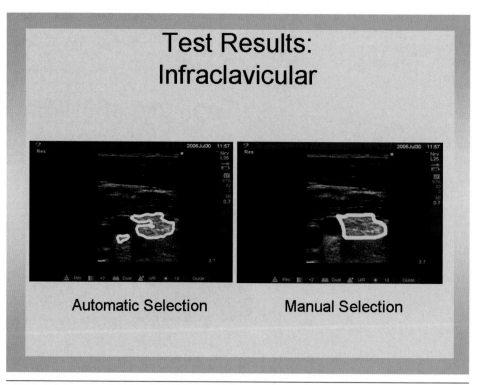

Figure 40-4. Comparison of machine vision versus human vision.

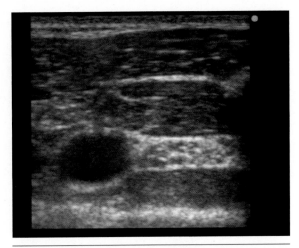

Figure 40-5. Infraclavicular plexus ultrasound.

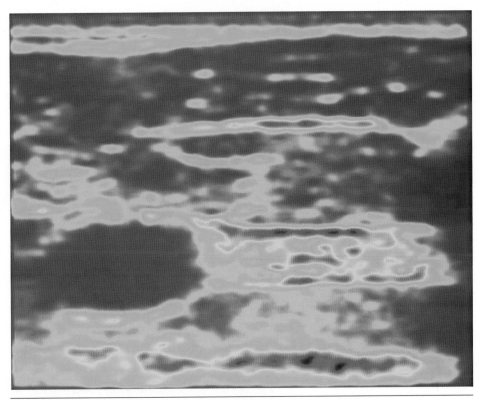

Figure 40-6. Texture energy analysis of Figure 40-5. Red, orange, and light blue regions are high probabilities for nerve tissue.

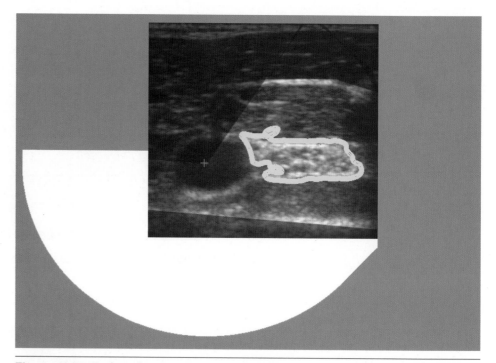

Figure 40-7. Fusion of texture energy map and search range yields machine identification of nerve tissue.

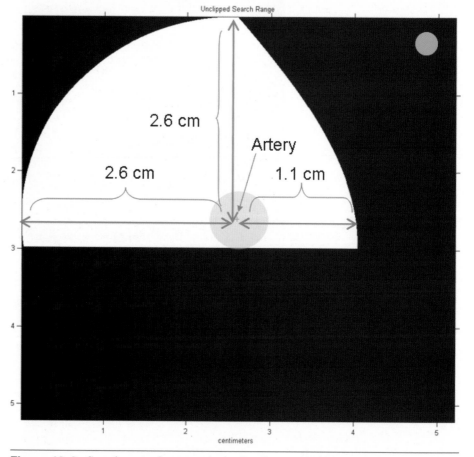

Figure 40-8. Search range for supraclavicular plexus relative to subclavian artery.

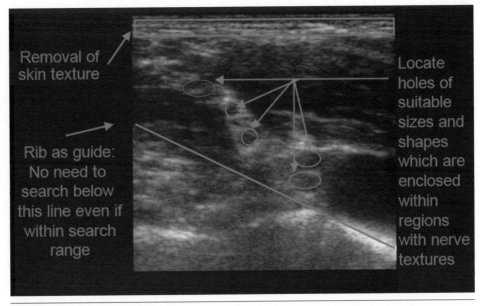

Figure 40-9a. Strategies for reducing the search range for supraclavicular plexus.

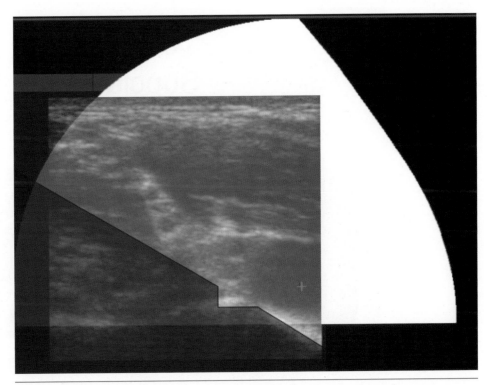

Figure 40-9b. Supraclavicular plexus superimposed on restricted search range.

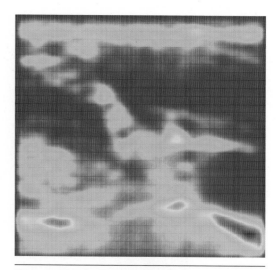

Figure 40-10. Texture energy plot of supracla- vicular plexus. Dark blue circles surrounded by light blue background are high probability for nerve tissue.

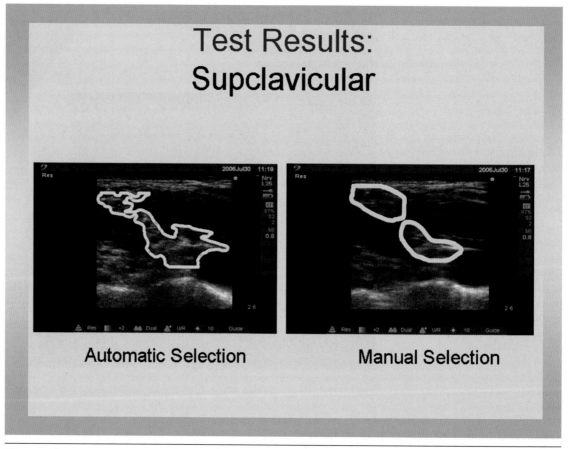

Figure 40-11. Comparison of machine vision identification of supraclavicular plexus with human vision.

References

1. Orebaugh SL, Bigeleisen P. Ultrasound Imaging in Brachial Plexus Blockade. Semin Anesth Perioperat Med Pain 2007;26:180–188.
2. Porter BC, Rubens DJ, Strang JG, et al. Three-dimensional registration and fusion of ultrasound and MRI using major vessels as fiducial markers. IEEE Trans Med Imaging 2001;20(4):354–359.
3. Jigang W, Neskovic P, Cooper LN. *Context-based tracking of object features.* Proceedings of the 2004 IEEE International Joint Conference on Neural Networks 2004(3):1775–1779.
4. Sauter AR, Smith HJ, Stubhaug A, et al. Use of Magnetic Resonance imaging to define the anatomical location closest to all three cords of the infraclavicular brachial plexus. J Anesth Analg 103;6:1574–1576.
5. Hegde UM, White JM, Hart GM, et al. Diagnosis of alpha-Thalasemia trait from Coulter Counter 's' indicies. J Clin Path 1977;30(9):884–889.
6. Laws K. *Textured Image Segmentation* [Ph.D. Dissertation]. University of Southern California; 1980.
7. Shigeo A. *Support Vector Machines for Pattern Classification.* Springer, 2005.
8. Theodoridis S, Koutroumbas K. Pattern recognition. *Academic* 2003.
9. Jain R, Kasturi R, Schunck BG. *Machine Vision* McGraw-Hill, 1995.
10. Gupta S, Chauhan RC, Saxena SC. Locally adaptive wavelet domain Bayesian processor for denoising medical ultrasound images using Speckle modeling based on Rayleigh distribution IEEE Proc Vis Image Signal Process 2005;152(1):129–135.
11. Poonguzhali S, Ravindran G. Performance Evaluation of Feature Extraction Methods for Classifying Abnormalities in Ultrasound Liver Images using Neural Network. Proceedings, 28th IEEE EMBS Conference Aug. 2006:4791–4794.

41

Acoustic Radiation Force Imaging in Regional Anesthesia

MARK PALMERI, STUART A. GRANT

Introduction: Currently, regional anesthesia using ultrasound guidance is performed using equipment developed for other medical specialties such as cardiology, obstetrics, and vascular surgery. B-mode imaging is used to help guide anesthetic injections during regional nerve blocks. B-mode imaging relies on acoustic impedance mismatches to scatter and reflect acoustic energy to generate images. Nerves can be difficult to visualize with B-mode imaging because they do not have appreciable ultrasonic contrast with adjacent soft tissues (muscle, fat, fascia). Additionally, problems can arise because the needles used for injection during regional anesthesia can be difficult to visualize once they move out of the plane of the beam and when the angle of needle insonation is increased.

Clinical palpation has been used for diagnosis of human pathology for centuries, and palpation has motivated the development of an imaging system capable of characterizing tissue elasticity (stiffness). This technology can differentiate tissue type based on mechanical properties. Tissues such as nerve and muscle may have similar density, making them impossible to differentiate using B-mode ultrasound. They may, however, have different elasticity or stiffness, and this provides a mechanical basis for contrast between different types of soft tissue (e.g., nerve, muscle, fat, fascia).

Acoustic force radiation imaging utilizes acoustic radiation force to impulsively excite tissues with a modified diagnostic ultrasound probe. The dynamic mechanical response of the tissue (movement) is monitored using conventional ultrasonic methods with the same transducer. Acoustic radiation force images display relative differences in tissue elasticity/stiffness that can provide improved contrast of soft-tissue structures over B-mode imaging.

Acoustic Radiation Force Imaging Methods: Focused acoustic energy can generate acoustic radiation force to reversibly deform soft tissues several microns.[1] Acoustic radiation force is applied to absorbing or reflecting materials in the propagation path of an acoustic wave resulting from a transfer of momentum. This radiation force can be described as[2]:

$$\vec{F} = \frac{2\alpha \vec{I}}{c},$$

where F is acoustic radiation force (in the form of a body force), c is the medium's sound speed, α is the medium's acoustic absorption coefficient, and I is the acoustic intensity at a given spatial location.

Acoustic radiation force impulse (ARFI) imaging has been used to image the mechanical properties of soft tissues for various clinical applications, including breast mass imaging, vascular imaging, ablation monitoring, liver, myocardial, and muscle stiffness mapping,

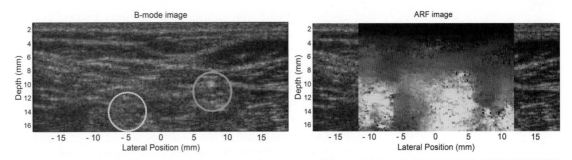

Figure 41-1. In vivo B-mode (*left*) and acoustic radiation force (*right*) images of the tibial and common peroneal nerves in a 29-year-old subject, just distal to their bifurcation from the sciatic nerve in the popliteal fossa. The ARFI image was generated using two excitation focal zones at 15 and 20 stiffer (darker) circular structures in cross-section; their location is not readily apparent in the B-mode image (they have been outlined in yellow [tibeal] and green [popliteal] based on the acoustic radiation force image boundaries). The improvement in nerve contrast is >600% in the acoustic radiation force image.

preoperative staging of rectal tumors, and prostate cancer imaging. The implementation of ARFI imaging described later represents the development of the first regional anesthesia-specific imaging modality.

Image Generation: Multiple excitation focal depths are utilized to optimize soft tissue structure contrast.[3] Displacements are estimated offline using Loupas' algorithm on IQ data acquired using 4:1 parallel receive beams.[4] The acoustic radiation force images utilize a copper colormap, wherein brighter pixels indicate greater displacement (and more compliant tissue) compared with darker pixels that represent stiffer tissue.

Imaging was performed using a modified Siemens Antares scanner, using linear arrays operating between 7 to 10 MHz. Multiple focal zone excitations ranging from 14 to 20 mm in depth were utilized with 35 μs radiation force excitations spanning a 20-mm lateral region of interest. Acoustic radiation force and B-mode image reconstructions were performed offline. Imaging was performed in situ on cadaveric sciatic nerves and in vivo in the brachial plexus and sciatic nerves. B-mode and acoustic radiation force images were acquired before, during, and after saline injections. Electrocardiogram (ECG) image acquisition triggering was utilized in vivo to limit motion artifacts.

Acoustic radiation force images demonstrate that nerves are relatively stiffer than their adjacent tissue. Improved nerve contrast up to 600% has been observed in acoustic radiation force images when compared with B-mode images (Fig. 41-1). Intraneural injection of nerves may also be recognized, because the stiffness of the nerve is reversed by injectate. This results in a reversal of acoustic radiation force image contrast.

Acoustic Radiation Force Imaging of Needles: Needles are very clearly delineated in B-mode images when they are (a) at shallow angles of approach (near parallel) relative to the transducer face, and (b) well-aligned 5 with the imaging plane. The *thickness* of an imaging plane in the depth of field is <1 mm; this small thickness can make needle alignment very challenging.

Needles are also difficult to visualize at steep insertion angles because most of the acoustic energy they reflect is directed away from the receiver aperture of the transducer, making them acoustically invisible. Needles cause an apparent stiffening of the adjacent tissue that can be visualized with acoustic force radiation imaging in situations where B-mode imaging fails (i.e., steep angles and misalignment). The ability to visualize needles in these orientations will allow an anesthesiologist to make more efficacious injections.

Experiments have been performed with needles in ex vivo beef muscle to evaluate the ability for acoustic force radiation images to localize needles at steep angles and in cross-section. Figure 41-2, left column, shows representative B-mode and acoustic force radiation images of an 18-gauge needle at a 50-degree angle relative to the transducer face; the right column shows the same needle realigned parallel to the transducer face at a depth of 18 mm, now in cross-section. Needles in cross-section can be difficult to visualize, because the hyperechoic reflections are small and can be mistaken for other small hyperechoic structures. Figure 41-3 shows how acoustic force radiation imaging can visualize needles and nerves concurrently in a cadaveric distal sciatic nerve in situ. An 18-gauge needle was intentionally inserted into the left upper quadrant of the nerve, causing significant ultrasound reflection and poor signal to noise deep to the needle that is very apparent in the ARFI image.

Acoustic Force Radiation Imaging of Injections: When soft tissues surrounding a nerve are infused with anechoic local anesthetic, there can be significant distortion of the preinjection B-mode image. This makes it difficult to evaluate the distribution of the anesthetic agent. The nerve itself may be displaced and distorted in the image. Knowledge of this motion/distortion of the nerve would be useful to an anesthesiologist, so that the needle could be repositioned to achieve a more effective nerve block where the entire nerve is bathed with

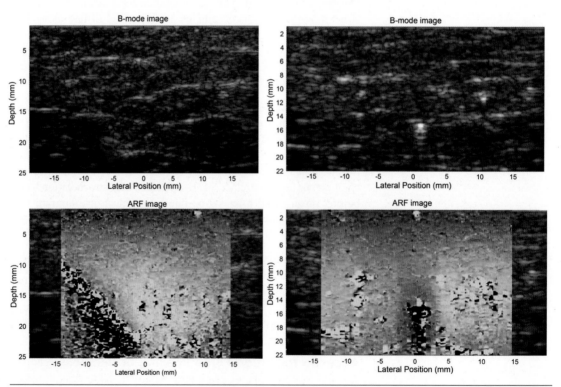

Figure 41-2. *Left, above,* and *below*: B-mode and acoustic radiation force images of an 18-g needle centered in the imaging plane at a 50-degree angle relative to the transducer face. Although the needle is not easily visualized in the B-mode image, it is clearly visible in the acoustic radiation image; however, there is significant decorrelation below the needle as a result of low signal-to-noise ratio. *Right, above,* and *below*: B-mode and acoustic radiation force images of an 18-g needle parallel to the transducer face in cross-section at a depth of 18 mm. The needle itself shows up as a black decorrelated circle with decorrelation deep to it. There is a ring of stiffened tissue extending an additional 2 mm from the needle that allows misaligned needle to be visualized in acoustic radiation force images.

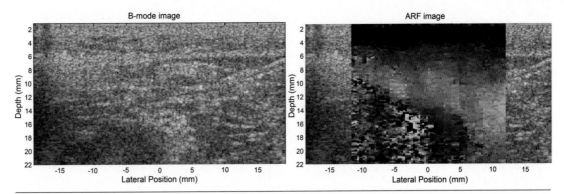

Figure 41-3. In situ distal cadaveric sciatic nerve with an 18-g needle intentionally piercing the upper left quadrant nerve sheath. There is significant decorrelation deep to the needle resulting from poor signal-to-noise ratio, but the tip of the needle and the edge of the decorrelation can be seen inside the sciatic nerve's left border, which appears dark (stiff) in the acoustic force radiation image. There is a 300% nerve contrast improvement in the acoustic radiation force image.

local anesthetic. Figure 41-4 shows how the nerves of interest can be translated and distorted by saline injections. This is more apparent in the acoustic force radiation images.

Summary: This preliminary data have demonstrated that nerves exhibit considerable mechanical contrast from their adjacent soft tissues. In the future, further optimized acoustic radiation force imaging beam sequences will be developed that can accommodate the array of nerve diameters and depths that may be encountered throughout the body based on anatomic location and body habitus.

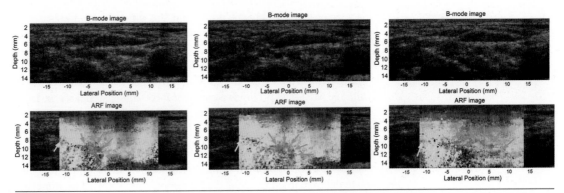

Figure 41-4. B-mode and acoustic radiation force images of the brachial plexus in vivo from an interscalene approach preinjection (*left*), after a 2-cc saline injection (*center*), and after an additional 4-cc saline injection (*right*). Preinjection, the needle (*yellow arrows*) was placed adjacent to the lower left aspect of the nerve bundle (*green arrows*). Notice that the substructures have displacement over 5 mm laterally in response to the injection, which is more apparent in the acoustic radiation force images.

References

1. Nightingale KR, Palmeri ML, Nightingale RW, Trahey GE. On the feasibility of remote palpation using acoustic radiation force. J Acoust Soc Am 2001;110(1):625–634.
2. Nyborg WLM. Acoustic streaming. In: Mason WP, ed. Physical Acoustics. Vol. IIB, Chap. 11. New York: Academic Press Inc; 1965:265–331.
3. Nightingale KR, Palmeri ML, Trahey GE. Analysis of contrast in images generated with transient acoustic radiation force. Ultrasound Med Biol 2006;32(1):61–72.
4. Dahl JD, Palmeri ML, Agrawal V, Nightingale KR, Trahey GE. A parallel tracking method for acoustic radiation force impulse imaging. IEEE Trans Ultrason Ferroelectr Freq Control 2007;54(2):301–312.
5. Palmeri ML, Dahl JJ, MacLeod DB, et al. On the feasibility of imaging peripheral nerves using acoustic radiation force impulse imaging. Ultrasonic Imaging 2009;31:172–189.

42

Impedance Neurography

PHILIP C. CORY, PAUL E. BIGELEISEN

There is a continuing need in anesthesia practice for technology that facilitates nerve location and the determination of the functional status of nerves. Impedance neurography is a noninvasive technique that enables the practitioner to construct two- and three-dimensional images of subcutaneous neural structures from skin surface impedance measurements. In addition, impedance neurography may demonstrate the functional status of peripheral nerves, including abnormalities, even at depth.

In 2002, Prokhorov et al reported that skin surface impedance measurements could identify the position of subcutaneous nerves. Additional work has improved our understanding of the underlying mechanism of impedance neurography so that deeper nerves can be imaged. The antenna is shown attached to the posterior of the thigh in Figure 42-1. A magnetic resonance imaging (MRI) scan and an impedance neurograph of the sciatic nerve in the popliteal fossa are shown in Figure 42-2.

Projecting a normal from the tibial portion of the sciatic nerve to the skin surface intersects the electrode array between dots 7 and 8. A normal from the peroneal portion of the sciatic nerve to the skin projects between dots 8 and 9. On the impedance neurograph, the peak intensity of the light contours (low impedance), running from top to bottom, track between columns 7 and 8. The predicted depth of the sciatic nerve on the impedance neurograph was 3.4 cm, which was similar to the MRI scan. The concordance of the depth prediction with the MRI data provides a basis for three-dimensional reconstructions and indicates the accuracy of our hypothesized mechanism enabling impedance neurography.

Impedance neurography may also have applications to pain management. A 150-kg patient sustained a left sacroiliac joint. An impedance neurograph was constructed from impedance data recorded over the sacral region (Fig. 42-3). The impedance map shows the six posterior primary divisions of the sacral nerve roots as they exit the neuroforamina (light-colored peaks) as well as two minima observed along the left margin of the image. These minima correspond to the articular branches of the posterior primary divisions supplying the injured sacroiliac joint. The left-sided (injured) structures generated lower impedances than did the right-hand structures. The relatively lower impedances shown in the articular branches may be a result of their smaller size or abnormal function. Confirmation of the structures was achieved with electrostimulations followed by the injection of local anesthetic. After generating an impedance neurograph, and employing electrostimulation and local anesthetic as targeting aids, radiofrequency lesioning of two left lateral minima resulted in 5 years of pain relief in the patient. Despite the depth from the skin to the articular branches (8 cm), we were able to identify the site of pathology with impedance neurography and efficiently treat the patient's pain.

Another patient presented with shoulder and neck pain. Impedance minima were associated with classic myofascial trigger points in the left levator scapulae muscle (Fig. 42-4).[4]

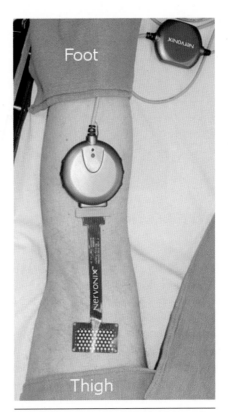

Figure 42-1. Antenna attached to the posterior thigh of a patient.

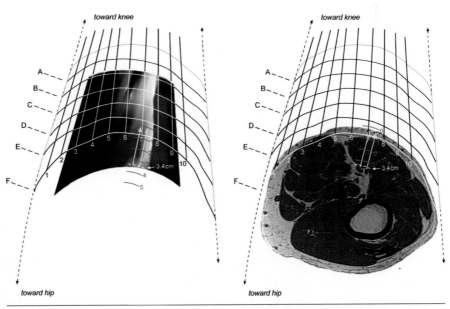

Figure 42-2. MatLab-based analysis of impedance neurography data (*left*) obtained during MRI scanning (*right*) with the electrode array visible as a series of white dots in the right superolateral position. Nerve imaging analysis predicted depth: 3.4 cm. MRI predicted depth: 3.2 cm. Note that the impedance neurograph image is rotated 90 degrees to the MRI image, and that MRI shows a slice through the long axis of the IN electrode array.

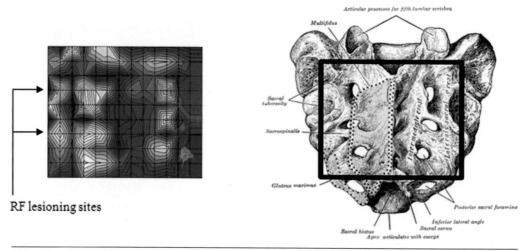

RF lesioning sites

Figure 42-3. Impedance data (*left*) corresponding to the boxed area (*right*) of the posterior sacral region of a patient with left-sided sacroiliac joint injury. Each square in the IN image is 0.5 cm on a side. The lesion sites are located 0.5 cm from the left edge at rows 1.5 cm and 3.0 cm from the top.

On clinical examination, a palpable nodule, tender to palpation, generated referred pain to the left occiput. Needle insertion at the impedance minimum, perpendicular to the skin surface, located the trigger point by pain provocation. Local anesthetic injection resulted in relief of approximately 2-week duration. With the aid of an impedance neurograph, a stimulating needle was inserted to the fascial layer of the levator scapulae muscle. Stimulation at this site generated a levator scapulae twitch. Advancement through the deep fascia generated a levator scapulae twitch plus a rhomboideus major twitch. These observations indicated that the line of low impedance readings on impedance neurograph, corresponded to the dorsal scapular nerve. Botulinum toxin was injected on the muscular side of the fascia at the trigger point, resulting in 3 months of pain relief without rhomboid weakness.[5]

In summary, the ability of impedance neurography to identify neural structures has been confirmed by electrostimulation, local anesthetic injection, and MRI. Impedance neurography

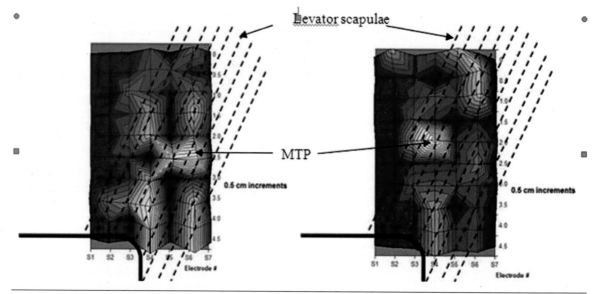

Figure 42-4. Myofascial trigger points (MTP) of the left levator scapulae, taken ahead of botulinum toxin injection of the MTP (*left*) and 3 months postbotulinum toxin injection when symptoms had recurred (*right*).

may detect neuromas, nerve contusions, and nerve entrapments because of the differential impedance between normal and abnormal nerve. Employing a simple and straightforward procedure, impedance neurography promises improvements in care and decreased cost for regional anesthesia, pain management, industrial medicine, as well as determining a patient's neuroanatomy prior to surgery.

References

1. Cory PC. Noninvasive, peripheral nerve mapping device and method of use. 190394(5560372). 10-1-1996. 2-2-1994.
2. Cory PC, Cory JC. Electrode array and skin attachment system for noninvasive nerve location and imaging device. 09912535(6609018). 8-19-2003. 7-6-2001.
3. Cory PC, Cory JC. Electrode array and skin attachment system for noninvasive nerve location and imaging device. 09624397(6564079). 5-13-2003. 7-27-2000.
4. Simons DG, Travell JG, Simons LS. Myofascial Pain and Dysfunction: The Trigger Point Manual. 2nd ed. Baltimore, MD: Williams & Wilkins; 1999:1–1038.
5. Lang AM. Am J Prev Med 2004;14:13–23.
6. Kwok G, Cohen M, Cosic I. Mapping acupuncture points using multi channel device. Australas Phys Eng Sci Med 1998;21:68–72.
7. Yamamoto T, et al. IEEE Trans Biomed Eng 1988;35:203–208.
8. McCarroll GD, Rowley BA. An investigation of the existence of electrically located acupuncture points. IEEE Trans Biomed Eng 1979;26:177–181.
9. Reichmanis M, Marino AA, Becker RO. Electrical correlates of acupuncture points. IEEE Trans Biomed Eng 1975;22:533–535.
10. Prokhorov E, Llamas F, Morales-Sánchez E, González-Hernández J, Prokhorov A. In vivo impedance measurements on nerves and surrounding skeletal muscles in rats and human body. Med Biol Eng Comput 2002;40:323–326.

43

Evaluation of Thoracic Paravertebral and Lumbar Plexus Anatomy Using a 3D Ultrasound Probe

SANJIB DAS ADHIKARY, SUGANTHA GANAPATHY

Introduction: Two-dimensional ultrasound has been used in defining anatomy and guiding needle insertion in different types of peripheral nerve blocks.[1,2] Lumbar plexus and paravertebral anatomy have been well described using two-dimensional ultrasound.[3] However, two-dimensional ultrasound has limited ability to visualize spatial relationships. This is mainly because of the varied course of neural and vascular structures as they traverse different tissue planes in these regions. Three-dimensional ultrasound has theoretical advantages of imaging the entire anatomy of any region. It may also give information regarding nerve thickness and three-dimensional relationships among different structures and may help in demonstrating the distribution and volume of anesthetic agents deposited around the nerve. The image of a three-dimensional ultrasound is generated from simultaneous reconstruction in the longitudinal and transverse planes.[4] Recently, three-dimensional ultrasound has achieved popularity among the obstetrical and cardiology fraternity, leading to commercial pressure to adopt these probes for peripheral neural block. To demonstrate this technology, we acquired three-dimensional ultrasound images of the lumbar plexus in the psoas muscle and the thoracic paravertebral area.

Methods: We used a 3D ultrasound probe (3D Ultrasound system 3D6-2 with × 3-1 with a curved array, Philips Medical systems; Markham, ON) for this procedure. Initially, a longitudinal sonogram was performed to identify the transverse processes of the region by placing the transducer approximately 3 cm parallel to the thoracic spinous process. To exclude any other structures such as ribs, or the articular process of vertebra producing these reflections, the transducer was moved laterally to confirm the position of the tip of the transverse process and to delineate underlying structures such as pleura. The exact level of the T3-T4 spaces was determined by scanning caudally from the transverse process of C7. After identifying the proper level, the transducer was rotated 90 degrees into a transverse plane. The probe was moved laterally until we could see the transverse process in the middle of the screen as a "hook-like" process. Thereafter, the probe was moved inferiorly until the hyperechoic image of the transverse process was lost and we could see the movement of the shimmering pleura laterally. The paravertebral area could be localized just deep to the transverse process. In that position, the three-dimensional ultrasound view was generated to visualize the paravertebral space. The image shows the paraveretebral region in three planes (longitudinal, transverse, and coronal) (Fig. 43-1). One can see the intervertebral nerve root as a linear hyperechoic shadow medial to the pleura and deep to the transverse process. Deep to the root, is a hyperechoic structure, which we believe is the costovertebral ligament. In the coronal view, when

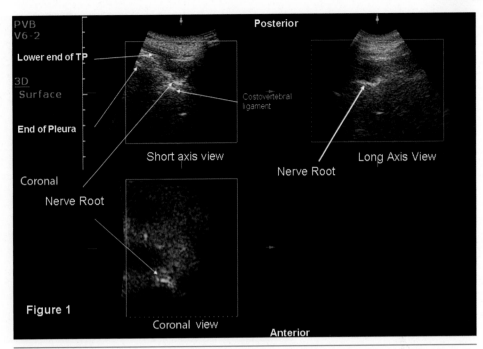

Figure 43-1. Demonstrates the three-dimensional reconstructed anatomy of the thoracic paraveretebral region in three different views.

one sees the reflection of the transverse process, the nerve root is not imaged. Because the probe was used to image more caudal planes, one could discern the nerve root and the hyperechoic structure of the costovertebral ligament ventral to this root (Fig. 43-1).

In the lumbar region, the transverse processes of the vertebral bodies were identified using a longitudinal transducer (2–6 MHz curved array) 3 cm lateral and parallel to the lumbar spinous processes. The exact localization of the levels was confirmed by counting the transverse process echoes upward from sacrum. The transverse plane scan was obtained by rotating the probe 90 degrees between two transverse processes. During two-dimensional imaging, when the transverse process is visualized as a hyperechoic horizontal linear structure, there was acoustic shadowing underneath the transverse process. When the probe was moved gradually inferior to the transverse process, one could visualize the psoas muscle and the peritoneum. The facet joints and the transverse process often were not visualized in the same plane because the facet joints are slightly superior to the transverse process. We could see the neural structure in the substance of the psoas muscle. The three-dimensional ultrasound view was generated to confirm the position of the lumbar plexus. The image demonstrated one of the components of the lumbar plexus in three planes (longitudinal, transverse, and coronal) (Fig. 43-2).

Discussion

Three-dimensional ultrasound is a recent advancement leading to improved cardiac and fetal sonographs.[5,6] The time required to reconstruct three-dimensional images has been reduced in newer machines. The main advantage of the three-dimensional imaging in regional anesthesia is the simultaneous visualization of the nerve in three different planes. Although the image quality was inferior to two-dimensional images, we were still able to identify the nerve in all three planes. We were also able to corroborate the nerve with other structures and virtual markers. Because of the larger size of the three-dimensional probe, its use in real time scenarios needs clinical testing.

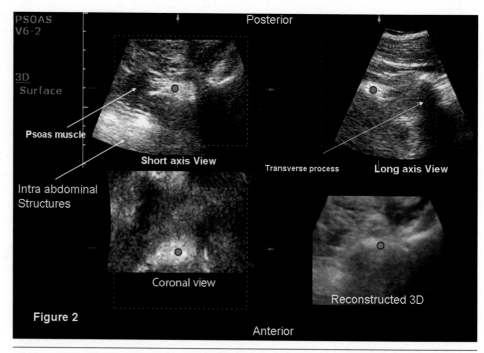

Figure 43-2. Demonstrates the three-dimensional reconstructed anatomy of lumbar plexus region. The marked structure corresponds to the neural structure in all the views.

References

1. Greher M, Scharbert G, Kamolz LP, et al. Ultrasound-guided lumbar facet nerve block: a sonoanatomic study of a new methodologic approach. Anesthesiology 2004;100:1242–1248.
2. Chan VW, Nova H, Abbas S, et al. Ultrasound examination and localization of the sciatic nerve: a volunteer study. Anesthesiology 2006;104:309–314, discussion 5A.
3. Karmakar MK, Ho AM, Li X, et al. Ultrasound-guided lumbar plexus block through the acoustic window of the lumbar ultrasound trident. Br J Anaesth 2008;100:533–537.
4. Feinglass NG, Clendenen SR, Torp KD, et al. Real-time three-dimensional ultrasound for continuous popliteal blockade: a case report and image description. Anesth Analg 2007;105:272–274.
5. Nemes A, Geleijnse ML, Krenning BJ, et al. Usefulness of ultrasound contrast agent to improve image quality during real-time three-dimensional stress echocardiography. Am J Cardiol 2007;99:275–278.
6. Kalache KD, Bamberg C, Proquitté H, et al. Three-dimensional multi-slice view: new prospects for evaluation of congenital anomalies in the fetus. J Ultrasound Med 2006; 25:1041–1049.

Optimum Design of Echogenic Needles for Ultrasound-Guided Nerve Block

ASSAD A. OBERAI, YUN JING, ROBERT E. BOCALA, PAUL E. BIGELEISEN

Introduction: In ultrasound-guided medical procedures involving a needle for injections (as in an ultrasound-guided nerve block), determining the location of the tip of the needle is of prime importance.[1] This is difficult because of low contrast between the needle and a noisy background in the ultrasound image. Classical reflection occurs at the surface of standard needles with a flat sound-hard outer surface, scattering the ultrasound away from the transducer. This results in poor contrast, because the transducer is simultaneously the source and the receiver of the reflection of ultrasound (a monostatic situation).

This study aims to optimize a grooved needle to maximize backscattering to the transducer (scattering the sound toward the transducer). Another needle that has been designed to produce backscattering to the transducer is the corner cube reflector (CCR) needle.[2] This needle utilizes the effects of reflection of a plane wave by a three-dimensional cube corner cut into a sound-hard surface. In the CCR case, the sound is reflected back to the observer because of the multiple reflections off of the mutually orthogonal surfaces (this may be verified by ray tracing). The grooved design studied here may have improved performance and/or lower cost of manufacture as compared to the CCR needle.

Background and Theory: We assume that the transducer, the path of the radiation, and the long axis of the needle are all in the same plane. The transducer is sufficiently far away from the needle, so we can assume that the wave front is planar. We define the insonation angle as the acute angle between the path of the sound from the transducer and the axis of the needle. We assume that the user of the needle will preserve this arrangement during the ultrasound imaging procedure. Physical, unoptimized, grooved needles were tested in this arrangement and were able to provide good imagery and contrast at the needle tip, but only for a single insonation angle (Fig. 44-1, qualitative results only).

Because of memory constraints of the computer, the method of numerical simulation with two-dimensional (2D) finite element analysis (FEA) was chosen (Fig. 44-2). Because of the restrictions placed on the path of the radiation above, this is a reasonable approximation. In addition, it has been suggested that analytical expressions for planar diffraction gratings can be used to approximate the scattering patterns produced by thin, cylindrical, elastic shells in water that have a repeating structure produced by reinforcing ribs.[3] Here, we study with finite elements of a cylinder with an open rectangular grating surface cut into a sound-hard substrate.

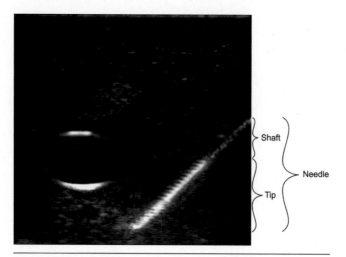

Figure 44-1. Ultrasound image of a grooved needle tip.

The repeated feature that composes the grating is the result of machining grooves into the surface of the needle by rotating the needle about its cylindrical axis. In profile, it is a rectangular cut with equal length groove and peak regions. Extending this profile into the page results in a planar grating.

The rectangular cut is described by the design variables of period and depth of groove. We are especially interested in finding the optimum depth of the cut made to produce the groove pattern in a needle. The lumen or open space within the inner diameter obviously cannot be breached, and the thinnest part of the needle wall cannot be below a certain limit because of manufacturing and strength constraints. From discussion with various needle manufacturers, the depth of cut should not exceed 150 μm.

We directed our design search using the grating equation to determine the period of a surface feature that would produce constructive interference back to the transducer. A formula to describe the location of maxima about a grating surface has been discussed in[4]:

$$\cos(\phi_n) = \cos(\phi_0) + n\lambda/\Lambda \tag{1}$$

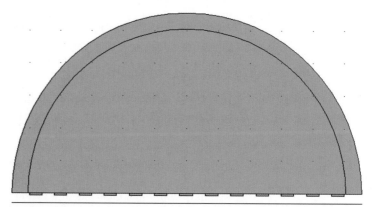

Figure 44-2. In the 2D meshed domain, the grating is visible along the bottom. The PML layer is the concentric subdomain along the upper edge.

Where Λ is the period of the surface grating, n is the order of a constructive interference maximum, ϕ_0 is the angle of insonation, and ϕ_n is the angle at which the constructive interference maximum is located. We assume the maxima are produced by virtual point sources that are produced by the grating along its surface with the same period as the grating period. The desired situation for backscattering and good imaging performance is when the incident angle and the angle at which a maximum is located from the normal are equal. The value of n for which the first maxima is backscattered rather than directed away is -1, and in the backscattering situation, $\phi_n = \pi - \phi_0$. The above equation is then rearranged to:

$$\Lambda = \lambda/(2\cos[\phi_0]) \tag{2}$$

Numerical Method and Results: The time-harmonic wave equation (Helmholtz equation) was solved using a commercially available FEA code. The finite elements were of the Lagrange quadratic type. The simulation was carried out with a minimum of six elements per wavelength.

A semicircular region about the needle was constructed with diameter equal to the total length of the grooved part of the needle. The design goal is to produce contrast at the tip of the needle, so the machined pattern is restricted to 1 cm of length at the tip of the needle. This limited the number of total repeats possible in the groove pattern. The outermost boundary on the semicircle is a radiation boundary condition from which the incident plane wave is emanated toward the sound-hard surface, which is the flat portion of the semicircle with an automatically generated rectangular groove pattern. The initial sound pressures are chosen as arbitrary values but are identical over all the simulations. A perfectly matched layer is present just before the radiation boundary to prevent reflections from the radiation boundary from contributing to the scattered sound field.

The sound pressure level (SPL) is calculated on a concentric 180-degree arc above the grating at a radius of 2.5 cm. This distance was chosen because it is a typical needle tip to transducer distance in medical procedures. First, the sound pressure at the boundary of the needle is obtained from the solution of the finite element problem, and then the Helmholtz-Kirchhoff Integral Theorem is applied, which allows calculation of the SPL at any location above the grating at any angular position.

Simulations were carried out at 13 MHz, which is a typical ultrasound frequency used in medical imaging. Insonation angles in the range of 20 to 75 degrees in steps of 5 degrees were examined. The difficult imaging situation occurs at these angles because of the oblique arrangement with the needle surface. In physical experiments, at higher angles (a broadside arrangement with the needle cylinder), the bulk of the needle is sufficient to produce a good image even with a flat surface geometry. The speed of sound is chosen as 1510 m/s, in this case the wavelength is 120 μm. The density of the medium is 1043 kg/m³.[5] In addition, attenuation is present in the medium and is modeled as 0.8 dB/cm/MHz.

Initial designs had periods guided by the grating equation as discussed previously (Table 44-1). In general, designs based on the grating equation produced a strong peak at the scattering angle corresponding to the location of the transducer and verified the 2D simulation was correctly computing the results as predicted by a planar grating. Figure 44-3 shows the peaks possible for needles configured according to the grating equation at an optimum groove depth (described next) at selected angles of insonation.

To investigate the effects of groove depth on the performance of designs with periods prescribed by the grating equation, a search for the best backscattering depth was performed by taking the mean of the backscattered SPL over all insonation angles for a range of possible

Table 44-1. Groove Periods Selected for Cackscatering via the First Maximum Predicted by the Grating Equation at 13 MHz

	Insonation Angle											
	20	25	30	35	40	45	50	55	60	65	70	75
Λ μm	62	64	67	71	76	82	90	101	116	137	170	224

grove depths (10–150 μm, in steps of 10 μm). There was periodicity in the dependence of scattered sound strength on grating depth. The depths that produced the largest mean sound pressure across all possible insonation angles were 20 μm, 80 μm, and 140 μm. These optimum depths were spaced by approximately half a wavelength (see Table 44-2).

Real-world use would require a needle with good performance at multiple insonation angles. A search of possible geometries by varying the design variables of period of groove and depth of groove was performed. Possible surface periods were 20 to 800 μm, in steps of 20 μm. Possible depths were 10 to 150 μm, in steps of 10 μm.

Iteratively, geometries were generated by a script, and the scattered sound field was determined with the same numerical simulation setup as before. For each geometry, the mean sound pressure was evaluated on a finite arc length (10 degrees), representing the transducer sensor surface centered on the insonation angle. This was done for all possible insonation angles (20–75 degrees in steps of 5 degrees, the critical range for medical imaging) for each geometry. Then, the minimum mean sound pressure out of all possible

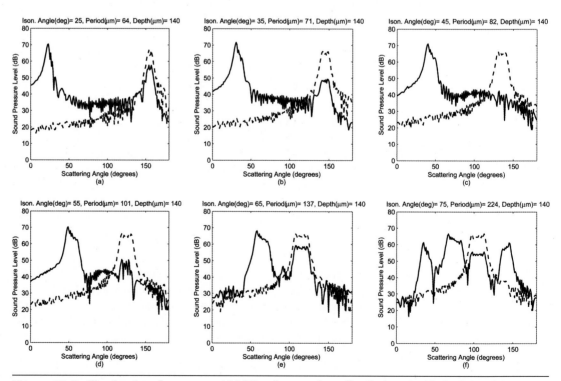

Figure 44-3. Simulated performance at 13 MHz of grooved needles designed with the help of the grating equation (*solid line*). The scattering profile of a perfectly flat needle is shown with a *dashed line*. Each period is specific for the current incident angle. The second maximum becomes visible at an insonation angle of 75 degrees (*f*).

Table 44-2. Dependence of Backscattered Sound Pressure Level* at 13 MHz on Depth of Groove

	Depth of Groove (µm)									
	10	20	30	40	50	60	70	80	90	100
S P L	62.0	65.5	65.4	63.1	54.1	54.4	63.7	65.7	65.2	62.0
	Depth of Groove (µm)									
	110	120	130	140	150					
S P L	52.4	57.0	64.1	65.6	64.0					

*Backscattered SPL means over all insonation angles; 20:5:75 degrees.

insonation angles for each geometry was determined. This resulting worst-case value was the output of the objective function. The purpose of this worst-case reasoning was to produce a design that provided the best performance in the worst-case application scenario.

A search across all possible geometries was used to maximize the objective function. Figure 44-4 shows the backscattering of an optimized configuration for selected angles. The improvement over a perfectly flat needle is clearly seen. Table 44-3 lists the parameters of the three best geometries.

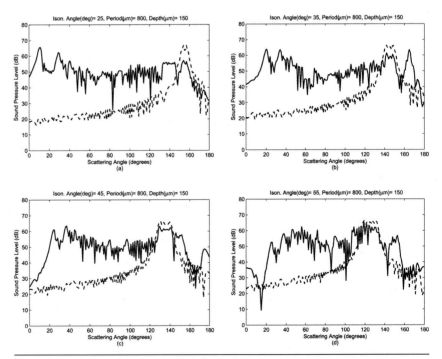

Figure 44-4. Simulated performance at 13 MHz of a groove design found to produce the strongest backscattering at multiple insonation angles 20:5:75 (25:10:55 shown). The scattering profile of a perfectly flat needle is shown with the *dashed line.*

Table 44-3. Optimum Backscattering Geometries at 13 MHz

Rank	Feature Period μm	Feature Depth μm	Minimum SPL for all angles of insonation(dB)
1	800	150	52.4
2	800	140	52.2
3	660	150	51.4

Discussion and Conclusion: This paper tries to optimize the design of a grooved needle for ultrasound-guided nerve block. The objective is to maximize the backscattering from the needle by varying the depth and the width of the groove. Simulations are done with 2D FEA and the guidance of the grating equation. The backscattered sound pressure of designs found to perform well at multiple insonation angles was much lower (on the order of 10 dB) than needles designed to perform well at a single insonation angle. Further work needs to be done to refine the surface geometry to perform well at many insonation angles.

The feature period found when searching for a design to work at multiple insonation angles is much wider than optimal grating widths for needles that work well at single angles of insonation. The current method may be augmented by generic algorithms applied to a more complex geometry.

References

1. Nichols K, Wright LB, Spencer T, et al. Changes in ultrasonographic echogenicity and visibility of needles with changes in angles of insonation. J Vasc Interv Radiol 2003;14:1553–1557.
2. Tamada T, Yasumura R, Takao R, et al. A quantitative comparative study of a new echogenic needle for nerve blocks. Paper presented at the 2008 annual meeting American Society of Anesthesiologists.
3. Brill D, Gaunaurd GC. Identification of cylindrical shells with sets of reinforcing ribs by their acoustic Bragg diffraction (grating) patterns. Applied Acoustics 1995;45:321–334.
4. Holford RL. Scattering of sound waves at a periodic, pressure-release surface: an exact solution. J Acoust Soc Am 1981;70:1116–1128.
5. Mast TD. Empirical relationships between acoustic parameters in human soft tissues. Acoutics Research Letters Online, 2000;1:37–42.

Medical Image Segmentation Using Modified Mumford Segmentation Methods

JUNG-HA AN, STEVEN BENJAMIN DAMELIN, PAUL E. BIGELEISEN

In this chapter we deal with methods developed in (An JH, Bigeleisen PE, Dannelin SB. Identification of Nerves in Ultrasound Scans Using Modified Mumford Shaw and Prior Information Methods. Mathematics, Fundamentals and Applications, proceedings, UKC 2009 [accepted for publication]) to perform medical image segmentation.

Introduction: Diagnostic medical imaging has developed rapidly in the last 3 decades. One widely used method in medical imaging is ultrasound, because it does not use ionizing radiation. Ultrasound-based imaging techniques can be used to recognize muscles, tendons, nerves, and other internal organs with many clinical applications. One application is to assist with conduction nerve blocks. To accomplish this, it is important to develop an efficient algorithm that recognizes the nerves, vessels, muscles, and bones. In this paper, we consider identifying nerve regions in ultrasound scans using a region-based image segmentation algorithm.

The most celebrated region-based image segmentation model was introduced by Mumford and Shah.[1] An image is decomposed into a set of regions within the bounded open set Ω, and these regions are separated by smooth edges Γ in this model. Because of the difficulties in numerical computation of the Mumford-Shah model, several numerical approximation methods have been developed. Chan and Vese proposed a piecewise constant Mumford-Shah model in by further Mumford Shah advances[2,3] by using a level set formulation.[4] Developments of variational level set implementation techniques are followed by applications of level sets to Mumford-Shah segmentation.[5,6,7] Another approach has been developed by Ambrosio and Tortorelli. They measured an edge-length term Γ in the Mumford-Shah model by a quadratic integral of an edge signature function.[8] The segmentation is represented by characteristic functions using phase fields in threshold dynamics for a Mumford-Shah functional[5,7], which are described in shape statistics for kernel space.[9,10,5,11,12–14]

These algorithms, however, have limited application to images with noise, artifacts, or loss of information. We have incorporated prior shape information into the segmentation process to overcome these problems.[9,15,16–21,22,25] The proposed model is motivated by the convergence and stochastic variational model for Mumford-Shah segmentation.[9,20,12,13] Using a Γ-approximation to a piecewise constant Mumford-Shah model is similar to region-based image segmentation,[9,12,13] and adding the prior shape information in the segmentation processing is similar to functional MR image registration.[11] However, our model also adds a nonrigid deformation for incorporating the prior information.

This paper is organized as follows: In section 2, a new region-based variational model is proposed. The suggested model uses a Γ-approximation to a piecewise Mumford-Shah model and prior shape information. Experimental results of the model that were applied to ultrasound images of a healthy human should be in section 3. Numerical results comparing our piecewise constant Mumford-Shah models and the results of expert clinicians are also shown in this section. Finally, the conclusion follows and future work is stated in section 4.

Description of the Proposed Model

In this section, a new region-based variational image segmentation model is introduced. The segmentation is attained using a modified Mumford-Shah model, along with the prior shape in formation. The model is aimed to find ϕ, u, μ, R, and T by minimizing the energy functional:

$$E(\phi, u, \mu, R, T) = \lambda_1 \int_\Omega H_\varepsilon^2(\phi)(I(\bar{x}) - c_1)^2 + (1 - H_\varepsilon(\phi))^2(I(\bar{x}) - c_2)^2 \, d\bar{x}$$

$$+ \int_\Omega \varepsilon_1 |\nabla H_\varepsilon(\phi)|^2 + \frac{\lambda_2 H_\varepsilon(\phi)^2(1 - H_\varepsilon(\phi))^2}{\varepsilon_1} \, d\bar{x}$$

$$+ \frac{\lambda_3}{2} \int_\Omega \delta_\varepsilon(\phi) d^2(\mu R\bar{x} + T + u) \left| \nabla\left(\frac{\phi}{\varepsilon}\right) \right| d\bar{x}$$

$$+ \lambda_4 \int_\Omega |\nabla u|^2 \, d\bar{x} + \lambda_5 \int_\Omega u^2 d\bar{x}, \tag{2.1}$$

where I is a given name image, Ω is domain, $\lambda_i > 0$, $i = 1, 2, 3, 4, 5$ are parameters balacing the influences from the five terms in the model, d is the distance function from the given prior shape, and ε and ε_1 are positive parameters. For the numerical computation,
$H_\varepsilon(\phi) = \left[\frac{1}{2}\left(1 + \frac{2}{\pi} \arctan\left(\frac{\phi}{\varepsilon}\right)\right) \right]^2$ and $\delta_\varepsilon(\phi) = H_\varepsilon'(\phi)$ are used.

The first term forces $H_2^\varepsilon(\phi)$ toward 0 if $I(\bar{x})$ is different from c_1 and toward 1 if $I(\bar{x})$ is close to c_1, for every $\bar{x} \varepsilon \Omega$. In a similar way, $(1 - H_\varepsilon[\phi])^2$, toward 0 if $I(\bar{x})$ is different from c_2 and toward 1 if $I(\bar{x})$ is close to c_2, for every $(\bar{x}) \varepsilon \Omega$. The second term is for measuring an edge-length term using Γ-approximation. In the theory of Γ-convergence, the measurement of an edge length term Γ in the Mumford-Shah model can be approximated by a quadratic integral of an edge signature function.[1] This model is combined with a double-well potential function, which is quadratic around its minima and is growing faster than linearly at infinity.[13,23,24] Here $\varepsilon_1 \ll 1$ controls the transition bandwidth. As $\varepsilon_1 \to 0$, the first term penalizes unnecessary interfaces, and the second term forces the stable solution to take one of the two-phase field values 1 or 0. For the details of phase-field models and double-well potential functions, please refer .[13,23–25] Prior information is incorporated with the distance function in the third term. The distance function consists of the global transformation and nonrigid deformation. Minimizing the magnitude of the nonrigid deformation term u is the fourth term. The final term smooths the nonrigid term u.

Euler-Lagrange of the Proposed Model: The evolution equations associated with the Euler-Lagrange equations in Equation (2.1) are

$$\frac{\partial \phi}{\partial t} = -2\lambda_1 H_\varepsilon'(\phi)\{H_\varepsilon(I - c_1)^2 - (1 - H_\varepsilon)(I - c_2)^2\}$$
$$+ 2\varepsilon_1\{\text{div}(\nabla\phi \, (H_\varepsilon'(\phi))^2) - |\nabla\phi|^2 \, H_\varepsilon'(\phi)H_\varepsilon''(\phi)\}$$
$$- \frac{2\lambda_2 H_\varepsilon(\phi)(1 - H_\varepsilon(\phi))(1 - 2H_\varepsilon(\phi))H_\varepsilon'(\phi)}{\varepsilon_1}$$

$$+ \delta_\varepsilon(\phi)\text{div}\left\{ \frac{\lambda_3}{2} d^2(\mu R\bar{x} + T + u) \frac{\nabla\left(\frac{\phi}{\varepsilon}\right)}{\left|\nabla\left(\frac{\phi}{\varepsilon}\right)\right|} \right\}, \text{ in } \Omega$$

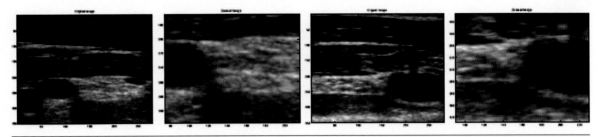

Figure 45-1 A, Ultrasound scan of the brachial plexus. **B,** Zoomed image of *A* showing noise and artifact. **C,** Another ultrasound scan of the brachial plexus. **D,** Zoomed image of *C* showing noise and artifact.

$$\frac{\partial \phi}{\partial n} = 0, \text{ on } \partial\Omega$$

$$\frac{\partial u}{\partial t} = \delta_\varepsilon(\phi)\lambda_3 d(\mu R\bar{x} + T + u)\nabla d(\mu R\bar{x} + T + u)\left|\nabla\left(\frac{\phi}{\varepsilon}\right)\right| + \lambda_4 |\Delta u| - \lambda_5 u, \text{ in } \Omega$$

$$\frac{\partial u}{\partial n} = 0, \text{ on } \partial\Omega$$

$$\frac{\partial \mu}{\partial t} = -\lambda_3 \int_\Omega \delta_\varepsilon(\phi)d(\mu R\bar{x} + T + u)\nabla d(\mu R\bar{x} + T + u)R\bar{x}\left|\nabla\left(\frac{\phi}{\varepsilon}\right)\right|d\bar{x}$$

$$\frac{\partial \theta}{\partial t} = -\lambda_3 \int_\Omega \delta_\varepsilon(\phi)\mu d(\mu R\bar{x} + T + u)\nabla d(\mu R\bar{x} + T + u)\frac{\partial R}{\partial \theta}\bar{x}\left|\nabla\left(\frac{\phi}{\varepsilon}\right)\right|d\bar{x}$$

$$\frac{\partial T}{\partial t} = -\lambda_3 \int_\Omega \delta_\varepsilon(\phi)d(\mu R\bar{x} + T + u)\nabla d(\mu R\bar{x} + T + u)\left|\nabla\left(\frac{\phi}{\varepsilon}\right)\right|d\bar{x},$$

where R is a rotation matrix with respect to θ.

Numerical Methods and Experimental Results: In this section, numerical methods to solve the Equation (2.1) are explained, and the experimental results of applications to the human neck ultrasound images are shown. The Equation (2.1) was solved by finding a steady-state solution of the evolution equations. The evolution equations are associated with the Euler-Lagrange equation. A finite difference scheme and the gradient descent method are applied to discretize the evolving equations. During the numerical experiments, $\lambda 1 = 0.05$, $\lambda i = 1$ with $i = 2,3,4,5$,

$$H_\varepsilon(\phi) = \left[\frac{1}{2}\left(1 + \frac{2}{\pi}\arctan\left(\frac{\phi}{\varepsilon}\right)\right)\right]^2 \text{ and } \delta_\varepsilon(\phi) = H'_\varepsilon(\phi) \text{ are used.}$$

To demonstrate our approach on an image with noise, artifacts, and loss of information, shoulder ultrasound scans with enlarged images are shown in Figure 45-1. Because it is difficult to find, the location of nerves without some prior knowledge about a region of interest (prior information) is incorporated with the distance function. This consists of the global transformation and local nonrigid deformation. The prior shape is also used as an initial contour during experiments.

In Figure 45-2, the proposed model segmentation result is compared with Chan-Vese model[5] and the suggested model without prior information,[2] which is $\lambda i = 0$ for $i = 3,4,5$ in Equation (2.1). The first image is the initial contour, the second image is segmented by Chan-Vese model as a red solid line and compared with an expert observer (white solid line). The third image is the segmented result without prior information shown as a red solid line and compared with an expert observer (white solid line). The fourth image is the segmented result of the proposed model shown as a red solid line and compared with an expert observer (white solid line).

In Figure 45-3, experimental results are shown with and without the nonrigid deformation term in the prior information. The first image is the original image, and the second image is given image with an initial contour. The third image is the segmented result without the nonrigid deformation term in prior information. It is shown as a red solid line and compared with an expert

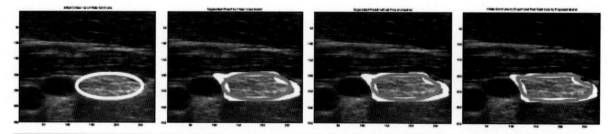

Figure 45-2. A, Ultrasound image from *A* with initial contour. **B,** Segmented result by Chan-Vese model (*red solid line*) and comparison with an expert (*white solid line*). **C,** Segmented result without prior information (*red solid line*) and comparison with an expert (*white solid line*). **D,** Segmented result of the proposed model (*red solid line*) and comparison with an expert (*white solid line*).

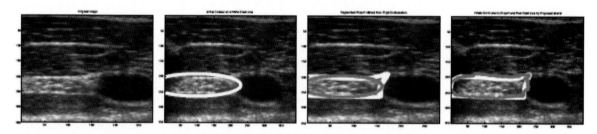

Figure 45-3. A, Ultrasound scan of the brachial plexus. **B,** Image in *A* with and initial contour. **C,** Segmented result with nonrigid deformation term in prior information (*red solid line*) and comparison with an expert (*white solid line*). **D,** Segmented result of the proposed model (*red solid line*) and comparison with an expert (*white solid line*).

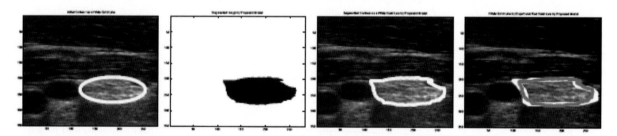

Figure 45-4. A, Ultrasound scan of the brachial plexus with and initial contour. **B,** Segmented image result using a Heaviside function. **C,** Segmented contour result (*white solid line*). **D,** Segmented result of the proposed model (*red solid line*) and comparison with an expert (*white solid line*).

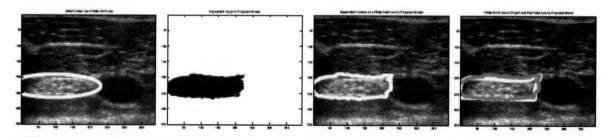

Figure 45-5. A, Ultrasound scan of the brachial plexus with and initial contour. **B,** Segmented image result using a Heaviside function. **C,** Segmented contour result (*white solid line*). **D,** Segmented result of the proposed model (*red solid line*) and comparison with an expert (*white solid line*).

observer (white solid line). The fourth image is the segmented result of the proposed model shown as a red solid line and compared with an expert observer (white solid line).

In Figures 45-4 and 45-5, numerical results are shown with segmented images. These images are created by using the Heaviside function. The first image is the given image with an initial contour. The second image is segmented by the Heaviside function. The third image is the segmented contour result (white solid line). Figure 45-6A shows an ultrasound image of the axillary and vein as well as the nerve before processing with the Mumford Shah model. Figure 45-6B shows the same images after processing with the Mumford Shah model. Notice that the boundary of the nerve is much clear, and that the needle is more visible after processing.

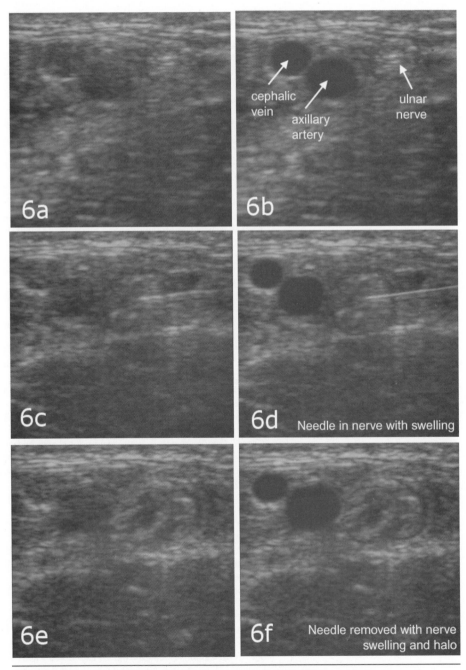

Figure 45-6. **A,C,E,** Original ultrasound scan. **B,D,E,** Ultrasound scan passed through a Mumford-Shaw filter.

Conclusions and Future Work: A new region-based image segmentation model is proposed. Image segmentation is obtained using Γ-approximation to a piecewise constant Mumford-Shah functional and prior information. The prior information is incorporated by the distance function, which consists of global rigid transformation and nonrigid deformation. The model is applied to healthy human neck ultrasound images and compared with existing piecewise constant Mumford-Shah models. The preliminary numerical results showed the effectiveness of the presented model against noise, artifact, and loss of information. Even though experiments were done on 2D ultrasound images, the proposed model can be applied to any type of images and dimension. However, the numerical result depends on an initial contour, and automatic parameter estimation will be continued in the future work. In addition, more numerical experiments will be done, and an extension to 3D is being considered.

References

1. Mumford D, Shah J. Optimal approximations by piecewise smooth functions and associated variational problems. Comm Pure Applied Math 1989;42:577–685.
2. Chan T, Vese L. Active contours without edges. IEEE Trans Image Proc 2001;10:266–277.
3. Chan TF, Vese LA. A level set algorithm for minimizing the Mumford-Shah functional in image processing. In Proceedings 1st IEEE Workshop on Variational and Level Set Methods in Computer Vision. Vancouver, B.C. Canada; 2001:161–168.
4. Osher S, Fedkiw R. Level set methods and dynamic implicit surfaces. New York: Springer Verlag; 2003.
5. Esedoglu S, Tsai R. Threshold dynamics for the piecewise constant Mumford-Shah fuctional. CAM Report 04-63 UCLA; 2004.
6. Gibou F, Fedkiw R. A fast hybrid K-means level set algorithm for segmentation. Stanford Technical Report, November 2002.
7. Lie J, Lysaker M, Tai X. A binary level set model and some applications to Mumford-Shah segmentation. CAM Report. Vol. 31; 2004.
8. Ambrosio L, Tortorelli V. Approximation of functionals depending on jumps by elliptic functionals via Γ-convergence. Comm Pure Applied Math 1990;43:999–1036.
9. An JH, Chen Y. Region based image segmentation using a modified Mumford-Shah algorithm. To appear in Scale Space Variational Methods (SSVM) in Computer Vision, 2007.
10. Baldo S. Minimal interface criterion for phase transitions in mixtures of Cahn-Hilliard fluids. Ann Inst Henri Poincare 1990;7:67–90.
11. Modica L. The gradient theory of phase transitions and the minimal interface criterion. Arch Rational Mech Anal 1987;98:123–142.
12. Shen. J. Γ-Convergence approximation to piecewise constant Mumford-Shah segmentation. Lec Notes Comp Sci 3708 2005;499–506.
13. Shen J. A stochastic-variational model for soft Mumford-Shah segmentation. Int J Biomed Imaging, special issue on Recent Advances in Mathematical Methods for the Processing of Biomedical Images, Vol. 2006(2006):1–14.
14. Wang M, Zhou S. Phase field: a variational method for structural topology optimization. Comput Model Eng Sci 2004;6(6):547–566.
15. Bresson X, Vandergheynst P, Thiran J. A variational model for object segmentation using boundary information and shape prior driven by the Mumford-Shah functional. Int J Comp Vis 2006;68:145–162.
16. Chen Y, Guo W, Huang F, et al. Using prior shapes and points in medical image segmentation. Proc Ener Mini Meth Comp Vis Pat Recog Lisbon Portugal; 2003;291–305.
17. Chen Y, Huang F, Tagare H, et al. Using prior shapes and intensity profiles in medical image segmentation. Proc Int Conf Comp Vis Nice France 2003;1117–1124.
18. Chen Y, Huang F, Wilson D, et al. Segmentation with shape and intensity priors. Proc Int Conf Image Graph Hefei China 2003;378–385.
19. Chen Y, Tagare H, Thiruvenkadam S, et al. Using prior shapes in geometric active contours in a variational framework. Int J Comp Vis 2002;50:315–328.
20. Chen Y, Thiruvenkadam S, Gopinath K, et al. Functional MR image registration using Mumford-Shah functional and shape information. Proc. the 6th World Multiconference on Systems, Cybernetics, and Informatic Orlando, 2002;580–583.
21. Cremers D, Kohlberger T, Schnorr C. Shape statistics in kernel space for variational image segmentation. Patt Recog 2003;36:1929–1943.
22. Huang X, Li Z, Metaxas D. Learning coupled prior shape and appearance models for segmentation. Proc 7th Ann Int Conf Med Image Comp Computer-Assi Interv MICCAI04 Vol. I LNCS-3216 2004;60–69.
23. Huang X, Metaxas D, Chen T. MetaMorphs: deformable shape and texture models. Proc. IEEE Comp. Soc. Conf. Comp. Vis. Pat. Recog. CVPR04, Vol. I 2004;496–503.
24. Leventon M, Grimson E, Faugeras O. Statistical shape influence in geodesic active contours. Proc IEEE Conf CVPR 2000;316–323.
25. Rousson M, Paragios N. Shape prior for level set representations. Comp Vis ECCV2002 7th Eur Conf Comp Vis Copenhgen Demark Proc 2002;78–92.

Index

Abdomen, cross section, 94*f*
Abdominal wall, anatomy, 93, 94*f*
Acoustic radiation force impulse (ARFI) imaging, 272–273
    injections, 274*f*, 275*f*
    nerves and, 273
    in regional anesthesia, 272–275
    tibial nerve, 273*f*
Adductor brevis, 116*f*
Adductor longus, 110*f*
Adductor magnus, 110*f*
Adductor muscles, 114
Agents. *See also* Bupivacaine; Bupivacaine with epinephrine; Epinephrine;
        Levobupivacaine; Morphine; Neurolytic agents; Ropivacaine;
        Sevoflurane
    intraneural injections and, 36–37
Anesthesia. *See* Local anesthetic; Pediatric(s); Regional anesthesia; Sacral
        plexus anesthesia; Total spinal anesthesia
Anesthetic
    injection, ultrasound-guided lumbar plexus block, 85*f*
    partial plexus block, 223
    toxicity
        intercostal blockade, 189
        pediatric anesthesia, 167–168
Anesthetic spillover, vocal cord paralysis, 224
Angle of insonation, 10
Ankle block
    anatomy and, 140, 141*f*–143*f*
    ultrasound-guided, 140–143
        background and indications, 140
Ankle, nerves of, 141*f*, 143*f*
Antecubital region, 72*f*
Anterior intercostal block, 189, 190*f*
Anterior interscalene block, 48*f*
Anterior scalene muscle, 53, 54*f*
Anterior sciatic nerve block, 123, 206*f*, 208–209
    ultrasound-guided, 123–126
        background and indications, 123
        summary of evidence, 126
        technique, 123, 124*f*, 125

Anterior sciatic scan, 124*f*, 125*f*
    with femoral and obturator nerves, 125*f*
Anticoagulated patient, peripheral nerve block, 8
Aorta, 233, 234*f*
ARFI imaging. *See* Acoustic radiation force impulse imaging
Arteries, 22
    identifying, 16
Articular process, 81
Artificial intelligence, 263–271
Axilla
    cross section, 12*f*, 66*f*
    histology of, 66*f*–67*f*
    schematic through, 13*f*
    ultrasound scan, 173*f*
Axillary nerve blocks, 7, 31
    needle/transducer position, pediatric, 172, 172*f*
    ultrasound-guided, 65–70
        anatomy, 65
        background and indications, 65
        technique, 68–69, 68*f*
Axillary plexus, bifid axillary artery and, 70*f*
Axons, 27
Azygous vein, 151*f*

Backscattered sound pressure level, depth of groove and, 287*f*
Backscattering
    depth of groove and, 287*f*
    grating equation, 285, 285*f*
    groove needle design, 288*f*
Beam attenuation, as function of frequency, 11*f*
Beam diffraction, near-field and far field, 18*f*
Beam direction, image *v.*, 13*f*–15*f*
Beam dispersion, near-field and far field, 18*f*
Biceps, 78*f*
Biceps femoris muscle, 110*f*, 111*f*, 133*f*, 135*f*
Bifid axillary artery, 69*f*
    axillary plexus and, 70*f*
Bifid axillary vein, 69, 69*f*
Bigeleisen, 34
    sonography, history/future, 261–262

Block cart, 2, 3*f*
Block needle, cervical sympathetic block, 230*f*
Blood flow, color, 16, 20*f*
B-mode ultrasound, 252
Bowel, 186*f*
Brachial artery, 72*f*
  gross anatomy, 77*f*
Brachialis, 78*f*
Brachial plexus, 58, 171
  anatomy, 40, 41*f*, 53
  infraclavicular approach, 176–179
    technique, 176–179
  interscalene approach, 174
    technique, 174–175
  microanatomy of, 48*f*
  roots of, 46*f*
    posterior approach, 40
  "sheath" of, 53
  supraclavicular approach, 176–179
  transverse section, 41*f*
  trunks of, 47*f*
  ultrasound scan
    initial contour, 292, 292*f*, 293*f*
    noise and artifact, 291, 291*f*
    segmented image, 293*f*
Brachial plexus blockade, ultrasound-guided, infants and children,
    171–180
Brachial plexus "sheath," evaluation of, 51
Brachioradialis, 78*f*
Bupivacaine, 208
  ankle block, 140, 141*f*–143*f*
  brachial plexus, infraclavicular approach, 176
  interscalene block, 40
    ultrasound-guided, 50
  lateral femoral cutaneous block, 104
  lower extremity blockade, 199
  mandibular nerve block, 217
  pediatric anesthesia, 166
  stellate ganglion block, 221
  supraclavicular brachial plexus block, 56
  TAP block, 182, 183
  toxicity, pediatric anesthesia, 167
  transverse abdominis plane block, 93
Bupivacaine with epinephrine
  anterior sciatic nerve block, 123
  IL-IH block, 187
  infraclavicular blocks, ultrasound-guided, 61
  inguinal nerve block, 89
  obturator nerve block, 118
  parasacral block, anatomy, 120
  paravertebral blocks, 192
  pediatric anesthesia, 166–167
  popliteal sciatic block, 133
  saphenous nerve block, 112
  supraclavicular brachial plexus block, 55
  ulnar block, above elbow, 79

Catheter(s). *See also* Indwelling catheter; Nonstimulating catheter; Para-
    vertebral catheter; Stimulating catheter; Subgluteal catheters
  bilateral paravertebral, 155*f*
  insertion, 4, 5*f*
  intercostal space injection, 154*f*
  in place, 44*f*
  ultrasound-guided peripheral nerve block, 2, 3*f*
Caudal canal, floor of, 211*f*
Caudal epidural block, 164, 167, 211–212, 211*f*
CCR needle. *See* Corner cube reflector needle

Celiac artery, 233, 234*f*
Celiac ganglion, anatomy, 232, 233*f*
Central neuroaxial block, pediatrics, 163
Cerebrospinal fluid (CSF), 27
Cervical 5 nerve roots, 43*f*
Cervical 6 transverse process, anterior tubercle, 43*f*
Cervical region, ultrasound-guided needle advancement, 222*f*
Cervical sympathetic block, ultrasound-guided, 225–231
  background and indications, 225
  technique, 229–231
Cervical sympathetic ganglia, 220, 221*f*
Cervical sympathetic trunk, anatomy, 225, 226*f*
Cesarean section, epidural anesthesia, 145
Chan-Vese model, 291*f*, 292
Child, 164*f*
Children. *See also* Infants and children
  brachial plexus blockade, 171–180
  TAP block, 182
Classical reflection, 283
Clavicle, 58
Color Doppler ultrasound, 16, 19*f*, 49*f*
  subgluteal sciatic block, 130
  synovial tissue and, 253
Common peroneal nerve, 135*f*, 209*f*
  acoustic radiation force imaging, 273*f*
    B-mode imaging and, 273*f*
Complex regional pain syndrome, stellate ganglion block, 220
Conduction nerve blocks, ultrasound and, 289
Continuous lumbar plexus block, postoperative pain, 87
Contrast. *See also* Radiocontrast injection
  low *v.* high, 17*f*
  normal, 16, 16*f*
Control top syringe, ankle block, 140, 141*f*–143*f*
Conventional radiograph, 254*f*
Coracoid block
  needle/probe position, 178, 178*f*
  ultrasound scan, 179*f*
Corner cube reflector needle (CCR needle), 283
Costal groove, 151*f*
Costotransverse ligament, 158, 158*f*
Crystal arthropathy, ultrasonography and, 257–258
CSF. *See* Cerebrospinal fluid

Deep peroneal nerve, injection, 141*f*
Deep radial nerve, 78*f*
Diabetic patients, popliteal sciatic block, 139
Diffraction, 10
Distal nerve block, in upper extremity, ultrasound-guided, 79
Doppler ultrasound, 252. *See also* Color Doppler ultrasound
  synovial tissue, 253
Dynamic range compression, 16, 16*f*

Echogenic needles, for ultrasound-guided nerve block, 283–288
Effusions, ultrasonography and, 253, 255*f*
Elbow
  above, gross anatomy, 72*f*
  below, gross anatomy, 73*f*
  blocks at, 71–79
Endoneurium, 29, 29*f*
Endoscopic celiac ganglion block, 232–236
  abdominal probe/needle, 235*f*
  background and indications, 232
  technique
    endoscopic approach, 232
    transabdominal approach, 232, 235*f*
    transabdominal sonogram, 235*f*
Endothoracic fascia, 150, 151*f*

Enthesitis, 256–257, 256f, 257f
Epidural analgesia
    labor and, 145
    longitudinal scan, 146f
    tips, 147
    transverse scan, 146f, 147, 147f
Epidural anesthesia, cesarean section and, 145
Epidural injections, 32
Epidural needle, placement, 145, 146f, 147f
Epinephrine, 208
    TAP block, 183
Epinephrine "test-dose," pediatric anesthesia, 168
Epineurium, 27–28, 29f
Epineurium rupture, 102f
Equipment
    regional anesthesia, infants and children, 164–166
    sterile procedures, 5f
    ultrasound-guided peripheral nerve block, 2–6
Erosive disease, 253, 255f
Euler-Lagrange equations, 290
External intercostal muscles, 151f, 190f
External oblique muscle, TAP block, 184f

Facet joint, 250f
    injection, 247f, 249, 250f
    visualizing, 281
Facet nerve block, 240
False femoral nerve, 101f
    ultrasound showing, 99f
Fascia iliac block, 100, 200
    needle/probe position for, 201f–202f
Fascicles, 27–30, 29f
Femoral artery, 110f, 111f, 203f
    local anesthetic, 209f
Femoral nerve, 98, 100f, 101f, 104, 105f, 125f, 195. See also Femoral
        nerve block; Lateral femoral cutaneous block
    after injection, 101f
    anatomy, 97, 98f, 198f, 199
    needle and probe position, 196f
    in psoas muscle, 98f
Femoral nerve block. See also Midfemoral block; Nerve stimulator
    ultrasound-guided, 97–103, 201
        anatomy, 97, 98f
        background and indications, 97
        probe/needle position, 99f
        technique, 97–100, 102
Femoral vein, 110f
    local anesthetic, 209f
Femoral vessels, 123, 124f. See also Femoral artery; Femoral vein
Femur, 135f
    ultrasound for, 207f
Flexor digitorum profundus, 73f
Flexor digitorum superficialis, 73f
Flow velocity, 16
"Flying bat" sign, 147, 147f
Focal zone, 16, 17f, 18f, 19f
    variable time delays and, 18f
Forearm, blocks at, 71–79
    background and indications, 71
Formalin, peripheral blocks, 37
Fresnel zone, 16, 17f

General anesthesia, paravertebral blocks, 26
Geniculate artery, 111f
Genitofemoral nerve, 105f
    inguinal nerve block and, 92
Gracilis muscle, 110f, 111f, 203f

Grating equation, 288
    backscattering and, 285, 285f
Greater trochanter, subgluteal sciatic block, 127, 128f
Groove needle design, 287f
    groove depth, 285–286, 286f
    optimum backscattering geometries, 288f

"Halo," anterior sciatic nerve block, 126
Halothane, epinephrine "test-dose," 168
Hamstring muscles, 123, 124f
Heart rate response, epinephrine "test-dose," 168
Hemlholtz equation, 285
Hydromorphone, pediatric neuroaxial block, 164
Hydrophilic opioids, pediatric neuroaxial block, 164
Hyperechoic cords of plexus, 59, 59f
Hyperechoic nerves, 13f, 22, 31
Hypoechoic nerves, 22, 25f, 31

Iliacus muscles, anatomy, 97, 98f
IL-IH block. See Ilioinguinal and iliohypogastric nerve block
Iliohypogastric nerve, 105f, 188f
    cross section, 90f
    ultrasound image, 90f
Ilioinguinal and iliohypogastric nerve block (IL-IH block), 89, 186–187
    transducer/needle position, 187f
Ilioinguinal nerve, 105f, 188f
    cross section, 90f
    ultrasound image, 90f
Image
    beam direction v., 13f–15f
    generation, 273
    identification process, schematic, 264, 265f
Image segmentation model, 290
Impedance neurography, 276–279, 278f
    MRI v., 276, 277f
Indwelling catheter
    interscalene block, ultrasound-guided, 51
    popliteal sciatic block, 135
    subgluteal sciatic block, 130
    supraclavicular brachial plexus block, 56
    ultrasound-guided, positions for, 62
Infants and children, 164–166
    brachial plexus blockade, 171–180
    equipment, 164–166
    local anesthetic, 166
    needles, 165
    nerve stimulator, 165–166
    probe, 165
    regional anesthesia, 164–166
    TAP block, 182
    transducer, 165
Inferior cervical ganglion, 220, 221f
Inferior trunk, position, 54f
Infraclavicular blocks, 8
    needle/probe position, 178f
    negative set identification, 264, 266f
    ultrasound-guided, 58–64
        anatomy, 58
        background and indications, 58
        medial approach, 62–64, 63f
        midinfraclavicular approach, 62–64
        positions for, 61, 61f
        technique, 61–62
    ultrasound scan, 179f
Infraclavicular brachial plexus, histology of, 58, 60f
Infraclavicular fossa, schematic, 20f
Infraclavicular plexus, ultrasound, 264, 267f

Infraclavicular region, search range for, relative to axillary artery, 264, 265*f*
Infragluteal block, with real-time ultrasound, 130
Infragluteal sciatic block, 127
Inguinal nerve block
  anatomy, 89
  tips, 92
  ultrasound-guided, 89–92
    background and indications, 89
    technique, 89–90, 92
Injection(s), 36–37, 153*f*, 258. *See also* Catheter(s); Intrafascicular
    injections; Intraneural injection; Intraneural sciatic injection;
    Zygapophysial injection
  agents, 36–37
  anesthetic, ultrasound-guided lumbar plexus block, 85*f*
  ARFI, 274–275, 274*f*, 275*f*
  deep peroneal nerve, 141*f*
  dog study, 36
  epidural, 32
  facet joint, 247*f*, 249, 250*f*
  femoral nerve, 101*f*
  innermost intercostal muscles, 153*f*
  internal intercostal muscles, 153*f*
  intracordal, catastrophic outcomes, 26
  intrafascicular, 36
  intraroot, 32
    catastrophic outcomes, 26
  local anesthetic
    intercostal space, 154*f*
    TAP block, 95, 96*f*
  nerve damage, 262
  paravertebral, 32
  pig study, 35, 36
  posterior tibial nerve, 142*f*
  saphenous nerve, 143*f*
  stellate ganglion block, 223*f*
  subepineurial, 29
  zygapophysial, spinal pain and, 240
In line block, 205*f*
Innermost intercostal muscles, 151*f*
  injection, 153*f*
Intercostal artery, 151*f*
Intercostal blockade, 187–189
  complications, 188–189
Intercostal nerve, 151*f*
Intercostal space
  gross and sonoanatomy, 151*f*
  needle position, 154*f*
Intercostal vein, 151*f*
Internal intercostal membrane, 151*f*
Internal intercostal muscles, 151*f*
  injection, 153*f*
Internal oblique muscle, 95, 95*f*
  TAP block, 184*f*
Interscalene block
  neck ultrasound scan, 175*f*
  patient position, 40
  study, 8
  technique, 40–44
  ultrasound-guided, 45–52
    anatomy, 45–46, 46*f*
    background and indications, 45
    clinical evidence summary, 51
    posterior approach, 40–44
    technique, 50–51
Interscalene region
  Color flow Doppler, 49*f*
  ultrasound scan, 49*f*

Interscalene space, anatomy, 45
Intracordal injections, catastrophic outcomes, 26
Intrafascicular injections, dog study, 36
Intraneural injection, 27, 28*f*, 35, 35*f*, 102*f*
  nerve damage and, 262
  ultrasound-guided, regional anesthesia and, 34–38
Intraneural sciatic injection, 135, 136*f*
Intraroot injections
  catastrophic outcomes, 26
  dura penetrations and, 32
In vivo B-mode images, tibial nerve, 273*f*
Ischial tuberosity, subgluteal sciatic block, 127, 128*f*
Isonification angle, 286–287, 286*f*, 287*f*

Joint effusion, 255*f*

Knee crease. *See also* Popliteal crease
  scanning, 134, 134*f*
Kulenkampff, paresthesia, nerve and, 7

Labor epidural placement
  technique, 146–149
  ultrasound for, 145–149
Labor, first/second stage of, analgesia for, 145
Large vessel vasculitis, 257
Lateral antebrachial cutaneous nerve, 72*f*
  gross anatomy, 77*f*
Lateral femoral cutaneous block
  needle and probe position, 105
  ultrasound-guided, 104–107
    anatomy, 104, 105*f*, 106*f*
    background and indications, 104
    technique, 104, 106–107
Lateral femoral cutaneous nerve, 105*f*, 195
  ultrasound scan, 106, 106*f*
Lateral infraclavicular block, 58, 59*f*
Lateral insertion approach, ultrasound-guided lumbar plexus block, 82, 84,
    84*f*, 87
Lateral out of plane block, 205*f*
Lateral "safe track," cervical sympathetic block, 230*f*
Lateral sciatic block
  needle/probe position, 209*f*
  ultrasound, 209*f*
Lateral vertebral foramina, 150, 151*f*
Law's texture analysis, images processed, 264
Leg, gross anatomy, 108, 109*f*
Lesser trochanter, 125
  cross section, 123, 124*f*
Levobupivacaine, TAP block, 95
Lidocaine, supraclavicular brachial plexus block, 56
Local anesthetic. *See also* Sedation
  ankle block, 140, 141*f*–143*f*
  anterior sciatic nerve block, 123, 126
  brachial plexus, infraclavicular approach, 176
  femoral nerve block, 97
  guidelines, infants and children, 166
  IL-IH block, 187
  inguinal nerve block, 89, 90
  injection
    intercostal space, 154*f*
    TAP block, 95, 96*f*
  labor epidural placement, 146
  lateral femoral cutaneous block, 104
  longus colli muscle, 228*f*
  lumbar plexus block, ultrasound-guided, 81
  mandibular nerve block, 217

musculocutaneous nerve and, 69f
obturator nerve block, 118, 118f
parasacral block, anatomy, 120
paravertebral blocks, 192
pediatric brachial plexus blockade, 173–174
pediatric lower extremity blockade, 197–198
pediatric shoulder joint surgery, 171
popliteal sciatic block, 133, 137, 138f
saphenous nerve block, 112
sciatic nerve and, 135, 136f
solution
  axillary block, 68
  infraclavicular blocks, 64
    ultrasound-guided, 61
  interscalene block, 40, 50
  supraclavicular brachial plexus block, 55, 56
  volume of, 4
stellate ganglion block, 221
subgluteal sciatic block, 130
superior hypogastric plexus block, 237
TAP block, 183
thoracic paravertebral blocks, 151, 156
transverse abdominis plane block, 93
ulnar block, above elbow, 79
Longitudinal lumbar plexus, needle and probe position, 196f
Lower extremities, sensory and motor innervation, 195
Lumbar 5 dorsal ramus, anatomy, 243f
Lumbar 5 dorsal ramus block, 240–251
  background and indications, 240
  probe position, 249f
Lumbar facet joints, anatomy, 240, 241f, 242f
Lumbar plexus, 81
  gross anatomy, 82f
  histological cross section, 83f
  roots of, 81
  ultrasound image, 83f
Lumbar plexus anatomy, evaluation of, three-dimensional ultrasound
    probe, 280–282
Lumbar plexus block, 8, 85f
  lateral insertion approach, 82, 84, 84f
  medial approach, 84, 86f
  sagittal approach, 84, 87
  techniques, 197–199
  transverse approach
    anatomy and, 81, 82f
    longitudinal scan, 88, 88f
    ultrasound-guided, 81–88
Lumbar plexus region, three-dimensional reconstructed anatomy, 281,
    282f
Lumbar zygapophysial joint pain, 250–251
Lumbar zygapophysial medial branch block
  background and indications, 240–251
  technique, 242, 244, 244f–247f, 247–249
Lymphatic vessels, 28

Machine vision
  human vision v., 264, 266f
  ultrasonography, 263–271
Magnetic resonance imaging. See MRI
Mandibular nerve
  alveolar vessels and, 217f
  anatomy, 217, 218
Mandibular nerve block
  linear transducer position, 217f
  technique, 217–218
  ultrasound guided, 217–219
Maxillary artery, 219f

Maxillary nerve, 219f
  anatomy, 214, 215
  ultrasound of, 216f
Maxillary nerve block, ultrasound-guided, 214–216
  probe/needle position, 215f
  technique, 214
Median nerve, 71, 72f
  above elbow, 75f
  gross anatomy, 77f
  ultrasound scan, 75f
Median nerve block
  above elbow, needle/probe position, 75f
  below elbow, needle/probe position, 75f
Middle trunk, 54f
Midfemoral block, 139
Midinfraclavicular region, ultrasound images of, 263–264
Modified Mumford-Shah model, nerve identification in, ultrasound scan,
    289–294
Monitors, ultrasound-guided peripheral nerve block, 2, 3f
Morphine
  pediatric neuroaxial block, 164
  TAP block, 182
MRI (Magnetic resonance imaging)
  erosive disease, 253
  impedance neurography v., 276, 277f
  X-ray v., ultrasound v., 254f
Musculocutaneous nerve
  local anesthetic and, 69f
  ultrasound scam, 25f
Musculocutaneous nerve block, axillary approach, 171–172, 172f
Musculoskeletal ultrasonography, 252–259

Neck
  axial view, 228f
  cross-section, 220, 221f
  dissection of, 225, 226f
  ultrasound, 223f
    interscalene block, 175f
Needle(s). See also Block needle; Echogenic needles; Epidural needle;
    Groove needle design
  acoustic radiation force imaging of, 273–274, 274f, 275f
  ankle block, 140, 141f–143f
  anterior sciatic nerve block, 123, 126, 126f
  axillary block, 65, 68, 68f
  design, groove depth and, 285–286, 286f
  endoscopic celiac ganglion block, 232
  femoral nerve block, 97–98
  guidance, aspiration and injection, 258
  imaging of, 23f
  infraclavicular blocks, ultrasound-guided, 60, 61–62
  inguinal nerve block, 89
  interscalene block, 40
    ultrasound-guided, 49
  labor epidural placement, 146
  lateral femoral cutaneous block, 104
  lumbar plexus block, ultrasound-guided, 81, 82
  and nerve roots, 43f
  oblique angle of insonation, 24f
  obturator nerve block, 114
  parasacral block, anatomy, 120
  pediatric brachial plexus blockade, 173–174
  popliteal sciatic block, 133, 135, 136f
  posterior interscalene block, 50f
  posterior popliteal approach, 134, 136f
  regional anesthesia, infants and children, 165
  superior hypogastric plexus block, 237
  supraclavicular brachial plexus block, 54f, 55

Needle(s), *(continued)*
  TAP block, 183*f*
  thoracic paravertebral blocks, 151, 156, 160*f*
  transverse abdominis plane block, 93
  type, nerve injury and, 36
  ulnar block, above elbow, 79
  ultrasound, and nerve roots, 43*f*
  ultrasound-guided lumbar plexus block, 82, 84, 84*f*, 85*f*, 87
Needle/probe position
  anterior intercostal block, 190*f*
  anterior sciatic nerve block, 125
  axillary nerve blocks, pediatric, 172, 172*f*
  brachial plexus
    axillary approach, 172, 172*f*
    interscalene approach, 174–175, 175*f*
  cervical sympathetic block, 225, 226*f*
  inguinal nerve block, 91*f*
  intercostal space, 154*f*
  lateral femoral cutaneous block, 105
  lateral sciatic block, 209*f*
  mandibular nerve block, 219*f*
  parasacral block, 121*f*
  paravertebral blocks, 193*f*
  popliteal sciatic block, supine lateral approach, 136–137, 138*f*
  posterior intercostal block, 191*f*
  subgluteal sciatic block, 127, 128*f*, 129*f*, 130
  supraclavicular block, 177, 177*f*
  thoracic paravertebral blocks, 160*f*
  ulnar nerve block, 72*f*
Needle tip, 25
  grooved, 283, 284, 284*f*
    grating equation and, 286
  SPL and, 285
Nerve(s). *See also specific nerves*
  acoustic radiation force imaging and, 273
  ankle, 141*f*, 143*f*
  identification of, 263–271
  injury, needle type, 36
  sonography, 261–262
  stimulated, 25
Nerve axis, ultrasound and, 164–165
Nerve block. *See specific nerve block*
  echogenic needles and, 283–288
  at wrist, 74*f*
Nerve damage
  intraneural injections, 262
    dog study, 36
  permanent, 32
Nerve roots, 43*f*
  ultrasound scan, 25*f*, 49*f*
Nerve stimulation
  anterior sciatic nerve block, 126
  popliteal sciatic block, 139
  subgluteal sciatic block, 127
Nerve stimulator, 4
  femoral nerve block, 98, 200
  interscalene block, ultrasound-guided, 50
  obturator nerve block, 118
  regional anesthesia, infants and children, 165–166
  subgluteal sciatic block, 130
  supraclavicular brachial plexus block, 56
Nerve tissue
  machine identification of, 264, 268*f*
  texture energy analysis, 264, 267*f*
Neuroaxial blocks, 7
Neurological complications, postoperative, 34
Neurolytic agents, obturator nerve block, 118

Neuromuscular blocking agents, pediatric anesthesia, 166
Neurostimulation, 7–9
  ultrasound-guided techniques *v.*, 7–8
Nonstimulating catheter, popliteal sciatic block, 135

Obese patient
  anterior sciatic nerve block, 126
  femoral nerve block, 99
Obturator nerve, 105*f*, 125*f*, 195
  cross-sectional anatomy, 115*f*
  gross anatomy, 115*f*
  ultrasound scan, 116*f*
Obturator nerve block, 118*f*
  anatomy and, 114, 115*f*
  ultrasound-guided, 114–119
    background and indications, 114
    needle/probe position, 117*f*
    technique and tips, 118–119
Oxygen, supplemental, ultrasound-guided peripheral nerve block, 2, 3*f*

Pain. *See also* Postoperative pain scores; Visceral pain syndromes
  lumbar zygapophysial joint, 250–251
  management, impedance neurography and, 276–278, 278*f*
  postoperative, continuous lumbar plexus block, 87
Pain therapy
  inguinal nerve block, 92
  lumbar plexus block, 81
Parasacral block
  anatomy and, 120
  background and indications, 120
  ultrasound-guided, 120–122
    technique, 120, 121*f*, 122
Parasacral sciatic nerve
  gross anatomy, 120, 121*f*
  ultrasound, 122, 122*f*
Paravertebral blocks, 192–193
  catastrophic outcomes, 26
  needle/probe position, 193*f*
  technique, 192–193
Paravertebral catheter, thoracic paravertebral blocks, 161
Paravertebral injections, 32
Paravertebral nerve blocks, 26–33
Paravertebral space, 159*f*
  anatomy, 156, 157*f*
Paresthesia, 7–9
Partial plexus block, 223
Patient-controlled regional anesthesia (PCRA), 44
PCRA. *See* Patient-controlled regional anesthesia
Pediatric(s)
  anesthesia
    agents for, 166
    anesthetic toxicity, 167–168
    plasma concentration levels, 167
  brachial plexus blockade, 171–180
    technique, 173–174
  lower-extremity blockade
    local anesthetic, 197–212
    ultrasound-guided, 195–212
  neuroaxial block, hydrophilic opioids and, 164
  peripheral nerve block, 164
  peripheral nerve blocks, 163
  regional anesthesia, 163–170
  shoulder joint surgery, 171
Perineurium, 27–28, 29, 29*f*
Peripheral nerve(s), 27–30, 35, 35*f*
  composition of, 27–30, 29*f*
  transverse scanning technique, 165

Peripheral nerve blocks, 7, 26–33, 262
    agents and, 36–37
    anesthesiologist, 2, 4
    anticoagulated patient, 8
    pediatrics, 163
    ultrasound and, 7
Peripheral nerve stimulation, 6
    supraclavicular brachial plexus block, 56
Peripheral nerve stimulation blocks, 57
Peripheral nerve stimulator, 22
Peripheral nervous system, microanatomy, 26–27, 26–33
Peripheral neuropathy, popliteal sciatic block, 139
Peritoneum, 93, 94f
Perivenous block of saphenous nerve, in calf, 112–113
Peroneal nerve, 111f, 132, 133f
Phenol, 118
Phrenic nerve block, 40
Phrenic/recurrent laryngeal nerve block, pediatrics and, 174
Pig study, intraneural injection, 35, 36
Plasma concentration levels, pediatric anesthesia and, 167
Pleura, longitudinal scan, 152f
Plexuses, 27–31, 32f
Plexus spinal roots, 30–31
Plexus trunks, 30–31, 32f
Pneumothorax, supraclavicular brachial plexus block, 53
Popliteal artery, 111f, 132, 133f, 135f
Popliteal crease, ultrasound image, 209f
Popliteal fossa block, 201
Popliteal fossa, probe position in, 132, 133, 133f
Popliteal sciatic block
    anatomy and, 132, 133f
    ultrasound-guided, 132–139
        background and indications, 132
        clinical evidence, 137, 139
        posterior popliteal approach, 134–136
        supine lateral approach, 136–137, 138f
        upper thigh posterior approach, 137, 138f
Popliteal vein, 111f, 132, 133f, 135f
Posterior abdominal wall, 233f
Posterior cervical block, probe/needle position, 42f
Posterior intercostal block, 189–192
    needle/probe position, 191f
    probe position, 191f
Posterior interscalene block, needle/probe position, 50f
Posterior tibial nerve, 142f
    injection of, 142f
Postoperative neural dysfunction, 34
Postoperative pain scores, TAP block, 182
Pressure monitoring device, 4
Prevertebral fascia, 220, 221f
Probe
    axillary block, 65, 68f
    endoscopic celiac ganglion block, 232, 233f
    movements, 13f–15f
    position
        anterior intercostal block, 190f
        anterior sciatic nerve block, 126f
        brachial plexus, interscalene approach, 174–175, 175f
        lateral femoral cutaneous block, 105
        lateral sciatic block, 209f
        longitudinal scan, 152f
        parasacral block, 121f
        paravertebral blocks, 193f
        popliteal sciatic block, supine lateral approach, 136–137, 138f
        posterior intercostal block, 191f
        subgluteal sciatic block, 128f, 129f
        supraclavicular block, 177, 177f
        ulnar nerve block, 72f

    posterior interscalene block, 50f
    regional anesthesia, infants and children, 165
    supraclavicular brachial plexus block, 54f
    TAP block, 183f
    toggling, 42–43, 43f
    transverse abdominis plane block, 93
    ulnar block, above elbow, 79
Profunda femoris artery, 110f
Profunda femoris vein, 110f
"Psoas compartment block," 197, 199
Psoas muscle
    anatomy, 97, 98f
    lumbar plexus and, 83f
    lumbar plexus block, 88

Quadratus femoris muscle
    nerve to, deep dissection, 100f
    subgluteal sciatic block, 127, 128f

Radial nerve, 72f, 77f
    gross anatomy, 77f, 78f
Radial nerve block, below knee, needle/probe position, 78f
Radial recurrent artery, 78f
Radiocontrast injection, sciatic nerve, dog, 30, 30f
Rectus abdominis block, 184–186
    probe/needle orientation, 185, 185f
    ultrasound scan, 185, 186f
Rectus abdominis muscle, 186f
Reflection, from needle, 23f, 24f
Regional anesthesia, 2, 3f. See also Sedation
    acoustic radiation force imaging, 272–275
    equipment, infants and children, 164–166
    intraneural injection, ultrasound-guided, 34–38
    transducer, 165
    transversus abdominis block, 181–184
    ultrasound-guided, 7–9
        anterior intercostal block, 189
        IL-IH block, 186–187
        intercostal block, 187–189
        paravertebral block, 192–193
        posterior intercostal block, 189–192
        rectus abdominis block, 184–186
        transversus abdominis block, 181–184
Region-based segmentation model, image and, 292
Resolution, wavelength v., 11f
Resuscitation, equipment for, 3f
Rheumatology, ultrasonography in, 252–259
Rib(s)
    longitudinal scan, 152f
    ninth/tenth, 151f
Ropivacaine, 208
    ankle block, 140, 141f–143f
    anterior sciatic nerve block, 123
    brachial plexus, infraclavicular approach, 176
    endoscopic celiac ganglion block, 232
    IL-IH block, 187
    infraclavicular blocks, ultrasound-guided, 61
    inguinal nerve block, 89
    interscalene block, 40
        ultrasound-guided, 50
    lateral femoral cutaneous block, 104
    lumbar plexus block, ultrasound-guided, 81
    mandibular nerve block, 217
    obturator nerve block, 118
    parasacral block, anatomy, 120
    paravertebral blocks, 192
    pediatric anesthesia, 166

Ropivacaine, *(continued)*
  peripheral blocks, 37
  popliteal sciatic block, 133
  saphenous nerve block, 112
  stellate ganglion block, 221
  superior hypogastric plexus block, 237
  supraclavicular brachial plexus block, 55
  TAP block, 95, 183
  thoracic paravertebral blocks, 151, 156
  ulnar block, above elbow, 79

Sacral plexus, 120, 202
Sacral plexus anesthesia, 197
Sacrum, 243*f*
Saphenous artery, 143*f*
Saphenous nerve, 108, 108*f*, 110*f*, 111*f*, 143*f*, 203*f*, 204
  gross anatomy, 203*f*
  injection of, 143*f*
Saphenous nerve block
  anatomy, 108, 109*f*–111*f*
  distal thigh approach, 112
  ultrasound-guided, 108–113
    background and indications, 108
    technique, 112–113
Saphenous vein, 111*f*
  of leg, 108, 109*f*
  and nerve, 108*f*
Sartorius muscle, 98, 110*f*, 111*f*, 203*f*
Scattering, 10
  irregular surface, 12*f*
Sciatic nerve, 123, 124*f*, 131, 132, 133*f*, 204
  local anesthetic with, 135, 136*f*
  popliteal sciatic block, supine lateral approach, 136–137, 138*f*
  scan, 204*f*
  subgluteal sciatic block, 127, 128*f*
  ultrasound for, 207*f*
Sciatic nerve block, 8, 204, 207
  at popliteal level, 134
Sedation, ultrasound-guided peripheral nerve block, 4
Semimembranosis muscle, 111*f*, 135*f*
Semitendonosis muscle, 135*f*
Sevoflurane, epinephrine "test-dose," 168
Signal processing modes, 22*f*
Sjögren syndrome, ultrasonography and, 257
Skin preparation, ultrasound-guided peripheral nerve block, 2, 3*f*
SLP. *See* Sound pressure gradient
Soft tissue structure contrast, 273
Software, project, 264, 265*f*
Sonography
  future of, 261–262
  principles of, 10–25
  supraclavicular brachial plexus block, 56
Sound pressure gradient (SLP), needle tip, 285
Sound, speed of, 10
Sound wave, frequency, 11*f*
Speculation, 10, 11*f*, 12*f*
Spinal blocks, catastrophic outcomes, 26
Spinous process, 81
Stellate ganglion block, 220–224
  injection, cervical-6, 223*f*
  procedure/tips, 221–224
Stimulating catheter, 131
  popliteal sciatic block, 135
  subgluteal sciatic block, 130
Stomach, endoscopic guidance, 233, 234*f*
"String of beads," 108

Subclavian artery, 53, 54*f*
Subclavian vein, 53, 54*f*
Subepineurial injection, 29
Subgluteal approach, 207
Subgluteal block, 204*f*
  needle/probe position, 204*f*
  ultrasound for, 205*f*
Subgluteal catheters, 131
Subgluteal sciatic block, 127–131, 129*f*
  anatomy, 127, 128*f*
  background and indications, 127
  clinical evidence, 130–131
  technique, 130
Subgluteal ultrasound, 205*f*, 206*f*
Sulcus ulnaris, 71, 72*f*
Superficial radial nerve, 72*f*, 78*f*
Superior hypogastric plexus, anatomy, 237, 238*f*
Superior hypogastric plexus block
  technique, 238, 239*f*
  ultrasound-guided, 237–239
Superior trunk, position, 54*f*
Supraclavicular brachial plexus block
  anatomy and, 53
  level of, microanatomy at, 55*f*
  needle/probe position, 177, 177*f*
  technique, 55–56
  ultrasound-guided, 53–57
Supraclavicular fossa
  focus and, 19*f*
  probe position in, 47*f*
  ultrasound scan, 178*f*
Supraclavicular plexus, 47*f*
  machine vision *v.* human vision, identification of, 264, 270*f*
  restricted search range, superimposed, 264, 269*f*
  search range, reduction of, 264, 269*f*
  subclavian artery *v.*, search range, 264, 268*f*
  texture energy plot, 264, 270*f*
Supraclavicular region, ultrasound images of, 263
Sympathetic nerve trunk, anatomy, 222*f*
Synovial tissue, ultrasonography and, 253
Synovitis, tenosynovitis *v.*, 256*f*

TAP block. *See* Transverse abdominis plane block
Tendinous sheath, ultrasound scan, 186*f*
Tenosynovitis, synovitis *v.*, 256*f*
Third lumbar nerve root, 98*f*
Thoracic nerves, 93, 94*f*
Thoracic paravertebral anatomy, evaluation of, three-dimensional ultrasound probe, 280–282, 281*f*
Thoracic paravertebral blocks, 160*f*
  anatomy and, 150, 151*f*, 156, 157*f*
  background and indications, 150
  probe/needle position, 153*f*
  probe position, 152*f*
  technique, 152
  ultrasonographic scanning, 158*f*
  ultrasound-guided, 150–155
    background and indications, 156
    classic approach, 156–161
    skin landmarks, 158*f*
    technique and tips, 158–159, 161
Thoracic spinal nerve roots, 150, 151*f*
Thoracic spinous processes, 158, 158*f*
Three-dimensional ultrasound, 281–282, 281*f*, 282*f*
Three-in-one block, 100
Tibial nerve, 111*f*, 132, 133*f*, 135*f*

acoustic radiation force imaging, 273*f*
  local anesthetic with, 209*f*
  scanning, 134, 134*f*
  in vivo B-mode images, 273*f*
Ting, axillary nerve blocks, 7
Toggling, 10, 13*f*
  of probe, 42–43, 43*f*
Total spinal anesthesia, 32
Transducer, 283
  ankle block
    saphenous, 140, 143*f*
    tibial, 140, 141*f*–142*f*
  anterior sciatic nerve block, 123
  axillary block, 65
  curved, mandibular nerve block, 219*f*
  elements, 16, 20*f*
    types, 21*f*
  endoscopic celiac ganglion block, 232
  femoral nerve block, 97
  frequency band, types, 22*f*
  infants and children, 165
  infraclavicular blocks, 63, 64
    ultrasound-guided, 60, 61–62, 61*f*
  inguinal nerve block, 89, 91*f*
  interscalene block, 40
    ultrasound-guided, 49
  labor epidural placement, 146
  lateral femoral cutaneous block, 104
  lumbar plexus block, ultrasound-guided, 81
  lumbar zygapophysial medial branch block, 242
  obturator nerve block, 114
  parasacral block, anatomy, 120
  pediatric brachial plexus blockade, 173–174
  popliteal sciatic block, 133–134
  position
    axillary approach, 172, 172*f*
    thoracic paravertebral blocks, 159*f*, 160*f*
    ultrasound-guided lumbar plexus block, 86*f*, 87*f*
  regional anesthesia, infants and children, 165
  saphenous nerve block, 112
  subgluteal sciatic block, 127
  superior hypogastric plexus block, 237
  supraclavicular brachial plexus block, 53, 54*f*, 55, 56
  thoracic paravertebral blocks, 151, 156
  ultrasound-guided lumbar plexus block, 82, 84, 84*f*, 85*f*
Transverse abdominis plane block (TAP block), 181–184
  anatomy, 93, 94*f*
  injections, 95, 96*f*
  probe/needle, 94*f*, 183*f*
  subcostal approach, 184*f*
  technique, 183, 185–186
  ultrasound-guided, 93–96
    background and indications, 93
    technique, 95
Transverse lumbar plexus block, needle/probe position, 196*f*
Transverse process, 81, 193*f*
Transverse scanning, 196*f*
  technique, peripheral nerves and, 165
Transversus abdominis muscle, 89, 93, 94*f*
  TAP block, 184*f*
Treatment response, ultrasonography and, 253

Triangle of Petit, 181
Trigeminal neuralgia, mandibular nerve block, 217
Tuohy needle, thoracic paravertebral blocks, 161
Two-dimensional meshed domain, 283, 284*f*
Ulnar artery, ultrasound scan, 75*f*
Ulnar nerve, 71, 72*f*, 73*f*
  gross anatomy, 77*f*
  at wrist, ultrasound scan, 74*f*
Ulnar nerve block
  above elbow
    patient position, 79
    technique, 79
  below elbow, 73*f*
  needle/probe position, 72*f*
Ultrasonography
  recovery on, stages of, 256*f*
  in rheumatology, 252–259
    indications for, 252–258
    publications in, 252, 253*f*
Ultrasound. *See also* Three-dimensional ultrasound
  beam
    reflection, 11*f*
    refraction of, 10, 11*f*
  blocks, 7
  epidural, infants and children, 164–166
  ilioinguinal and iliohypogastric nerve, 188*f*
  image, 10
  MRI, X-ray *v.*, 254*f*
  needle, and nerve roots, 43*f*
  nerve identification in, modified Mumford-Shah model, 289–294
  platform, 5*f*
  rectus abdominis block, 185, 186*f*
  system, choice, 4, 5*f*
  TAP block, 184*f*
Ultrasound-guided techniques, neurostimulation *v.*, 7–8
Upper extremity, mid infraclavicular approach, 62

VACTERL syndrome, TAP block, 182
Vastus lateralis, 111*f*
Vastus medialis, 111*f*
Veins, 22
  identifying, 16
Velocity gates, 16
Visceral pain syndromes, endoscopic celiac ganglion block, 232
Vocal cord paralysis, anesthetic spillover, 224

Wavelength, resolution *v.*, 11*f*
Wrist
  gross anatomy, 74*f*, 76*f*
  median nerve block at, needle/probe position, 75*f*
  ultrasound scan, 76*f*, 77*f*

X-ray, MRI *v.*, ultrasound *v.*, 254*f*

Zygapophysial injection, spinal pain and, 240Abdomen, cross section, 94*f*
Abdominal wall, anatomy, 93, 94*f*
Acoustic radiation force impulse (ARFI) imaging, 272–273
  injections,
    274*f*, 275*f*
  injections, 274*f*, 275*f*
    injections, 274*f*, 275*f*